Pathology of Asbestos-Associated Diseases

Second Edition

Springer
New York
Berlin
Heidelberg
Hong Kong
London
Milan
Paris
Tokyo

Pathology of Asbestos-Associated Diseases

Second Edition

Victor L. Roggli, MD
Professor of Pathology, Duke University and Durham VA Medical
Centers, Durham, North Carolina
Tim D. Oury, MD, PhD
Assistant Professor of Pathology, University of Pittsburgh Medical
Center, Pittsburgh, Pennsylvania
Thomas A. Sporn, MD
Assistant Professor of Pathology, Duke University Medical Center,
Durham, North Carolina

Editors

With 130 Illustrations in 191 Parts

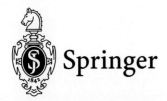

Springer

Victor L. Roggli, MD
Professor of Pathology
Duke University and Durham
    VA Medical Centers
Durham, NC 27710
USA

Tim D. Oury, MD, PhD
Assistant Professor of Pathology
University of Pittsburgh Medical
    Center
Pittsburgh, PA 15213
USA

Thomas A. Sporn, MD
Assistant Professor of Pathology
Duke University Medical Center
Durham, NC 27710
USA

Library of Congress Cataloging-in-Publication Data
Roggli, Victor L.
    Pathology of asbestos-associated diseases / Victor L. Roggli, Tim D. Oury, Thomas
A. Sporn.—2nd ed.
        p. ; cm.
    Includes bibliographical references and index.
    ISBN 0-387-20090-8 (hard cover : alk. paper)
    1. Asbestosis—Complications—Cytopathology.   2. Asbestosis—Complications—
Cytodiagnosis.   3. Asbestos—Carcinogenicity.   4. Asbestos fibers—Analysis.
I. Oury, Tim D.   II. Sporn, Thomas A.   III. Title.
    [DNLM: 1. Asbestosis—pathology.   2. Asbestos—adverse effects.   3. Lung
Neoplasms—pathology.   4. Mesothelioma—pathology.   5. Pleural Diseases—
pathology. WF 654 R733p 2003]
RC775.A8R64 2003
616.2′44—dc22   2003056816

First edition © 1992 Little, Brown and Company, Boston/Toronto/London.

ISBN 0-387-20090-8   Printed on acid-free paper.

Printed in the United States of America.   (BS/MVY)

9 8 7 6 5 4 3 2 1   SPIN 10944332

Springer-Verlag is a part of Springer Science+Business Media

springeronline.com

Dedicated to the memory of
S. Donald Greenberg and Philip C. Pratt
and to the loving memory of
Louis and Anna Roggli

Contents

Preface

It has been more than a decade since the publication of the first edition of *Pathology of Asbestos-Associated Diseases*. Since that time, some things have changed very little relative to our knowledge of these diseases, whereas in other areas, considerable progress has been made. The purpose of this second edition is to update pathologists, pulmonologists, radiologists, occupational medicine practitioners, industrial hygienists and others with an interest in the field regarding progress in our understanding of these diseases.

A great deal of information has been published in the past decade on methods for diagnosing mesothelioma. This area can be quite intimidating to those who do not deal with this question on a daily basis, and a summary of the more recently published data is therefore deemed to be of some utility. As a result of the explosion of diagnostic techniques, the correct diagnosis of mesothelioma is rarely a problem for the practicing pathologist. Nonetheless, pathologists are being pressed to make the diagnosis on ever-smaller biopsies or on cytologic specimens. A discussion of the latest diagnostic criteria for mesothelioma is presented in Chapter 5, and the limitations of cytologic diagnoses in this regard are emphasized in Chapter 9.

Considerable information has also been published in the medical literature during the past several years regarding the relationship between asbestos exposure and carcinoma of the lung. This information is updated in Chapter 7. This is an area where there is still considerable controversy, and physicians are frequently asked to determine whether asbestos contributed to one or more of the 170,000 lung cancer deaths that occur in the United States annually. Guidelines for making this assessment are provided based on the latest literature on the subject.

The explosion of research in the area of molecular biology has provided us with an abundance of information bearing on the mechanisms by which asbestos causes disease. Studies of cells from both humans and experimental animals have provided further insight in this regard. This information is updated in Chapter 10. We still do not understand all of the steps leading in the transformation, say, of mesothelial cells into a malignant mesothelioma. Nonetheless, many pieces have been added to the puzzle, and many more are expected in the next decade.

A tremendous amount of information has been accumulated in the past decade regarding the numbers and types of fibers accumulating in the lung and their relation to various asbestos-related diseases and exposures. This information is summarized in Chapter 11. Considerably less information is available concerning fiber burdens in extra-pulmonary tissues, and it is expected that advances in this area will occur in the near future. Because the fiber levels in these tissues is expected to be quite low relative to those in the lung, very careful studies utilizing appropriate controls will need to be done if our knowledge of this area is to be advanced significantly.

Since the publication of the first edition of this book, thousands of workers have died of asbestos-related diseases, and more than a dozen manufacturers have filed for bankruptcy. The judicial and legislative branches have refused to provide any relief to the burden these cases impose on civil courts. Hundreds of thousands of cases are still pending. Legal strategies have necessarily changed as a consequence, and the viewpoints of plaintiff and defense attorneys with considerable experience in the field are presented in Chapters 12 and 13, respectively. Although the reduction of workplace exposures will eventually result in the virtual eradication of asbestos-related diseases, it is anticipated that cases will continue to occur during the next two decades or more. Hopefully, this volume will assist those involved with the treatment, care, and diagnosis of these cases.

Durham, North Carolina   *Victor L. Roggli, MD*
Pittsburgh, Pennsylvania   *Tim D. Oury, MD, PhD*
Durham, North Carolina   *Thomas A. Sporn, MD*

Preface to the First Edition

The purpose of *Pathology of Asbestos-Associated Diseases* is to give a detailed description of the pathologic abnormalities associated with exposure to asbestos fibers. The past decade has witnessed substantial advances in our understanding of the pathology of asbestos-associated diseases, as a result of observations using both human and animal tissue samples. A book with this information summarized in a single volume is a valuable resource for pathologists, pulmonologists, radiologists, occupational medicine practitioners, industrial hygienists, and others with an interest in this subject.

Knowledge of asbestos-associated diseases has been derived primarily from three lines of investigation: (1) observations and detailed descriptions of pathologic changes in tissues of individuals exposed through their occupations to airborne asbestos fibers, including quantification of asbestos content; (2) reproduction of these diseases in animals exposed to asbestos fibers under controlled conditions; and (3) epidemiologic observations made of asbestos workers examined as part of either cross-sectional or longitudinal studies. Because these latter two lines of investigation have contributed to knowledge of the pathology of asbestos-associated diseases, they are also summarized in this volume. The chapters dealing with specific diseases include a review of pertinent epidemiologic studies. One entire chapter is devoted to a review of the contributions of experimental animal studies to knowledge of asbestos-associated diseases.

The book is organized into thirteen chapters, each dealing with a specific aspect of asbestos-associated diseases. The first chapter is designed to tell the reader what asbestos is and includes a simplified description of asbestos mineralogy, its sources, and the methods used to detect and identify asbestos fibers. The second chapter describes how individuals are exposed to asbestos, both in the workplace and in the home environment. Chapter 3 gives a detailed description of asbestos bodies, how they are formed, and how they can be distinguished from ferruginous bodies lacking an asbestos core.

The first three chapters give the background for the chapter on asbestosis, a form of pneumoconiosis that has been recognized since the early decades of this century. This is followed by a chapter dealing with the pathologic features of malignant mesothelioma, a signal neoplasm occurring with alarming regularity in populations exposed to asbestos. An explosion of information regarding the specific features of this neoplasm has greatly increased the reliability of the pathologist's diagnostic armamentarium for distinguishing from other malignancies with which it may be confused. The sixth chapter is devoted to the nonneoplastic alterations in the pleura that may occur in individuals exposed to asbestos.

Chapter 7 is a review of the pathologic and epidemiologic features of carcinoma of the lung related to asbestos exposure. This is a particularly difficult and controversial area, mainly due to the strong and confounding association of the various lung carcinomas with cigarette smoking. Other asbestos-related neoplasms are the topic of the following chapter, an area of investigation that is badly in need of more detailed studies. Chapter 9 reviews the contributions of cytopathology to the diagnosis of asbestos-associated diseases, a source of valuable information often neglected in the past.

A book on the pathology of asbestos-associated diseases would be incomplete without a discussion of the contributions of experimental animal studies. Chapter 10 shows how these models of asbestos-related disease have greatly expanded our understanding of the interactions of asbestos with the respiratory system and the resulting changes that ultimately lead to disease. In addition, they have in a more general sense increased our knowledge of pulmonary pathobiology. With the current rapid progress in molecular biology research, the coming decade should witness even greater progress in understanding the mechanisms at the molecular level, whereby asbestos is able to induce pulmonary fibrosis or effect neoplastic transformation of cells of the lung and pleura.

A great deal of information has also been gained in the past decade with regard to the tissue asbestos levels associated with various asbestos-induced diseases. Although these analytic and quantitative techniques have yet to be standardized, the information provided by different laboratories has been surprisingly consistent. This information is summarized in Chapter 11, including a considerable amount of previously unpublished data from the authors' own laboratories.

The medicolegal repercussions of asbestos-related diseases have affected a large segment of our population through asbestos litigation, and Chapters 12 and 13 deal with the pathologic aspects of asbestos-associated diseases from an attorney's perspective. Both the plaintiff's and the defendant's points of view are presented by prominent attorneys with extensive experience in this litigation.

Each of the chapters also contains a brief historic review to place the discussion in proper perspective. The information in these reviews is largely derived from a few excellent and detailed sources on the historic perspective of asbestos and asbestos-related diseases.

Due to increasing public awareness of asbestos and its effects on health, as well as increasing concern of public health officials on the prevention of future disease, it is important that pathologists have a working knowledge of the various manifestations of asbestos-related tissue injury. It is hoped that this volume will provide pathologists and other health-care workers with this necessary information.

Durham, North Carolina
Houston, Texas
Durham, North Carolina

Victor L. Roggli, MD
S. Donald Greenberg, MD
Philip C. Pratt, MD

Contributors

Tony Alleman, MD
Fellow, Department of Occupational Medicine, Duke University Medical Center, Durham, NC 27710, USA

Kelly J. Butnor, MD
Assistant Professor, Department of Pathology, University of Vermont College of Medicine, Burlington, VT 05405, USA

Charleen T. Chu, MD, PhD
Assistant Professor of Pathology, University of Pittsburgh Medical Center, Pittsburgh, PA 15213, USA

Patrick Coin, PhD
Program Director of Environment, Health and Safety Technology, Durham Technical Community College, Durham, NC 27703, USA

Dennis J. Darcey, MD, MSPH
Assistant Clinical Professor of Occupational Medicine, Duke University Medical Center, Durham, NC 27710, USA

Cheryl L. Fattman, PhD
Department of Pathology, University of Pittsburgh Medical Center, Pittsburgh, PA 15213, USA

Anne McGinness Kearse
Attorney, Ness Motley, P.A., Mt. Pleasant, SC 29465, USA

Ronald L. Motley, JD
Attorney, Ness Motley, P.A., Mt. Pleasant, SC 29465, USA

Tim D. Oury, MD, PhD
Assistant Professor of Pathology, University of Pittsburgh Medical Center, Pittsburgh, PA 15213, USA

Albert H. Parnell, JD
Attorney, Hawkins & Parnell, Atlanta, GA 30308, USA

Charles W. Patrick, Jr., JD
Attorney, Richardson, Patrick, Westbrook & Brickman, L.L.C., Charleston, SC 29402, USA

Victor L. Roggli, MD
Professor of Pathology, Duke University and Durham VA Medical Centers, Durham, NC 27710, USA

Raj Rolston, MD
Department of Pathology, University of Pittsburgh Medical Center, Pittsburgh, PA 15213, USA

Anupama Sharma, MD
Assistant Professor, Department of Interdisciplinary Pathology, H. Lee Moffitt Cancer Center, Tampa, FL 33612, USA

Thomas A. Sporn, MD
Assistant Professor of Pathology, Duke University Medical Center, Durham, NC 27710, USA

1

Mineralogy of Asbestos

Victor L. Roggli and Patrick Coin

Introduction

The term *asbestos* refers to a group of mineral fibers that share the properties of thermal and chemical resistance, flexibility, and high tensile strength. The word derives from the Greek σασβεστοσ, signifying "unquenchable" or "indestructible."[1] Asbestos is actually a commercial term rather than a mineralogic one. Because of its many useful properties, asbestos has been incorporated into some 3000 different products in our industrialized society.[2] Indeed, it has been referred to as the "magic mineral" and, for many applications, substitutes with similar properties and equally as inexpensive are extremely difficult to find.[3] This chapter's purpose is to describe what asbestos is, where it is found, and what analytical techniques are available for its identification and characterization. A description of the means by which one may be exposed to asbestos in the workplace, at home, or in the environment is given in Chapter 2, and techniques used for the analysis of asbestos in tissue samples are referred to in Chapter 11.

Historical Background

The usage of asbestos dates back to at least 2500 BC, when asbestos was used in the manufacture of Finnish pottery. One of the earliest historical accounts of the use of asbestos describes its incorporation into the wick of a gold lamp for the goddess Athena in the fourth to fifth centuries BC. Records from this same period note the use of asbestos cloth for retaining the ashes of the dead during cremation, and Pliny in the first century AD refers to asbestos cloth as the funeral dress of kings.[1] Both the Chinese and the Egyptians wove asbestos into mats.[4] The Emperor Charlemagne around 800 AD is said to have displayed a tablecloth made from asbestos. After a great feast, the cloth and its contents would be thrown into a fire and the cloth then removed unharmed, to the amazement of his guests. Marco Polo in his travels around 1250 AD also referred to a cloth in one of the northern provinces of the Great Khan with the property of being unconsumed and even purified by fire.[1,3]

The discovery of substantial deposits of asbestos in the Ural Mountains around 1720 led to the establishment of the first factory for making asbestos products, including textiles, socks, gloves, and handbags. This factory operated for approximately 50 years beginning during the reign of Peter the Great, but eventually closed because of a lack of demand.[1,4] Chevalier Aldini constructed an asbestos suit for protection against fire, which was exhibited in the Royal Institution of London in 1829.[3] Chrysotile asbestos was discovered in Quebec, Canada, in 1860, a specimen of which was exhibited in London in 1862.[1,3,4] Mining of Quebec chrysotile deposits was started in 1878, with 50 tons produced during the first year of operation. Crocidolite asbestos was discovered in South Africa in 1815,[4] but mining of substantial amounts did not begin until 1910.[1] Amosite was discovered in the central Transvaal in 1907, with mining operations commencing about 1916.[4] Thus, with the institution of mining operations in the latter half of the 19th century and the early decades of the 20th century and with the advent of the Industrial Revolution, the stage was set for the widespread exploitation of asbestos. The industrial application of asbestos in the manufacture of various products is recounted in greater detail in Chapter 2.

Geological Features of Asbestos

Asbestos is a naturally occurring mineral, which is conventionally divided into two mineralogic groups. The *amphiboles* include crocidolite (blue asbestos), amosite (brown asbestos), tremolite, anthophyllite, and actinolite. Among the amphiboles, only crocidolite and amosite have received widespread commercial utilization. The noncommercial amphiboles (tremolite, anthophyllite, and actinolite) are the most commonly occurring amphibole asbestos minerals and are widely distributed,[4] but they are primarily important as contaminants of other minerals, such as chrysotile, vermiculite, and talc.[5] The other group of asbestos minerals is the *serpentine* group, of which chrysotile (white) asbestos is the sole variety. As of the year 2000, chrysotile accounted for virtually 100% of the asbestos used commercially in the United States.[6]

Asbestos deposits occur in four types of rocks: (I) alpine-type ultramafic rocks including ophiolites (chrysotile, anthophyllite, and tremolite); (II) stratiform ultramafic intrusions (chrysotile and tremolite); (III) serpentinized limestone (chrysotile); and (IV) banded ironstones (amosite and crocidolite). Type I deposits are by far the most important, with the best known commercial deposits of this type located in Quebec and Russia. Type II and Type III deposits are found mostly in South Africa. These are of limited commercial importance. Type IV deposits are found only in the Precambrian banded ironstones of the Transvaal and Cape Province regions of South Africa and the Wittenoom Gorge area of Western Australia. Only the South African deposits are still actively mined. Geologic evidence indicates that asbestos deposits form where there is a favorable stress environment, as where folding or faulting occurs.

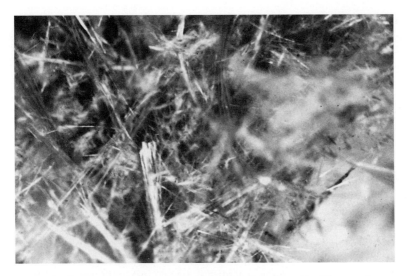

Figure 1-1. Crude chrysotile asbestos from Quebec. Note the fibrous character of the mineral. (Reprinted from Greenberg SD: Asbestos-Associated Pulmonary Diseases, Medcom, Inc., 1981, with permission.)

The amphibole and serpentine minerals occur both as asbestiform (fibrous) varieties (Figure 1-1) and as nonasbestiform (massive) varieties of identical chemical composition. The nonasbestiform counterpart of crocidolite is known as riebeckite, and the nonasbestiform counterpart of amosite is cummingtonite-grunerite. The nonasbestiform counterparts of tremolite, anthophyllite, and actinolite have the same names as their asbestiform varieties. Nonasbestiform serpentines include antigorite and lizardite. Amphibole crystallization is believed to occur initially as the massive form under conditions of moderate temperature and pressure, and transformation to the fibrous form occurs when the unstable massive form is submitted to rock stresses. Similarly, serpentine minerals first crystallize as the massive form and chrysotile is formed subsequently by recrystallization.[4] The best known geographic locations of the various asbestiform minerals are summarized in Table 1-1.

Table 1-1. Geographic locations of best-known deposits of asbestiform minerals

Asbestos variety	Geographic locations
Chrysotile	Quebec (Canada), Rhodesia, Russia (Ural Mountains), China, Italy, United States (California, Vermont)
Crocidolite	South Africa (Northwestern Cape Province, Transvaal), western Australia, Bolivia, northern Rhodesia
Amosite	South Africa (Transvaal), India
Tremolite	Turkey, Cyprus, Greece, Italy, Pakistan, South Korea
Anthophyllite	Finland, United States
Actinolite	South Africa (Cape Province), India

Source: Adapted from Refs. 1, 4

Table 1-2. Chemical composition of asbestiform minerals

Asbestos variety	Chemical formula	
Chrysotile	$Mg_3Si_2O_5(OH)_4$	
Crocidolite	$Na_2Fe_3^{++}Fe_2^{+++}Si_8O_{22}(OH)_2$	
Amosite	$(Fe—Mg)_7Si_8O_{22}(OH)_2$	$Fe > 5$
Tremolite	$Ca_2Mg_5Si_8O_{22}(OH)_2$	
Anthophyllite	$(Mg—Fe)_7Si_8O_{22}(OH)_2$	$Mg > 6$
Actinolite	$Ca_2MgFe_5Si_8O_{22}(OH)_2$	

Physicochemical Properties of Asbestos

Chrysotile is a hydrated magnesium silicate with chemical composition as indicated in Table 1-2. Individual fibrils of chrysotile have diameters of 20 to 40 nm (0.02–0.04 μm).[4] Crushing of chrysotile ore produces fiber bundles consisting of variable numbers of aggregated individual fibrils. These fibers have varying lengths but may exceed 100 μm. Typically, chrysotile fibers have a curved, curly, or wavy morphology, which is particularly apparent in fiber bundles exceeding 10 μm in length (Figure 1-2). In addition, the ends of chrysotile fiber bundles often have a splayed appearance because of the separation of the individual fibrillar units. This curly morphology influences the interceptive deposition of chrysotile fibers, which in turn, affects the depth of penetration into the lower respiratory tract[7,8] (see Chapter 10). However, inhalational studies in rats have shown that substantial numbers of chrysotile fibers 5 μm or greater in length can penetrate into the lung periphery.[7,9–11] The diameter of chrysotile fibers tends to increase with increasing fiber length; however, some very long chrysotile fibers may be extremely thin.

The amphiboles are a group of hydrated silicates with a wide range of cation substitutions within the silicate backbone of the crystal struc-

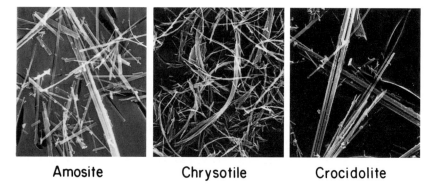

Amosite   Chrysotile   Crocidolite

Figure 1-2. Scanning electron micrographs contrast the curved fibers of chrysotile asbestos (*center*) with the straight fibers of amosite (*left*), and crocidolite (*right*) asbestos. Magnified ×2000. (Reprinted from Greenberg SD: Environmentally Induced Pulmonary Disease, Medcom, Inc., 1987, with permission.)

ture. The idealized chemical formulas of the asbestiform varieties of amphibole minerals are summarized in Table 1-2. The diameters of individual fibers vary considerably with substantial overlap among the members of the amphibole group. However, crocidolite generally has the finest fiber diameters, especially dust obtained from the North-western Cape Province in South Africa or the Wittenoom Gorge in Western Australia. Amosite fibers are on average somewhat thicker, and the noncommercial amphiboles (tremolite, anthophyllite, and acti-nolite) tend to be the coarsest fibers. Fiber diameters may vary consid-erably depending on the source. For example, tremolite fibers from South Korea or the Metsovo region of Greece may be very fine with high aspect (length-to-diameter) ratios. The amphibole fibers have varying lengths, but the authors have observed amosite fibers with diameter less than one micron and length in excess of 200 μm. The amphiboles are typically straight fibers with parallel sides and often have readily identified longitudinal grooves (Figure 1-2). They do not have splayed ends or the tendency toward longitudinal splitting which is typically observed with chrysotile. The diameters of amphibole fibers generally tend to increase with increasing fiber length.

Crystallographic Structure

Serpentine Asbestos

Chrysotile is a phyllosilicate or sheet silicate, in which a silica layer is joined to a brucite (Mg $[OH]_2$) layer. The silica layer consists of a pseudohexagonal network of linked silica tetrahedra. There is consid-erable mismatching between the silica and brucite layers, resulting in substantial strain in the crystal lattice and curvature of the sheet struc-ture. This is the result of the fact that the brucite layer is slightly larger than the silica layer. When viewed end on, chrysotile fibers have the appearance of a sheet rolled up into a scroll. The scroll or tubule of an individual chrysotile fiber thus has a central capillary with a diameter of 2 to 4.5 nm (Figure 1-3). Selected area electron diffraction (SAED) pat-terns obtained from chrysotile fibers have a characteristic appearance consisting of smearing of the dot patterns along the layer lines and a layer line spacing of 5.3 Å (Figure 1-4). A schematic diagram of the crystal structure of chrysotile is illustrated in Figure 1-5.[12,13] Chrysotile occurs as three distinct polymorphs referred to as clinochrysotile, orthochrysotile, and parachrysotile. Of these three polymorphs, clino-chrysotile is by far the most common.[4]

Amphibole Asbestoses

The amphiboles are inosilicates or chain silicates,[14] in which the silica tetrahedra are arranged linearly and wrap around each other like the strands of a rope. The crystalline structure of the amphiboles displays a perfect prismatic cleavage. The structure of the amphiboles is in

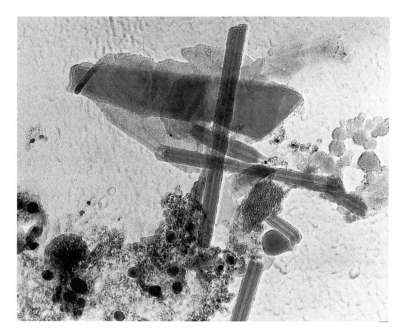

Figure 1-3. Transmission electron micrograph of individual chrysotile fibrils in longitudinal section showing the distinct central capillary characteristic of chrysotile. Magnified ×60,000. (Courtesy Mr. Frank D'Ovidio, Manville Sales Corp., Denver, CO.)

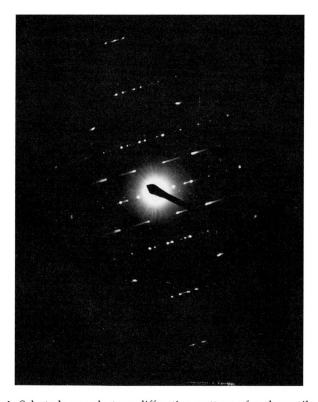

Figure 1-4. Selected area electron diffraction pattern of a chrysotile asbestos fiber showing the 5.3Å interlayer line spacing. Note the very prominent "streaking" along the layer lines, a feature which is characteristic of chrysotile asbestos. (Courtesy Dr. Neil Rowlands, JEOL USA Inc., Peabody, MA.)

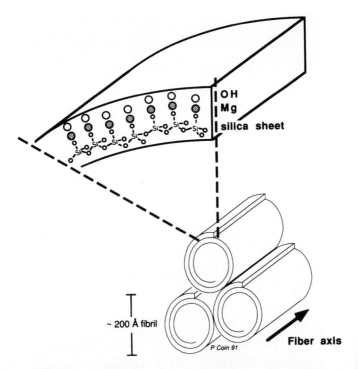

Figure 1-5. Schematic diagram of the crystalline structure of chrysotile asbestos. Modified after Refs. 12 and 13.

the monoclinic class, with the exception of anthophyllite, which is orthorhombic. Thus the diffraction patterns of the various amphibole asbestoses are indistinguishable, consisting of discrete dots along the layer lines and a layer line spacing of 5.3 Å (Figure 1-6). End-on views of amphibole fibers reveal a rectangular or rhombic shape, with a ratio of width to thickness varying from 1:1 to 10:1.[15,16] This appearance is in contrast to the characteristic tubular morphology of chrysotile. A schematic diagram of the crystal structure of amphibole asbestos is illustrated in Figure 1-7.[12,13]

Techniques for Identification of Asbestos

A variety of techniques have been devised for the identification of asbestos fibers,[17] taking advantage of the various features characterizing asbestos, including morphology, crystalline structure, and chemical composition. Each of these techniques has its own advantages and limitations (Table 1-3). A brief discussion of the more common techniques used for the identification of asbestos fibers is presented in the following sections.

Phase-Contrast Microscopy

Phase-contrast light microscopy takes advantage of phase optics to increase the resolution and hence the sensitivity with regard to the size

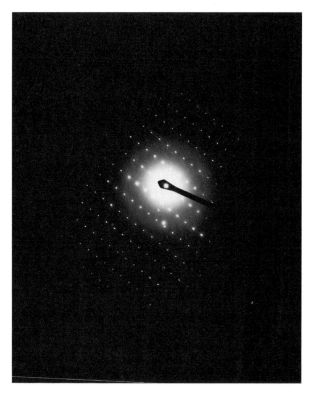

Figure 1-6. Selected area electron diffraction pattern of a crocidolite asbestos fiber showing the 5.3 Å interlayer line spacing. Note the discrete localization of the dots (representing diffraction maxima) along the layer lines (compare with Figure 1-4). (Courtesy Dr. Neil Rowlands, JEOL USA Inc., Peabody, MA.)

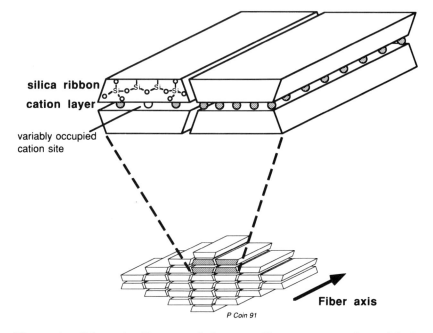

Figure 1-7. Schematic diagram of the crystalline structure of amphibole asbestos. Modified after Refs. 12 and 13.

Table 1-3. Techniques for identification of asbestos

Analytical Technique	Specificity	Limitations	Advantages	Disadvantages
Phase Contrast Microscopy	Nonspecific	Fiber detection only	Inexpensive, ease of sample preparation	Resolution limited to fibers $\geq 0.2\,\mu m$ in diameter
Polarizing Microscopy with Dispersion Staining	Relatively Specific	Bulk samples	Inexpensive, minimal sample preparation, reproducible	Resolution limited, inaccuracies especially for biological samples
Infrared Spectroscopy	Relatively Specific	Bulk samples	Relatively inexpensive, simple operation	Inaccuracies in presence of mixed particle population, interference from organic residues
Magnetic Alignment and Light Scattering	Nonspecific	Bulk samples	Rapid; simple; relatively inexpensive	Does not allow determination of specific mineral fiber types
X-ray Diffraction	Highly specific	Bulk samples	Rapid, simple	Relatively insensitive
Selected Area Electron Diffraction (SAED)	Specific for chrysotile	Individual fiber analysis	Crystallographic information regarding individual fiber	Tedious; time-consuming, expensive
Transmission Electron microscopy with EDS	Highly specific	Individual fiber analysis	Specific identification of individual fibers by EDS/ SAED; superior resolution	More complex sample preparation; tedious; expensive
Scanning Electron microscopy with EDS	Highly specific	Individual fiber analysis	Specific identification of individual fibers, minimal sample preparation	Tedious, time-consuming, expensive

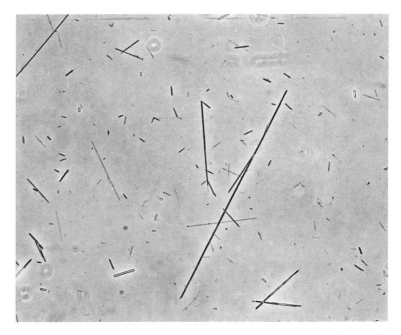

Figure 1-8. Phase-contrast light micrograph of U.I.C.C. amosite asbestos fibers. Magnified ×375.

of fibers that can be detected. Fibers with diameters as small as 0.2 μm may be identified by means of this technique. Information that can be obtained with this approach is limited to morphologic features, such as size (length and diameter), shape, and aspect ratio (Figure 1-8). However, information regarding specific fiber composition cannot be obtained so that one cannot readily distinguish among the various types of asbestos fiber, nor can asbestos fibers be distinguished from nonasbestos mineral fibers. Furthermore, fibers with diameters less than 0.2 μm are beyond the resolution of phase contrast light microscopy and therefore cannot be detected with this technique. Today phase contrast is seldom used for the detection or identification of asbestos in environmental or tissue samples.[17,18]

Polarizing Microscopy with Dispersion Staining

Polarizing microscopy takes advantage of the property of rotation of polarized light by anisotropic (i.e., crystalline) substances. This technique thus provides information regarding the relative crystallinity of a fibrous particle, and if immersion oils are also used, information regarding its index of refraction. The latter procedure is referred to as dispersion staining, and by careful selection of immersion oils, it can be used to distinguish among the various asbestos fiber types as well as making the distinction between asbestos and nonasbestos mineral fibers.[17,18] For example, asbestos fibers are birefringent when viewed with polarizing microscopy because of their crystalline nature, whereas fibrous glass (which is amorphous) is nonrefringent. According to some authorities, polarizing microscopy with dispersion staining is the method of choice for the identification of asbestos fibers in bulk samples and may also be useful in the analysis of air samples.[19,20] Its advantages include low cost, minimal sample preparation, simplicity of the analytical procedure, and reproducibility of results. Disadvantages include limitations of light microscopy for detection of the finest diameter fibers and some inaccuracies in the determination of specific mineral types based on indices of refraction because of overlapping values for the bulk of the asbestos mineral types.[18]

Infrared Spectroscopy

Asbestos minerals produce characteristic spectra when examined by means of infrared spectrophotometry (IR).[17,18,21] IR is a bulk analytical technique and thus cannot be used for the identification of individual fibers. The advantages of this procedure include its relative low cost and simple operation. Disadvantages include inaccuracies in the presence of a mixed particulate population (e.g., chrysotile mixed with clay minerals or talc) and interferences from organic debris. This technique is seldom used for the detection or identification of asbestos in environmental or tissue samples.

Magnetic Alignment and Light Scattering (MALS)

The MALS method of estimating asbestos content in a sample involves the use of a magnetic field to achieve alignment of fibers in a thin transparent film, which is then examined by light scattering. The fibers are suspended in an agar solution within a shallow brass ring mounted on a glass slide, which is supported in the air gap of an electromagnet. When such a film is illuminated orthogonally with a parallel beam of white light, scattering by the fibers produces a distinctive bright band which, when measured photometrically, provides information regarding fiber mass, fiber number, and median fiber length and diameter.[22,23] Fiber surface area can also be estimated with this technique. The MALS method has been used to measure the fiber content of lung tissue and compare various fiber parameters with severity of fibrosis among patients with asbestosis. Comparison of individuals exposed to a wide variety of asbestos fiber types showed that the fibrosis score estimated by light microscopy correlated best with the relative fiber surface area per unit weight of tissue.[24] The fibrosis score correlated less well with relative fiber number or mass per unit weight of tissue. The advantages of this technique are that it is rapid, simple, and relatively inexpensive. However, it is a bulk analytical technique and must be calibrated by means of transmission electron microscopy. It does not provide information about the range of particle dimensions in a sample or allow determination of specific mineral fiber types.

X-Ray and Electron Diffraction

When x-rays or electrons pass through a crystalline material, they are diffracted by the regularly spaced atomic planes within the crystal according to Braggs' law.[25] The diffraction pattern resulting from this interaction provides useful information with regard to the three-dimensional structure of the substance under consideration. For x-ray diffraction, the diffraction pattern can be recorded on x-ray sensitive film or as peaks on a strip chart using an x-ray diffractometer. For electron diffraction, the pattern appears as a series of dots on the CRT of a transmission electron microscope and can be recorded on photographic film (Figures 1-4 and 1-6).

X-ray diffraction is a bulk analytical technique and is therefore suitable for the analysis of macroscopic samples. The diffraction pattern often appears as a series of concentric rings on the x-ray film, and the distance from any one ring to the center of the film is inversely proportional to the distance d between the planes of atoms in the crystal giving rise to that particular x-ray intensity maxima. The peaks of x-ray intensity maxima on a strip chart are presented as angular deviation 2θ from center which in turn can be related to interplanar spacing d (given in angstrom units, Å). An x-ray diffraction tracing for amosite asbestos is shown in Figure 1-9 with major peaks at 3.07, 3.21, and 8.33 Å. Although x-ray diffraction is generally considered a qualitative technique, methods have been devised whereby x-ray diffraction may be used to quantitatively measure the amounts of asbestos present in a sample.[26] By comparing the integrated peaks of the x-ray tracing

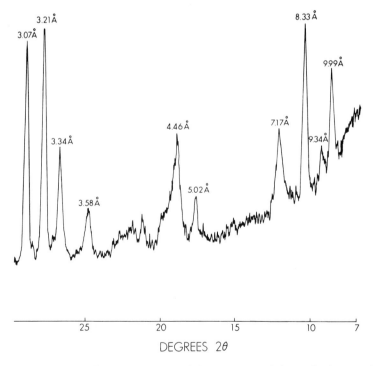

DEGREES 2θ

Figure 1-9. X-ray diffraction tracing of dust recovered from the lungs of an asbestos worker with asbestosis (Same case as Figure 4-5). The tracing shows several prominent peaks correlating with diffraction maxima for amosite asbestos (see text).

from known standards of chrysotile asbestos with those of unknown samples and correcting for x-ray absorption by the matrix and the filter, investigators have been able to measure chrysotile asbestos with detection limits as low as $3\mu g/cm^2$ of filter when chrysotile is present in small quantities (1% by weight of matrix material). In addition, concentration methods have been described that permit the detection of as little as 0.01% to 0.05% (100–500 ppm) tremolite in chrysotile by quantitative XRD.[5]

Whereas x-ray diffraction is a bulk analytical method, electron diffraction is a microanalytical technique, capable of providing a diffraction pattern from a particle or area as small as 1 µm or less in diameter.[27] Thus using this technique, often referred to as selected area electron diffraction (SAED), one can obtain crystallographic data from an individual asbestos fiber. Some investigators consider electron diffraction to be the method of choice for separating the six asbestos minerals from most other nonasbestos minerals.[28] The diffraction pattern is formed by weakening the first projector lens in the transmission electron microscope, bringing the backfocal plane of the objective lens into focus on the viewing screen.[25] This results in the imaging of the diffraction pattern as a series of dots on the CRT, and the distance R between the individual spots of the diffraction pattern and the central spot is inversely related to the interplanar spacing d of the planes of atoms in the crystal giving rise to that particular electron intensity maximum. As noted in a previous section, chrysotile has a particularly characteristic diffraction pattern (Figure 1-4). However, diffraction patterns cannot be obtained from all fibers, and in practice, the technique is tedious and time-consuming.

Analytical Electron Microscopy

Although there are a wide variety of techniques for the identification of asbestos, most investigators prefer some form of analytical electron microscopy.[17,18] The analytical electron microscope has the ability to provide high resolution images of the smallest of fibers, detailing their finest morphologic features, and spectral information regarding chemical composition by means of energy dispersive spectrometry (EDS). The basic components of an analytical electron microscope are shown schematically in Figure 1-10.

Perhaps the most widely used instrument for the detection and analysis of asbestos fibers is the analytical transmission electron microscope (TEM). This technique has the advantages of superior resolution as well as the ability to obtain both crystallographic and elemental compositional data for an individual fiber by means of SAED (see above) and EDS, respectively.[29] The latter technique involves focusing the electron beam on an individual particle and observing the x-ray spectra produced by the interaction of the electrons of the primary beam with the atoms within the specimen. The resultant spectrum consists of peaks distributed according to the energy (KeV) of the x-rays generated, which is in turn related to the elements composing the particle (or fiber). The spectra generated can then be visually compared with

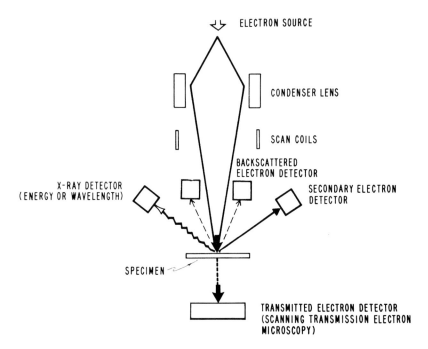

ELECTRON SOURCE

CONDENSER LENS

SCAN COILS

BACKSCATTERED
ELECTRON DETECTOR

X-RAY DETECTOR
(ENERGY OR WAVELENGTH)

SECONDARY ELECTRON
DETECTOR

SPECIMEN

TRANSMITTED ELECTRON DETECTOR
(SCANNING TRANSMISSION ELECTRON
MICROSCOPY)

Figure 1-10. The basic components of the scanning electron microscope, equipped with back-scattered electron and x-ray detectors, are illustrated. Such an instrument is extremely valuable in the characterization of inorganic particulates such as asbestos fibers. (Reprinted from Garner and Klintworth: Pathobiology of Ocular Disease, Marcel Dekker, Inc., NY, 1982.)

known samples of asbestos (e.g., the U.I.C.C. standard asbestos samples), or can be subjected to discriminate function analysis. The latter is a more objective method which can differentiate among the various amphiboles with a high degree of confidence.[30] Analytical TEM has been used for the analysis of asbestos in dust recovered from human lung samples for at least three decades.[31,32] However, preparatory techniques for TEM are often complex, and the method is expensive and time-consuming.

Analytical scanning electron microscopy (SEM) has also been employed by various investigators for the detection and identification of asbestos.[30,33] This technique has been used to detect as little as 0.002% (20 ppm by weight) of tremolite in chrysotile samples in which the chrysotile was removed by treatment with acids and bases.[34] Analytical SEM has the advantages of less complicated preparatory steps and larger sample size (e.g., an entire filter) as compared to TEM. Although it is generally acknowledged that TEM has superior resolution, state-of-the-art SEMs have resolutions approaching that of the TEM and are thus capable of resolving fine asbestos fibrils.[33] A potential disadvantage of the SEM is that electron diffraction cannot be readily performed with this technique. However, in the authors' experience, most fibers can be unequivocally identified based on their morphologic characteristics and energy dispersive spectra.[33] A further advantage of analytical SEM is the potential for automation. Automated image x-ray analyzers are commercially available with capabilities of completely analyzing more than one thousand individual particles per hour under optimal conditions.[35] Although such systems have great potential for biological analyses, application has thus far been extremely limited. As is the case for analytical TEM, analytical SEM is an expensive and time-consuming technique.

References

1. Lee DHK, Selikoff IJ: Historical background to the asbestos problem. *Environ Res* 18:300–314, 1979.
2. Craighead JE, Mossman BT: Pathogenesis of asbestos-associated diseases. *N Engl J Med* 306:1446–1455, 1982.
3. Murray R: Asbestos: A chronology of its origins and health effects. *Br J Ind Med* 47:361–365, 1990.
4. Pooley FD: Asbestos Mineralogy. Ch. 1 In: *Asbestos-Related Malignancy* (Antman K, Aisner J, eds.), Grune & Stratton, Inc: Orlando, 1987, pp. 3–27.
5. Addison J, Davies LST: Analysis of amphibole asbestos in chrysotile and other minerals. *Ann Occup Hyg* 34:159–175, 1990.
6. Virta RL: Asbestos. In: *Minerals Yearbook–2000*, Reston, VA: U.S. Geological Survey, 2000, pp. 9.1–9.3.
7. Brody AR, Hill LH, Adkins B, O'Connor RW: Chrysotile asbestos inhalation in rats: Deposition pattern and reaction of alveolar epithelium and pulmonary macrophages. *Am Rev Respir Dis* 123:670–679, 1981.
8. Lee KP: Lung response to particulates with emphasis on asbestos and other fibrous dusts. *CRC Crit Rev Toxicol* 14:33–86, 1985.
9. Roggli VL, Brody AR: Changes in numbers and dimensions of chrysotile asbestos fibers in lungs of rats following short-term exposure. *Expl Lung Res* 7:133–147, 1984.
10. Coin PG, Roggli VL, Brody AR: Deposition, clearance, and translocation of chrysotile asbestos from peripheral and central regions of the rat lung. *Environ Res* 58:97–116, 1992.
11. Coin PG, Roggli VL, Brody AR: Persistence of long, thin chrysotile asbestos fibers in the lungs of rats. *Environ Health Persp* 102 [Suppl 5]:197–199, 1994.
12. Hodgson AA: Chemistry and physics of asbestos. In: *Asbestos: Properties, Applications, and Hazards* (Vol. 1) (Michaels L, Chissick SS, eds.), New York: John Wiley and Sons, 1979, pp. 67–114.
13. Zussman J: The mineralogy of asbestos. In: *Asbestos: Properties, Applications, and Hazards* (Vol. 1) (Michaels L, Chissick SS, eds.), New York: John Wiley and Sons, 1979, pp. 45–65.
14. Roggli VL, Mastin JP, Shelburne JD, Roe MS, Brody AR: Inorganic particulates in human lung: Relationship to the inflammatory response. In: *Inflammatory Cells and Lung Disease* (Lynn WS, ed.), Boca Raton, FL: CRC Press, Inc., 1983, pp. 29–62.
15. Crawford D: Electron microscopy applied to studies of the biological significance of defects in crocidolite asbestos. *J Microscopy* 120:181–192, 1980.
16. Franco MA, Hutchison JL, Jefferson DA, Thomas JM: Structural imperfection and morphology of crocidolite (blue asbestos). *Nature* 266:520–521, 1977.
17. Langer AM, Ashley R, Baden V, Berkley C, Hammond EC, Mackler AD, Maggiore CJ, Nicholson WJ, Rohl AM, Rubin IB, Sastre A, Selikoff IJ: Identification of asbestos in human tissues. *J Occup Med* 15:287–295, 1973.

18. Berkley C, Langer AM, Baden V: Instrumental analysis of inspired fibrous pulmonary particulates. *NY Acad Sci Trans* 30:331–350, 1967.
19. McCrone WC: Asbestos monitoring. *Amer Lab* 17:20–28, 1985.
20. McCrone WC: Evaluation of asbestos in insulation. *Amer Lab* 11:19–31, 1979.
21. Coates JP: IR analysis of toxic dusts: Analysis of collected samples of quartz and asbestos. *Amer Lab* 9:105–111, 1977.
22. Timbrell V: Measurement of fibres in human lung tissue. In: *Biological Effects of Mineral Fibres*, (Vol. 1) (Wagner JC, ed.), IARC Scientific Publications No. 30, Lyon: 1980, pp. 113–126.
23. Timbrell V: Deposition and retention of fibers in the human lung. *Ann Occup Hyg* 26:347–369, 1982.
24. Lippmann M: Asbestos exposure indices. *Environ Res* 46:86–106, 1988.
25. Roggli VL, Ingram P, Linton RW, Gutknecht WF, Mastin P, Shelburne JD: New techniques for imaging and analyzing lung tissue. *Environ Health Persp* 56:163–183, 1984.
26. Lange BA, Haartz JC: Determination of microgram quantities of asbestos by x-ray diffraction: Chrysotile in thin dust layers of matrix material. *Anal Chem* 51:520–525, 1979.
27. Geiss RH: Electron diffraction from submicron areas using STEM. *Scanning Electron Microsc* 11:337–344, 1976.
28. Ruud CO, Barrett CS, Russell PA, Clark RL: Selected area electron diffraction and energy dispersive x-ray analysis for the identification of asbestos fibers—a comparison. *Micron* 7:115–132, 1976.
29. Churg A: Quantitative methods for analysis of disease induced by asbestos and other mineral particles using the transmission electron microscope. Ch. 4 In: *Microprobe Analysis in Medicine* (Ingram P, Shelburne JD, Roggli VL, eds.), New York: Hemisphere Pub. Corp, 1989, pp. 79–95.
30. Millette JR, McFarren EF: EDS of waterborne asbestos fibers in TEM, SEM and STEM. *Scanning Electron Microsc* 111:451–460, 1976.
31. Langer AM, Rubin IB, Selikoff IJ: Chemical characterization of asbestos body cores by electron microprobe analysis. *J Histochem Cytochem* 20:723–734, 1972.
32. Langer AM, Rubin IB, Selikoff IJ, Pooley FD: Chemical characterization of uncoated asbestos fibers from the lungs of asbestos workers by electron microprobe analysis. *J Histochem Cytochem* 20:735–740, 1972.
33. Roggli VL: Scanning electron microscopic analysis of mineral fibers in human lungs. Ch. 5 In: *Microprobe Analysis in Medicine*, (Ingram P, Shelburne JD, Roggli VL, eds.), New York: Hemisphere Pub. Corp, 1989, pp. 97–110.
34. Tossavainen A, Kotilainen M, Takahashi K, Pan G, Vanhala E: Amphibole fibres in Chinese chrysotile asbestos. *Ann Occup Hyg* 45:145–152, 2001.
35. Johnson GG, White EW, Strickler D, Hoover R: Image analysis techniques. In: *Symposium on Electron Microscopy of Microfibers: Proceedings of the First FDA Office of Science Summer Symposium* (Asher IM, McGrath PP, eds.), Washington, DC: U.S. Government Printing Office, 1976, pp. 76–82.

2

Occupational and Environmental Exposure to Asbestos

Dennis J. Darcey and Tony Alleman

Introduction

The usefulness of asbestos as an industrial material must be considered to understand the breadth of its consequent public health impact. Since its discovery as an indestructible material centuries ago, it has been used in countless applications, often because no identified substance rivals its engineering or commercial performance.

Asbestos applications result from its many unique physical attributes. Its high tensile strength stabilizes mixtures with concrete, asphalt, and plastic. Asbestos also offers a stable material for frictional use, that is, as a brake surface. Because of the length and pliability of its fibers, it has been incorporated into specially manufactured products, including gaskets, pads, fabric sheets, and asbestos paper with intrinsic properties of resistance and strength. Because it blocks heat transfer and is itself fireproof, it represents an ideal insulation material. Mixed into a slurry, it has been applied in economical fashion to building surfaces for fire protection and heat retention. In both its fabric and compacted-brick forms, it has been used to encase furnaces and kilns.

Economic advantages of asbestos must also be considered in explaining its widespread application. As a natural (mined) rather than a manufactured substance, it was more available and its use not as closely evaluated by producers or consumers. Present in natural deposits on several continents, it has remained easily available for construction and industrial exploitation by all nations, both industrialized and developing. Its production cost, as a truly raw material, has always been far less than substitute agents, which require manufacture and even technology licensing.

Historical Origin and Applications

Preindustrial Applications

The first recorded use of asbestos is as a wick material for oil lamps in ancient times. The material's name originates from the Greek for "inextinguishable" or "indestructible."[1] Woven into cloth, asbestos provided nearly miraculous resistance to fire, especially impressive for shrouds of the deceased whose cremation was open to public display.

Combining asbestos with clay and other malleable materials is also cited as one of the earliest applications of the material. In Finland in 2500 BC, asbestos was added to clay pots for greater strength. Asbestos as a fortifying additive remains its major present-day use as a component of cement, concrete, paint, vinyl, and tar mixtures, accounting for 70% of current applications worldwide.

The Modern Period

The past decades have witnessed a drastic change in America's patterns of asbestos use. Regulatory and health issues, rather than direct economic and engineering factors, now dominate. In the United States, regulatory concern regarding asbestos' use and continued presence has continually grown. A ban on the use of asbestos was proposed by the U.S. Environmental Protection Agency (EPA) in 1989 to prohibit the manufacture, importation, processing and distribution, and commerce of certain asbestos-containing products.[2] The provision also called for labeling requirements. However, in October 1991, the United States Court of Appeals for the 5th Circuit vacated and remanded most of the EPA Asbestos Rule. The legal implications of the court's decision forced the EPA to revise its rule under the Clean Air Act (CAA) and Toxic Substances Control Act (TSCA). The ban under the TSCA includes (1) corrugated paper, (2) roll board, (3) commercial paper, (4) specialty paper, (5) flooring, and (6) new uses of asbestos. Products not currently banned include asbestos cement products, roofing felt and coatings, asbestos cement shingle, millboard, asbestos automatic transmission components, clutch facings, friction materials, disc brake pads, and brake linings. Under the Clean Air Act most spray-applied surfacing asbestos containing materials that have more than 1% asbestos are banned, as are wet-applied and preformed asbestos pipe insulation.[3]

The Collegium Ramazzini, an international, nongovernmental organization that promotes public policy on occupational and environmental issues, has proposed an international ban on asbestos. The members believe substitutes for asbestos exist that are safer and note that many European countries have already banned asbestos use.[4] However, others have criticized their proposal arguing that the risks of continued asbestos use have been exaggerated and that health studies have not yet determined the risk of substitute materials.[5]

The late Dr. Irving J Selikoff, whose scientific, clinical, and public affairs careers are synonymous with asbestos and its health effects, categorized the societal impact of asbestos disease into three population "waves" of asbestos exposure and consequent clinical disease. Because of the well-documented latent interval for asbestos-related disease, the public health impact from each period of asbestos disease trails the period of exposure by 30 to 50 years.

The first wave of asbestos exposure comprises the workers whose activities actually generate asbestos for use, including the miners and packagers who transformed an ore into an industrial material. This exposure period, involving relatively few workers, extends from the initial use of the mineral into the early twentieth century. These workers, in countries where asbestos was first processed, Canada and South Africa, prompted the initial recognition of the diseases that required a latent period of decades to manifest themselves.[6]

The second wave of asbestos-induced disease represents the impact of the manufacturing and construction use of the material. The most important peak in Western society's exposure to asbestos occurred during the period of rapid economic expansion surrounding World War II. Intense and high-volume ship construction, structural insulation, and the industrial fabrication of asbestos-containing products created a huge cohort of exposed workers during the mid-twentieth century. The ensuing period of public health impact manifested itself from the 1970s through the 1990s.

The third wave of asbestos exposure and disease generates the most controversy and conjecture regarding both its size and the intensity of its public health impact. This comprises the cohort of citizens exposed to asbestos already in place. This population is likely to be exposed during the disruption of preapplied asbestos insulation in homes and commercial buildings. Specific groups exposed to the highest dose of the mineral during this phase include building maintenance workers, construction workers, electricians, custodians, and the workforce employed specifically for asbestos abatement. The public health impact is seen at the present time. Disasters such as the collapse of the World Trade Center on September 11, 2001, raise concerns regarding the release of in-place asbestos into the ambient air and possible health effects of such exposures (Figures 2-1 and 2-2).

Worldwide production of asbestos declined between 1980 and 2000, but worldwide use of asbestos remains sizable despite the increased recognition of its health consequences. In the United States, use of asbestos had markedly diminished even before the U.S. Environmental Protection Agency (EPA) ban in July 1989. Although the present rule still allows significant uses of asbestos, U.S. consumption of asbestos dropped from a high of 801,000 metric tons in 1973 to minimal amounts recently (Figure 2-3).

Occupational Exposure to Asbestos

Asbestos Processing

In the United States, for geological reasons, asbestos production has never been an important commercial enterprise. Even before restrictions for asbestos use, the combined workforce involved in mining and milling was known to be fewer than 600 people.[7] Mining creates exposure levels that are surprisingly low when compared to those of materials manufactured, averaging 0.9 fibers/ml.[1] Because of the way the ore is handled, the fibers remain consolidated and have not yet become individualized. In contrast, the subsequent operation of mineral refining and milling (usually designed to "open" the bundles

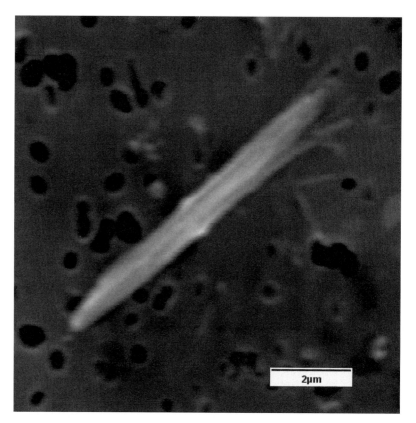

Figure 2-1. Scanning electron micrograph of chrysotile bundle isolated from bronchoalveolar lavage fluid from a New York City firefighter working on site for two weeks after the World Trade Center towers collapsed on September 11, 2001. Nuclepore filter preparation, magnified ×14,000.

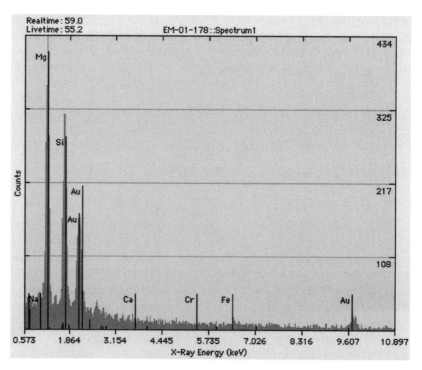

Figure 2-2. Energy dispersive spectrum from fiber shown in Figure 2-1. Note the large peaks for magnesium and silicon, characteristic for chrysotile asbestos.

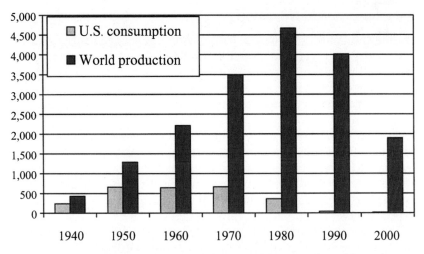

Figure 2-3. Asbestos consumption in the United States and world production of asbestos, which is used as a guide to world consumption. Peak U.S. consumption of asbestos was 801,000 metric tons in 1973. Peak world production was 5.09 million metric tons in 1975. Data from Minerals Yearbook, v. 1 (published by the U.S. Bureau of Mines until 1995 and by the U.S. Geological Survey after 1995, with permission).

into individual fibers) generates worker exposure levels of 6.0 to 12.1 fibers/ml.[1]

Asbestos is shipped in bags, historically made of porous cloth but recently of paper and plastic. The handling of this material in secondary industries routinely begins with cutting open these bags and manually emptying them into hoppers, for example, for mixture with concrete. Because this material is both dry and nonaggregated, the likelihood of dispersal is then at its maximum. The waste packaging material constitutes a source of exposure separate from the intended construction or industrial application.

Manufacture of Asbestos-Containing Products

The exposures that occur during the manufacture of asbestos products are extremely variable. Production of asbestos textiles involved higher exposure than other products. Carding and conventional spinning produced extreme air concentrations, resistant to environmental controls. Methods of manufacture utilizing liquid dispersion rather than dry asbestos are more successful at controlling potential exposure.

Work with material where the asbestos fibers were already entrapped (e.g., in roofing materials, floor tile, or cement pipe) presented considerable exposure opportunities, but only when such products are broken, thereby releasing respirable fibers. The job title sometimes provides information that offers some basis for assessing actual exposure, but it is often incomplete or misleading in estimating the degree of exposure. Certain jobs are more variable than others; for example, exposures for "inspectors" in manufacturing depend on the amount of loose asbestos dust remaining on the finished product.

Asbestos Insulation Materials

During the 1940s, 1950s and 1960s, covering boilers and furnaces with asbestos was universal. Before the health effects of asbestos exposure were well recognized, the use of asbestos insulation material was considered an effective safety practice, preventing burns, heat release, and fire. Boilermakers and pipe coverers constitute the most important and widely evaluated cohort of exposed workers. Selikoff's 1964 study of New York insulation workers unionists was one of the earliest U.S. reports of the health consequences of this work. Among the 255 deaths evaluated in this mortality study, 18% were the result of lung cancer, 11% of direct pulmonary damage from the dust, and 1.2% of mesothelioma. This staggering impact was an early demonstration of asbestos exposure risk.[8]

The construction industry application of asbestos coating to structural steel beams increased the societal scope of this exposure. The spraying of asbestos-cement mixtures was initiated in 1935, and from 1958 through 1978 was widely employed for railway carriages, naval ships, and newly constructed buildings. By one estimate, 1.2 billion square feet of asbestos-containing insulation (averaging 14% in concentration) is present in 190,000 American buildings.[9] The process was actually employed more—rather than less—frequently in the final years of this period, until the practice was halted when health issues became widely known.

Friction Materials

The use of asbestos for vehicular brakes takes advantage of its heat resistance and material strength. Asbestos concentrations in these materials are sizable, ranging from 30–80%. Because manufacture and repair of automotive wheels is geographically widely distributed, this application exposes individuals in a wide variety of trades and geography. The number of workers exposed as a consequence of asbestos brake and clutch work is estimated at 900,000. The practices of "blowing out" brake surfaces and beveling or grinding brake shoes produce modest airborne fiber concentrations for considerable periods of time and at distances extending many feet from the actual operation. The dispersion of asbestos dust particles from brake surfaces (even in situations of automotive traffic) remains a distinct possibility.[10]

Construction Materials

In floor tile and in roof shingles and coatings, asbestos mixtures utilize the flexibility and strength of the mineral additive as an important stabilizing feature. Because these materials are popular for home improvement activities, this application provides additional opportunity for exposure to nonprofessional workers, who lack specific occupational monitoring or training. Ordinarily, exposures are quite low and require considerable disruption of the product's integrity to release respirable particles with asbestos content.

Shipyards

Shipbuilding makes unusually intense use of insulation materials because of the nature of the construction. Ships have greater vulnerability to fire because of their isolation and the confined spaces. Noise and heat from the immediate proximity of a shipboard power plant create an important need for effective thermal and acoustic insulation, which must also be fireproof. In addition, preparing ships brings workers not necessarily directly involved with asbestos work (e.g., electricians, metal workers) into an asbestos-containing closed environment for the entire duration of the project. This closed-space exposure is, by its nature, difficult to control by the usual industrial measures, such as ventilation, wetting of the fiber sources, and containment.

Because workplace safety efforts were relaxed during the establishment of the wartime economy of the 1940s, the massive shipbuilding effort of that period put the largest segment of workers at risk for subsequent asbestos-related disease. The conditions of enclosed, poorly ventilated, and unmonitored assignments produced prolonged and heavy exposure to all interior ship workers.

Asbestos Removal

As a result of the regulatory recommendation that asbestos must be removed from schools, industrial work sites, and residences, the most significant and identifiable current exposure to asbestos occurs during asbestos abatement.[11] In the removal of pure asbestos lagging, for example, potential exposures of 62 to 159 fibers/ml have been reported.[12] This process often takes place in considerable disorder, because the surfaces are no longer easily accessible, and the work site is either in demand or in current use. Geographic isolation, soaking of the asbestos source, and personal containment represent the most important strategies for reduction of exposure.

The safety advantage in this process is that workers are required to be trained and to become aware of the nature of the task and its hazards. Current regulations for asbestos exposure provide detailed rules for these workers that contrast dramatically with the historically careless handling of the same material.

The administrative demands of asbestos worker protection are extensive. Currently, workers involved in asbestos abatement are required to undergo a pre-employment evaluation of their ability to work wearing a HEPA (high-efficiency-particulate air) filter respirator and impermeable (thus hot and humid) disposable clothing.[13] Baseline and periodic chest radiographs are taken, and measurement of pulmonary function. Before initiation of asbestos work, these individuals receive mandatory instruction regarding the health effects of asbestos-related disease and the means of dust and exposure control. Educational opportunities regarding the multiplicative effect of tobacco smoking on the risks from asbestos exposure are now a required component of asbestos worker training.

The area for asbestos removal is enclosed with a plastic barrier of specified 6-mil-thick polyethylene sheeting and by toxic-hazard

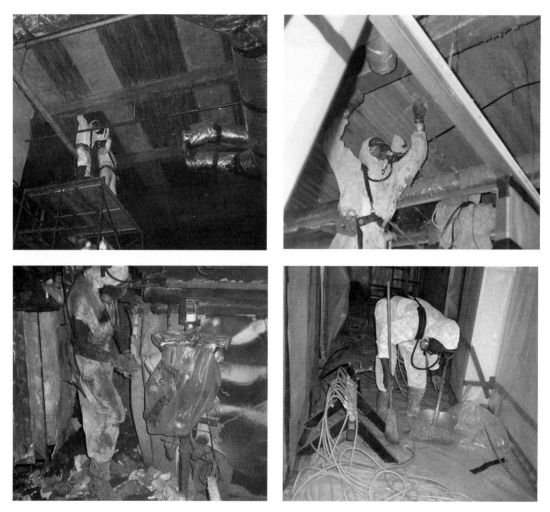

Figure 2-4. Workers in the North Carolina Asbestos Abatement Program. Asbestos removal occurs within confined spaces. Note the respiratory equipment and special protective clothing.

warning signs. The site is kept at negative barometric pressure (relative to the surrounding area) by having fans blow air outward through HEPA filters. If possible, asbestos-containing material is covered in plastic bags to encase escaping fragments. Additionally, workers wear personal protective gear (mask, gown, and gloves, as in Figure 2-4). Throughout removal, every effort is made to keep the material soaked so that respirable dust is minimized. Waste products are labeled and are handled with special care. Monitoring for airborne asbestos concentration is performed outside the confined asbestos-abatement area. Following each work period, workers are required to discard all outer clothing and shower, to prevent secondary contamination from work clothes. Periodic medical monitoring is also required, although the decades-long latency of asbestos-related disease makes these sessions more appropriately an opportunity for discussions of health risk and for counseling on smoking cessation.

Nonoccupational Exposure to Asbestos

Exposure to asbestos in the ambient indoor and outdoor environments results from many sources, both natural and manufactured. Chrysotile asbestos, which accounts for more than 90% of the asbestos used in the United States, has become a ubiquitous contaminant of ambient air. It has been noted that asbestos fiber can be found in the lungs of almost everyone in the American population.[14] Natural sources of asbestos fiber release include weathering and erosion of asbestos-containing rock and of road surfaces composed of asbestos ores. If the primary areas of source rock are compared with high population density, the most critical areas for emissions from natural sources appear to be eastern Pennsylvania, southeastern New York, southwestern Connecticut, and greater Los Angeles and San Francisco.

Manufactured sources of exposure in the past have included off-site releases from mining, milling, and manufacture of asbestos products, exposing residents in nearby communities. Before occupational work practices improved in the 1970s, secondary contamination of homes occurred when employees brought home asbestos-laden work clothes. Weathering of asbestos cement wall and roofing materials is a relatively minor environmental source of exposure from man-made construction materials. However, off-site release from construction sites (primarily from sprayed-on asbestos fireproofing) have resulted in ambient asbestos levels 100 times background.[15]

Asbestos brake and clutch pads in automobiles contribute to the environmental load of asbestos. However, it is uncertain how much respirable fiber is released, because thermal degradation occurs at the high temperatures generated during braking. Waste disposal has become a growing source of potential exposure to asbestos fibers, and promises to continue as removal, abatement, and renovation occur in the existing building stock. Consumer products, water supplies, and food sources have been contaminated with asbestos-containing materials in the past. These manufactured sources of exposure have been significantly reduced by regulatory activity over the past 30 years and will continue to decline.

Currently, the most important source of nonoccupational exposure is the release of fibers from existing asbestos-containing surface materials in schools, residences, and public buildings or from sprayed asbestos-containing fireproofing in high-rise office buildings. The greatest potential for future exposure will be determined by the asbestos released during the maintenance, repair, and removal of these structures. The implementation of the Asbestos Hazard Emergency Response Act (AHERA), requiring inspection of the nation's public and private schools for asbestos, has resulted in an explosive commercial growth of the industry involved in asbestos identification and removal.

Some have argued that removal itself presents more of an exposure hazard than leaving the materials undisturbed or encapsulated.[16]

Measuring Exposure

Different techniques have been developed for measuring the concentration of asbestos in ambient air and in the workplace. The phase-contrast light microscope for counting fibers in the workplace has been less useful in the ambient environment, where fiber identity and character are usually unknown, fibers are too small to be seen by light microscopy, and concentrations expressed as mass are usually hundreds or thousands of times lower than those in the workplace.

Fiber concentrations in the workplace have generally been measured as the number of fibers longer than 5 microns. Ambient concentrations are now determined by transmission electron microscopy and usually are expressed as mass per unit volume (nanogram per cubic meter). Because of intrinsic variability in the unit weight of individual fibers, the conversion factors relating mass concentration to optical fiber concentration range from 5 to $150 \mu g/m^3/f/ml$. These conversion factors have been adopted by the EPA[15] and other scientific bodies.

Measurements acquired through transmission electron microscopy have established background concentrations of asbestos in urban ambient air at generally less than 1 nanogram per cubic meter (0.00003 fibers per ml) and rarely more than 10 nanograms per cubic meter (0.00033 fibers per ml).[17] Table 2-1 summarizes fiber concentration data from a variety of studies in both urban and rural areas.

Asbestos concentrations in buildings, on the other hand, are more variable, revealing threefold variability among arithmetic mean concentrations.[17] Earlier studies often focused on buildings in which asbestos surface materials were visibly damaged and friable, which were not representative. In buildings with evidence of severe damage or deterioration, the probability of detecting excessive asbestos levels

Table 2-1. Summary of asbestos exposure samples in different environments

Sample set	Sample No.	Measured concentration (ng/m^3)		Equivalent concentration (fibers/cc)*	
		Median	90th %ile	Median	90th %ile
Air of 48 U.S. cities	187	1.6	6.8	0.00005	0.00023
Air in U.S. school rooms without asbestos	31	16.3	72.7	0.00054	0.00242
Air in Paris bldgs with asbestos surfaces	135	1.8	32.2	0.00006	0.00107
Air in U.S. bldgs with cementitious asbestos	28	7.9	19.1	0.00026	0.00064
Air in U.S. bldgs with friable asbestos	54	19.2	96.2	0.00064	0.00321

Source: Modified from Ref.17. *Based on conversion factor of $30 \mu g/m^3 = 1$ fiber/cc.

Table 2-2. Summary statistics for average airborne fiber concentrations in U.S. schools and buildings

Statistic	Schools (71)	Outdoor air (48)	Public buildings		
			Category 1 (6)	Category 2 (6)	Category 3 (37)
Median		0.00000	0.00010	0.00040	0.00058
Mean	0.00024*	0.00039	0.00099	0.00059	0.00073
Standard Deviation	0.00053	0.00096	0.00198	0.00052	0.00072

Source: From Ref. 18, with permission.
*80th percentile = 0.00045; 90th percentile = 0.00083.
The data used in the calculation of each statistic are the average concentrations (expressed as number of fibers greater than 5 μm in length per cubic centimeter of air) in a building (for indoor samples) or the concentration outside each building (for outdoor samples). By visual inspection, category 1 buildings contained no asbestos-containing material (ACM), category 2 buildings contained ACM in primarily good condition, and buildings in category 3 showed at least one area of significantly damaged ACM. In the study on public buildings, 387 indoor and 48 outdoor air samples were evaluated. No asbestos fibers were detected in 83% of the 387 samples. The sample size is given in parentheses below each heading.

over background was high. If the asbestos-containing surface materials or thermal insulation was undamaged or encapsulated, lower air concentrations were observed.

Table 2-2 shows summary statistics for average airborne fiber concentrations near schools and buildings Levels are comparable to outdoor air and are several orders of magnitude lower than current workplace standards (OSHA permissible exposure level (PEL) of 0.1 fibers per ml).

Asbestos abatement work is a significant potential source of asbestos exposure, particularly in schools and public buildings. While abatement procedures already specified by the EPA should minimize building contamination following renovation, removal, enclosure, or encapsulation of asbestos materials, these procedures may be violated.

The EPA has monitored the efficacy of the specified controls and cleanup procedures. Table 2-3 presents the results of one study of five schools where removal and encapsulation of asbestos-containing surfaces followed EPA procedures.[17] Although escape of asbestos fibers did occur during encapsulation and removal, there appeared to be a net reduction in fiber levels after encapsulation. Little improvement occurred in asbestos fiber levels following physical removal, with pre- and postabatement fiber levels being virtually the same. These results have brought into question both the health risk/benefit and the cost-benefit considerations of removal versus encapsulation. Currently, widespread removal of asbestos is not frequently recommended, and encapsulation is preferred in many situations.

Table 2-3. Geometric mean of chrysotile fiber and mass concentrations before, during, and after asbestos abatement

	Before abatement		During abatement*		Immediately after abatement		After school resumed	
Sampling location	(f/l)[†]	(ng/m³)	(f/l)	(ng/m³)	(f/l)	(ng/m³)	(f/l)	(ng/m³)
Encapsulation								
Rooms with un-painted asbestos	1423.6	6.7	117.2	0.6	13.7	0.1	248.1	1.2
Rooms with painted asbestos	622.9	2.7	—	—	0.8	0.0	187.2	0.8
Asbestos-free rooms	250.6	1.2	0.5	0.0	9.3	0.0	30.7	0.2
Outdoors	3.5	0.0	0.0	0.0	6.5	0.0	2.8	0.0
Removal								
Rooms with asbestos	31.2	0.2	1736.0	14.4	5.6	0.1	23.9	0.2
Asbestos-free rooms	6.1	0.1	12.0	0.1	1.6	0.0	18.1	0.1
Outdoors	12.6	0.1	1.3	0.0	20.0	0.1	7.9	0.0

Source: Reprinted from Ref. 17, with permission.
*Measured outside work containment areas.
[†]Fibers of all lengths.

Regulatory Activity

Public health concern over the occupational and nonoccupational sources of asbestos exposure has created a vast array of governmental regulatory activity and the phasing out of asbestos production and its use in consumer products. This marked reduction in use is the result of regulatory activities in the 1970s and 1980s, during which time five government agencies invoked statutory authority to regulate asbestos.

The Occupational Safety and Health Administration (OSHA) regulates workplace exposure to asbestos and has set a PEL (an 8-hour time-weighted average for a 40-hour-per-week work shift) for occupational exposures. The PEL has been steadily lowered, as concern over health hazards and better monitoring methods have become established (Table 2-4). The first permanent standard, set in 1972, was 5 fibers/ml. This was lowered in 1976 to 2 fibers/ml and in 1986 to the lowest agreed to be technologically feasible at that time, 0.2 fibers/ml. The National Institute for Occupational Safety and Health (NIOSH) recommended a PEL of 0.1 fibers/ml, and this was also proposed as a regulatory standard by OSHA in 1990 and adopted in 1993.

The Mine Safety and Health Administration regulates the mining and milling of asbestos ore. The Food & Drug Administration (FDA) is responsible for regulating asbestos in food, drugs, and cosmetics. Consumer product bans on the use of asbestos in garments, dry-wall patching compounds, and fireplace-emberizing materials have been implemented by the Consumer Product Safety Commission. Despite these selected events, most of the regulatory activity has emanated from the Environmental Protection Agency.

Table 2-4. Regulatory exposure levels in the workplace

Date	U.K. Advisory Committee on Asbestos	British Occupational Hygiene Soc.	National Institute of Occupational Safety and Health	OSHA (proposed)	OSHA (regulation)	EPA
1969		2 fibers/ml. TWA chrysotile				
March 1971						Asbestos listed as hazardous air pollutant
1972					5 fibers/ml STEL	
April 1973						No visible emissions, milling and manufacturing Ban: Spray application of friable materials containing more than 1% asbestos
Oct. 1975				0.5 fibers/ml TWA		
July 1976					2 fibers/ml TWA 10 fibers/ml STEL	
Dec 1976			0.1 fibers/ml TWA			
1979	0.5 fibers/ml TWA chrysotile 0.5 fibers/ml TWA amosite 0.2 fibers/ml crocidolite					

Continued

Table 2-4. *Continued*

Date	U.K. Advisory Committee on Asbestos	British Occupational Hygiene Soc.	National Institute of Occupational Safety and Health	OSHA (proposed)	OSHA (regulation)	EPA
1983		0.5 fibers/ml TWA chrysotile				
June 1986					0.2 fibers/ml TWA	
Sept 1988					1.0 fibers/ml STEL	
July 1989						Ban: cloth, felt, tile, gaskets, brakes, after-market brakes, air conditioning, pipe, shingles, roof materials to be phased out over several years[†]
July 1990				0.1 fibers/ml TWA		
July 1993					0.1 fibers/ml TWA	
Nov 1993						Revision of ban on asbestos, vacating and remanding most of 1989 rule
Nov 2000						Asbestos Worker Protection Rule, cross reference to OSHA standards to protect state and local government employees[‡]

[†] Federal Register, Vol. 54, No. 132, July 12, 1989
[‡] Federal Register, Vol. 65, No. 221, November 15, 2000

Through the National Emissions Standards for Hazardous Air Pollutants (NESHAP) program, the EPA regulates external emissions from asbestos mills and from manufacturing and fabrication operations. The EPA also regulates the use of asbestos in roadway surfacing and in insulation materials, and has banned most uses of sprayed-on asbestos materials and pipe wrapping. These standards also require specific work practices during demolition and renovation involving asbestos materials, and regulate the removal, transport, and disposal of asbestos-containing materials. The EPA has also established programs to evaluate and certify asbestos-removal contractors and established work rules to protect workers during asbestos-abatement activities.

Since 1982, when the EPA issued the Asbestos and Schools Identification and Notification Rule, the agency has required all local education agencies to inspect for friable asbestos materials; to notify parents and teachers if such materials are found; to place warning signs in schools where asbestos is found; and to keep accurate records of their actions eliminating this problem. With Congressional approval of the Asbestos School Hazards Abatement Act of 1984, the EPA was given responsibility for providing both financial and technical assistance to local education agencies.

Assessing Nonoccupational Risk

Asbestos-related disease resulting from nonoccupational exposure to asbestos has been recognized in published reports of mesothelioma among household contacts of asbestos workers and in residents living near asbestos mines and factories. An increase in the prevalence of malignant mesothelioma and asbestos-related disease has been reported in nonoccupationally exposed populations in Turkey, Cyprus, the Metsovo region of Greece, and Northeast Corsica. The causal factor for at least some of the excess mesothelioma in Turkey may be due to the geologic presence of a nonasbestos mineral fiber, erionite (see Chapter 5).

A metaanalysis of eight published studies conducted in populations with relatively high household and neighborhood exposure to asbestos showed significantly elevated relative risks for developing pleural mesothelioma. In the neighborhood exposure groups, the risk ranged between 5.1 and 9.3. In the household exposure groups the risk ranged between 4.0 and 23.7.[19]

However, these study populations were exposed to ambient concentrations much higher than those observed in U.S. homes and public buildings, and these data are insufficient to estimate the magnitude of the excess risk for pleural mesothelioma at levels of environmental exposure commonly encountered by the general population in industrialized countries.

In an effort to assess the health risk of nonoccupational exposure to asbestos in buildings and schools, numerous international panels have been convened. In the absence of undisputed evidence, several mathematical models have been proposed to assess the lifetime risk of lung cancer and mesothelioma. Underlying these varying risk assessment models are assumptions and uncertainties that make the interpretation of these risk estimates inherently difficult.

The estimation of risk is based upon extrapolation from high-dose workplace exposures in the past to low doses found in buildings and the ambient environment. Modern ambient exposures are orders of magnitude less than even today's OSHA permissible exposure level of 0.1 fibers per ml. Estimates of exposure assigned to these retrospective worker cohorts cannot be fully characterized, due in part to poor sampling and analytical methodology and the use of surrogate exposure categories based on job title. Mass-to-fiber conversions utilized in these models add substantial uncertainty. Models that include an assumption of a linear dose-response assume that exposure to one fiber of asbestos carries an inherent and finite risk for lung cancer and mesothelioma, and that the risk is cumulative for each fiber to which an individual is exposed. There appears to be no evidence of a threshold level below which there is no risk of mesothelioma.[20] This hypothesis is still debated.

In a review of the potential health risk associated with working in buildings constructed of asbestos-containing materials, the lifetime risk for premature cancer death was estimated to be 4 per million for those exposed for 20 years working in office buildings (estimated exposure levels ranging from 0.0002–0.002 fibers per ml). For those exposed for 15 years in schools the risk was estimated to be 1 per million (estimated exposure levels ranging from 0.0005–0.005 fibers per ml).[21] In comparison, the risk associated with the OSHA permissible exposure level of 0.1 fibers per ml for 20 years was estimated at 2000 per million exposed. The risk estimates associated with building exposure to asbestos are orders of magnitude lower than some commonplace risks from drowning, motor vehicle accidents, and household accidents. They are also far less than the background estimate of mesothelioma of 1 to 2 cases per million population per year.

Calculations of unit risk for asbestos at the low concentrations measured in the environment must also be viewed with great caution. The World Health Organization proposed a range of cancer risks based on an exposure of 0.0005 fibers/ml. The predicted lifetime cancer risk per 100,000 (smokers and nonsmokers) for the general population is 1–10 for mesothelioma and 0.1–1 for lung cancer.[22] The EPA's best estimate of the risk to the U.S. general population for a lifetime of continuous exposure to 0.0001 fibers/ml is 2.8 mesothelioma deaths and 0.5 excess lung cancer deaths per 100,000 females; and for males, 1.9 mesothelioma and 1.7 excess lung cancer deaths per 100,000. The risk assessment model used by the EPA was recently called into question in a study by Camus et al. of nonoccupational exposure to chrysotile asbestos.[23]

Some studies of asbestos workers have observed an increased risk of cancer at other sites, including the gastrointestinal tract, larynx, esophagus, and kidney (see Chapter 8). However, these findings have not been consistent and there is still considerable controversy as to whether these cancers are associated with asbestos exposure. All reviews regarding asbestos risk considered asbestosis to be of little importance at levels now typical in the ambient environment and buildings.[15]

References

1. Gilson JC: Asbestos. In: *Encyclopedia of Occupational Health and Safety* (Parmeggiani L, ed.), Geneva: International Labour Office, 1983, pp. 185–187.
2. Federal Register, Vol. 54, No. 132, July 12, 1989.
3. EPA Asbestos Material Bans, 1999, http://www.epagov/opptintr/asbestos/asb-bans2.txt.
4. Collegium Ramazzini: Call for an international ban on asbestos. *J Occup Environ Med* 41:830–832, 1999.
5. Camus M: A ban on asbestos must be based on a comparative risk assessment. *Can Med Assoc J* 164:491–494, 2001.
6. Nicholson WJ, Selikoff IJ, Seidman H, Lilis R, Formby P: Long-term mortality of chrysotile miners and millers in the Thetford Mines, Quebec. *Ann NY Acad Sci* 330:11–21, 1979.
7. U.S. Department of Health Education and Welfare, Public Health Service: Asbestos: An information resource (Levine RJ, ed.). 1980, DHEW Publication No. 78–1681, pp. 41–60.
8. Selikoff IJ, Churg, J, Hammond EC: Asbestos exposure and neoplasia. *JAMA* 188:142–146, 1964.
9. U.S. Environmental Protection Agency. Asbestos Fact Book, USEPA Office of Public Affairs (A-107), 1985, p. 5.
10. Kohyama N: Airborne asbestos levels in non-occupational environments in Japan, IARC Scientific Publications No 30: Lyon, 1989, pp. 262–276.
11. Report to the Congress, Study of Asbestos-Containing Materials in Public Buildings, U.S. Environmental Protection Agency, February 1988, p. 5.
12. Dement JM: Asbestos. In: *Occupational Respiratory Diseases, National Institute for Occupational Safety and Health, U.S. Department of Health and Human Services* (Merchant JA, ed.), 1986, p. 288.
13. Code of Federal Regulations. Title 29 Chapter XVII, Subpart 1926.58, 1986.
14. Churg A: Current issues in the pathologic and mineralogic diagnosis of asbestos-induced disease. *Chest* 84:275–280, 1983.
15. Airborne Asbestos Health Assessment Update. U.S. Environmental Protection Agency, Office of Health and Environmental Assessment, EPA/600/8-84/003F, June 1986.
16. Whysner J, et. al.: Asbestos in the air of public buildings: a public health risk? *Prev Med* 1:119–125, 1994.
17. Nicholson WJ: Airborne mineral fiber levels in the non-occupational environment, In: *Non-Occupational Exposure to Mineral Fibers* (Bignon J, Peto J, Saraccci J, eds.), IARC Scientific Publication No. 90: Lyon, 1989, pp. 239–261.
18. Mossman BT, et al: Asbestos: Scientific developments and implications for public policy. *Science* 247: 294–301, 1990.
19. Bourdes V, Bofetta P, Pisani P: Environmental exposure to asbestos and risk of pleural mesothelioma: Review and meta-analysis. *Eur J Epidemiol* 16:411–417, 2000.
20. Hillerdal G: Mesothelioma: Cases associated with non-occupational and low dose exposures. *Occup Environ Med* 56:505–513, 1999.
21. Health Effects Institute—Asbestos Research. 1991. *Asbestos in Public and Commercial Buildings: A Literature Review and Synthesis of Current Knowledge.* Cambridge, MA: Health Effects Institute.
22. World Health Organization, Air Quality Guidelines, Copenhagen, 1987.
23. Camus M, Siemiatycki J, Meek B: Nonoccupational exposure to chrysotile asbestos and the risk of lung cancer. *N Engl J Med* 338:1565–1571, 1998.

3

Asbestos Bodies and Nonasbestos Ferruginous Bodies

Victor L. Roggli

Introduction

Asbestos bodies are the histologic hallmark of exposure to asbestos.[1-4] These structures are golden brown, beaded or segmented, dumbbell-shaped objects that have a characteristic microscopic appearance that is readily recognized by the pathologist. Their identification in histologic sections is an important component of the pathologic diagnosis of asbestosis (See Chapter 4), and their presence serves to alert the pathologist that the patient has been exposed to airborne asbestos fibers. This chapter discusses the structure and development of asbestos bodies, as well as their occurrence and distribution within human tissues. In addition, techniques for the quantification of asbestos bodies are reviewed, along with the relationship of asbestos body formation to the various types of asbestos fibers. Finally, the distinction of asbestos bodies from other ferruginous bodies based on light microscopic and analytical electron microscopic observations is emphasized. The identification and significance of asbestos bodies in cytologic specimens is discussed in Chapter 9, and the relationship between asbestos body concentrations in pulmonary tissues and the various asbestos-associated diseases is reviewed in Chapter 11.

Historical Background

Asbestos bodies were first described in the lung by Marchand in 1906.[5] He called them peculiar "pigmented crystals" and did not recognize their relationship to asbestos fibers. Eight years later, the German pathologist T. Fahr also took note of peculiar crystals in the lungs of an asbestos worker with pulmonary interstitial fibrosis.[6] W.E. Cooke described these structures as "curious bodies,"[7] and by 1929 Stewart and Haddow had coined the term "asbestosis bodies."[8] By this time Cooke[9] and Gloyne[10] recognized that these curious bodies had asbestos fibers at their core, but as late as 1930 in this country the fibers were confused with fungal hyphae.[11] The term asbestosis body was changed to asbestos body when it was discovered that the bodies also occurred in the lungs of workers who did not have asbestosis.[12,13] Experimental animal studies in the 1960s showed that structures resembling asbestos bodies were formed when a number of different types of fibrous dusts (fibrous aluminum silicate, silicon carbide whiskers, cosmetic talc, and fibrous glass) were instilled intratracheally into the lungs of hamsters.[14] As a result, it was suggested that the noncommittal term "ferruginous body" be used when the precise nature of the fibrous core was not known.[14,15] It then remained for Churg and Warnock[16,17] to show by means of energy dispersive spectrometry and electron diffraction that ferruginous bodies isolated from human lungs and having a thin, translucent fibrous core were virtually always true asbestos bodies.

[handwritten: other to substances for bodies]

Structure and Development of Asbestos Bodies

Asbestos bodies form when an asbestos fiber is inhaled and deposited in the distal regions of the lung parenchyma.[13] Here the free alveolar macrophages phagocytose the fiber (Figure 3-1). Subsequently, through a process that is poorly understood, the fiber becomes covered with a layer of iron-protein-mucopolysaccharide material.[18-20] It has been proposed that this process is a means of host defense, since in vivo[21] as well as in vitro[22] studies have shown that asbestos bodies are nonfibrogenic and noncytotoxic in comparison to uncoated asbestos fibers. Furthermore, the iron coating is bound in such a way that it does not efficiently

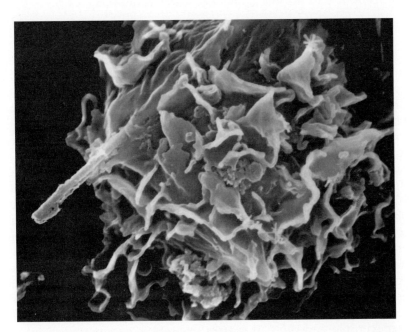

Figure 3-1. Scanning electron micrograph of a human free alveolar macrophage phagocytizing an amosite asbestos fiber. Magnified ×2000. (Reprinted from Greenberg SD, Asbestos-Associated Pulmonary Diseases, Medcom, Inc., 1981, with permission.)

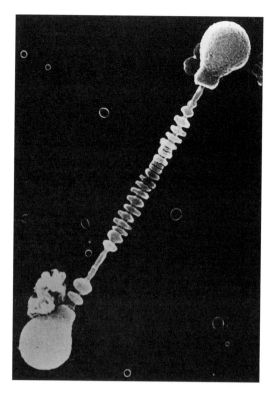 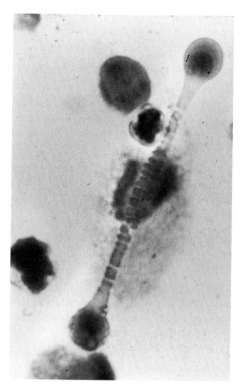

Figure 3-2. Side-by-side scanning electron micrograph of an asbestos body to the left with bronchoalveolar lavage recovered asbestos body and free alveolar macrophage to the right. (SEM, magnified ×2000; Papanicolaou, magnified ×600). (Reprinted from Ref. 2, with permission.)

participate in the generation of reactive oxygen species.[23,24] The coated asbestos fiber, or asbestos body, has a characteristic golden-brown appearance, which is the result of the iron component of the coating. These structures thus give a strong positive reaction with the Prussian blue stain. In histologic sections, asbestos bodies have a beaded, segmented, dumbbell or lancet shape, which is especially well appreciated in cytologic preparations (Figure 3-2) and in Nuclepore filter preparations of lung tissue digests (Figure 3-3). Branched forms, which result from the deposition of coating material on a splayed fiber, may also occur (Figure 3-4). Curved or circular asbestos bodies may also be observed (Figure 3-5), and these are usually found to have very thin core fibers (average core diameter of 0.2 μm).[17] Asbestos bodies are generally 20 to 50 μm in length,[20] with an average length of about 35 μm.[25] However, they may exceed 200 μm in length and some examples approaching 0.5 mm (500 μm) have been reported.[26] Asbestos bodies are usually 2 to 5 μm in diameter,[20] although by scanning electron microscopy, the author has observed rare bodies which were only 0.5 μm in diameter (Figure 3-6).[13]

Only a small percentage of asbestos fibers found within the lung at any single point in time are coated, and a number of factors determine whether an individual fiber will become coated to form an asbestos

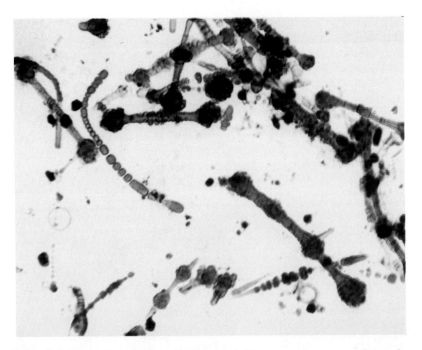

Figure 3-3. Asbestos bodies on a Nuclepore filter show the range of morphologic appearances, including dumbbell shapes, beaded structures, lancetforms, and so on Note the variable quantity of iron coating and the visible asbestos core fibers.

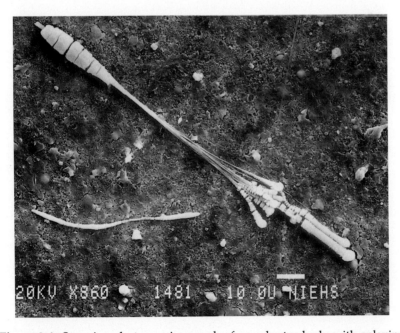

Figure 3-4. Scanning electron micrograph of an asbestos body with splaying of one end of the core fiber. Each splayed fiber has its own ferroprotein coating. Magnified ×860.

body. These factors include both characteristics of the inhaled dust and characteristics pertaining to the host. Regarding the former, fiber dimensions are important factors in asbestos body formation. Morgan and Holmes[27] found that in humans, fibers less than 20 μm in length

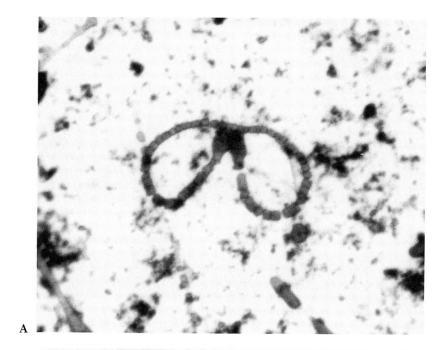

A

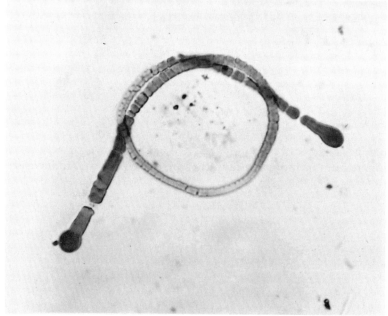

B

Figure 3-5. Examples of curved asbestos bodies with thin amphibole cores. **(A)** Pair of asbestos "spectacles." **(B)** This asbestos body isolated from bronchoalveolar lavage fluid appears to be tied in a knot.

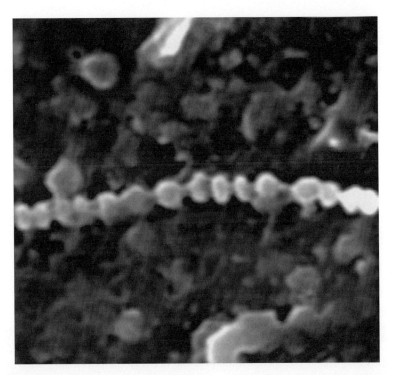

Figure 3-6. Scanning electron micrograph of an asbestos body with very thin coating, measuring approximately 0.5μ in diameter. The core fiber is less than 0.2μ in diameter. Such a body would be difficult to visualize with light microscopy. Magnified ×14,000.

rarely become coated, while virtually all fibers $80\mu m$ or greater in length are coated. Fiber diameter is also an important factor, with thicker fibers being more likely to become coated than thinner fibers.[28] Dodson et al.[29] suggested that fiber surface irregularities, such as etching, fracture, fraying, and multifibrillar composition, may also influence the coating process, with uncoated fibers having much smoother surface features. The type of fiber is also important (vide infra), with the vast majority of asbestos bodies isolated from human lungs possessing an amphibole asbestos core.[13,16,17,20,28] The proportion of fibers $5\mu m$ or more in length that are coated appears to increase as the tissue fiber burden increases (Figure 3-7). The presence of other dusts in the lung may also influence the coating process. For example, the author has observed that welders, who have heavy burdens of iron-oxide particles in their lungs, tend to have a high percentage of coated fibers (median value of 26% for 9 welders, as compared to 10.8% for 254 other asbestos-exposed individuals).

With regard to host factors, coating efficiency depends on the animal species exposed to the asbestos fibers. Humans, hamsters, and guinea pigs form asbestos bodies efficiently, whereas cats, rabbits, and mice do so much less readily, and rats and dogs are poor asbestos body formers.[21] Individual variability also is present in coating efficiency, with some individuals appearing to be poor asbestos body formers.[30,31]

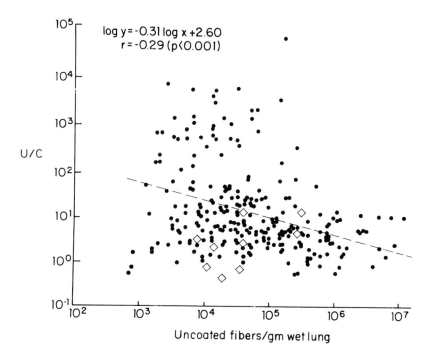

Figure 3-7. Graph showing the relationship between the pulmonary burden of uncoated fibers 5 μm or greater in length and the ratio of uncoated to coated fibers (U/C) isolated from the lung, as determined by scanning electron microscopy of 263 cases. The percentage of fibers which are coated increases significantly as the pulmonary asbestos burden increases. Welders (◇) tend to have especially low U/C ratios (i.e., high percentage of coated fibers).

Considerable variation in coating efficiency has even been observed in different areas of the lung from a single individual.[28] In the author's laboratory, the percentage of fibers 5 μm or greater in length which are coated (as determined by scanning electron microscopy) has ranged from 0.002% to 72%, with a median value of 11.8%. This latter value is very similar to the 11% coated fibers reported by Morgan and Holmes[28] using phase-contrast light microscopy. Finally, fiber clearance may be reduced in individuals with asbestosis, so that increased numbers of short fibers are retained and the proportion of fibers which become coated is greatly reduced.[28]

The mechanism of formation of asbestos bodies was studied in detail by Suzuki and Churg.[32] Asbestos fibers deposited in the distal regions of the lung parenchyma are phagocytosed by free alveolar macrophages. Those fibers that are approximately 20 μm or greater in length cannot be completely ingested by a single cell, and by poorly understood mechanisms this "frustrated phagocytosis" then triggers the coating process. Within 16 days of initial exposure, the iron micelles appear in the cytoplasm of the macrophages in close proximity to the ingested fibers, and by continuous accretion of these micelles embedded in a homogeneous matrix material, the typical asbestos bodies recognizable by light microscopy are eventually formed.[32] The asbestos fiber is separated from the cytoplasm of the macrophage by a lysosomal limiting membrane. Koerten et al. demonstrated that the process of asbestos body formation may occur extracellularly and is analogous to the process of bone resorption by osteoclasts.[33] The source of the iron which coats the fiber is unknown, but is probably derived from either hemoglobin or plasma transferrin. In experimental animals, asbestos bodies can be recognized by light microscopy within two or three months of exposure.[28] The finding of asbestos bodies in lung tissue digests of infants from three to twelve months of age[34] suggests that the time course for the formation of asbestos bodies is similar in humans. It has been suggested that the peculiar segmentation of asbestos bodies is due to the fragmentation of the rigid, sheath-like coating, and that further "weathering" and dissolution of the coating eventually occurs.[35,36] This sequence of events has been supported by scanning electron microscopic observations of asbestos bodies isolated from human tissues (Figure 3-8).[37] However, Koerten et al. have shown that typical, segmented asbestos bodies can be formed in vitro in a mouse peritoneal macrophage culture system,[38] casting doubt on the "weathering" mechanism of asbestos body segmentation.

It should be noted that not all asbestos bodies have a ferruginous coating. De Vuyst et al.[39] described a case in which amosite asbestos fibers coated with calcium oxalate crystals were recovered by bron-

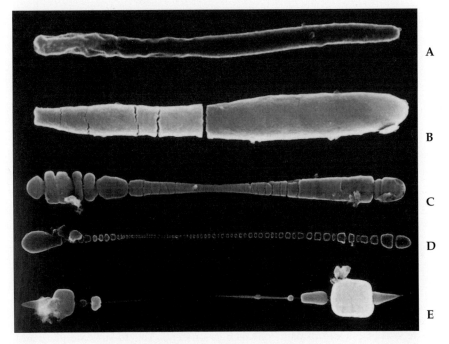

Figure 3-8. A composite SEM demonstrating the proposed sequence of events in asbestos body segmentation. **(A)** Membrane limited smooth coating. **(B)** Partial and complete cracks in a coated fiber. **(C)** Erosion of the sharp edges of cracked regions to form a smooth contour along an asbestos body. **(D)** Extensive beading along the axis of an asbestos body. **(E)** A bizarre form, with an extensive central uncoated fiber region capped by heavily eroded ends. (Reprinted from Ref. 37, with permission.)

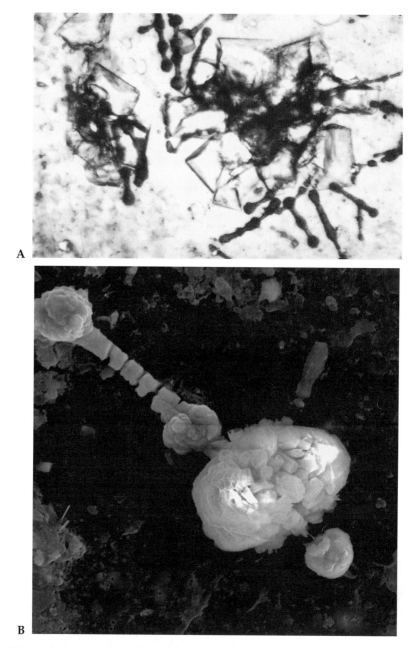

Figure 3-9. Calcium oxalate bodies. **(A)** Light micrograph of cluster of asbestos bodies in sputum associated with numerous crystals of calcium oxalate dihydrate. (Courtesy of Dr. Robert Moore of the Richmond, Virginia, VA Medical Center.) **(B)** Scanning electron micrograph of asbestos body with a bulbous deposit of calcium oxalate crystals near one end. The crystals are platy and yielded peaks for calcium only by EDXA. Magnified ×1900.

choalveolar lavage. Similar observations were reported by Le Bouffant et al.,[40] who described "enrobant" forms in which entire asbestos bodies are encased within an oxalate crystal. The author has observed similar cases (Figure 3-9), including one with longstanding renal failure.

However, systemic disturbance in oxalate metabolism cannot be identified in some cases.[38,39] Coating of asbestos fibers with spherules of calcium phosphate has also been observed in humans and experimental animals (Figure 3-10).[33,41] The formation of calcium phosphate salts

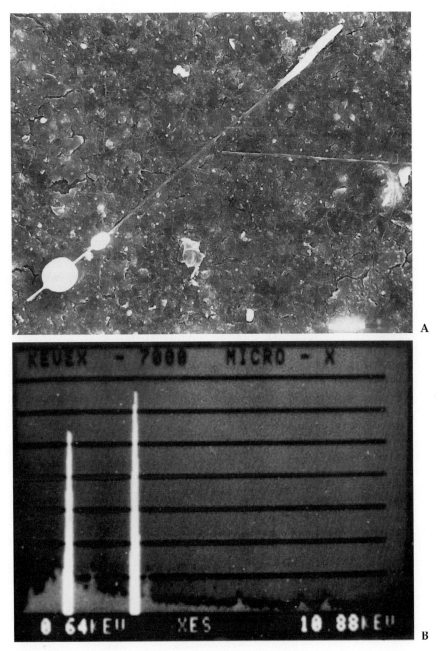

Figure 3-10. (A) Calcium phosphate coated asbestos fiber isolated from the lungs of a construction worker with asbestosis and squamous carcinoma of the lung. Note the uncoated fibers. Magnified ×1100. (B) Energy dispersive X-ray spectrum of the large spherical globule in A shows peaks for calcium and phosphorus but not for iron. Reprinted from Ref. 41, with permission.

in association with interstitial asbestos fibers appears to be a common reaction to injury in the white rat.[42] The calcium phosphate coatings are distinctive by virtue of their large size, spherical shape, and wide separation between deposits on an individual fiber. Intraalveolar calcium carbonate concretions (pulmonary "blue bodies") have also been reported in association with asbestos exposure,[43] but have not been described as a coating material on asbestos fibers. It must be emphasized that calcium phosphate and calcium oxalate bodies are rare occurrences, and that ferruginized asbestos fibers are by far the most common form of asbestos body.

Occurrence and Distribution of Asbestos Bodies

In 1963, Thomson et al.[44] reported that asbestos bodies could be found in scrapings of autopsy lungs in 24% of urban residents in South Africa. Since that time, a number of studies have demonstrated that when digestion-concentration techniques are employed to analyze sufficient quantities of lung tissue, some asbestos bodies can be recovered from the lungs of virtually all adults in industrialized nations.[1,45–55] The percentage of patients from a general autopsy adult population with asbestos bodies in their lungs has ranged from as low as 21% in East Texas in a study using 0.3 gm samples of lung tissue[54] to as high as 100% in a study from the United States employing 5 gram samples.[46] The median value for the 12 cited studies is 90% (Table 3-1). Correlations with occupational data indicate that "blue-collar" men tend to have the highest counts,[50] reflecting some occupational exposure to asbestos for many of these individuals. Lower counts are often found in women as compared to men,[47,50,51,56,57] indicating that men are more likely to have jobs with some asbestos exposure. In addition, smokers appear to have higher lung asbestos body counts than nonsmokers.[50,57] Environmental asbestos contamination is not confined to urban areas, since rural dwellers are found to have asbestos bodies in their lungs just as often

Table 3-1. Occurrence of asbestos bodies in the general population as determined by tissue digestion

Authors	Year	Country	No. cases	Percentages[a]
Bignon et al.[43]	1970	France	100	100%
Smith and Naylor[44]	1972	United States	100	100%
Rosen et al.[45]	1972	United States	86	90%
Breedin and Buss[46]	1976	United States	124	93%
Bhagavan and Koss[47]	1976	United States	145	91%
Churg and Warnock[48]	1977	United States	252	96%
Roggli et al.[1]	1980	United States	52	92%
King and Wong[55]	1996	United States	135	80%
Steele and Thomson[49]	1982	United Kingdom	106	80%
		New Zealand	248	75%
Rogers[50]	1984	Australia	128	37%
Kobayashi et al.[51]	1986	Japan	656	33%
Dodson et al.[54]	1999	United States	33	21%

[a] Percent indicates the percentage of cases in which asbestos bodies were recovered from autopsy lung tissue by digestion

as urban dwellers (95% vs. 91%), although the levels tend to be higher in urban areas.[48,57,58] An increasing prevalence and concentration of asbestos bodies in autopsy lungs during the past several decades has also been reported. Bhagavan and Koss reported an increase in asbestos body prevalence in the United States from 41% in the 1940s to 91% of cases in 1970 to 1972.[49] Arenas-Huertero et al. reported an increase in average asbestos body concentration in lung samples from Mexico from 4.2/gm in 1975 to 42.5/gm in 1988.[57] Bhagavan and Koss also found a significant increase in the proportion of lungs containing asbestos bodies with increasing age,[49] although others have found no increase in asbestos body content with age.[47,50,51] Indeed, studies by Haque et al.[34] who reported the isolation of asbestos bodies from the lungs of infants indicate that exposure to asbestos in our industrialized society begins within the first year of life.

A few studies have examined the topographic distribution of asbestos bodies within the lung. Sebastien et al.[59] examined autopsy lung tissue from six patients with no known asbestos exposure and found no consistent relationship between the concentration of asbestos bodies in the upper versus lower lobes or central versus peripheral lung parenchyma. Rosen et al.[47] reported on results from 14 cases in which lung tissue was analyzed for asbestos body content from more than one site and again found no consistent relationship between asbestos body content in the upper versus lower lobes or right versus left lung. Gylseth and Baunan[60] described the asbestos body content in two asbestos workers and found considerable variation from site to site within the lungs. These observations are consistent with the data from the author's laboratory involving 41 cases for which tissue was available for digestion from two or more sites. The asbestos body concentration in the upper lobe exceeded that in the lower lobe in 17 instances, whereas the reverse was true in 15 instances. Similarly, the asbestos body concentration in the right lung exceeded that in the left lung in 24 cases, whereas the opposite was found in 17 cases. This variability in asbestos body concentration from one site to another within the lung was dramatically demonstrated in the studies of Morgan and Holmes,[61,62] who extensively sampled lung tissue from one insulator and two Finnish anthophyllite mine workers. Their data show a five-to tenfold variation in asbestos body concentration in adjacent blocks of tissue. Experimental animal studies suggest that this site-to-site variability in asbestos content may be related to airway path lengths and branching patterns.[63]

Quantification of Asbestos Bodies

Because a few asbestos bodies can be found in the lungs of virtually everyone in industrialized nations, quantitative studies are required to draw inferences relative to exposure and various disease processes. A number of techniques have been devised for quantification of asbestos bodies in tissues, and these are reviewed in the following sections. They include quantification in histologic sections, lung tissue digests, lymph nodes, and extrapulmonary tissues.

[handwritten margin note: A few asb bodies found in virtually everyone in industrialized nations]

Histologic Sections

Paraffin sections are routinely used by pathologists for diagnostic purposes, so it is only natural that histologic sections have played an important role with respect to identification and quantification of asbestos bodies in tissues. In early studies investigating the prevalence of asbestos bodies in the general population, 30 μm thick paraffin sections were employed.[64] Selikoff and Hammond used basal smears and ashed tissue sections to study the prevalence of asbestos bodies in the lungs of New York City residents.[65] However, there was little attempt to actually quantitate the numbers of asbestos bodies in histologic sections. A semiquantitative study was reported in 1980 by Roggli et al.,[1] who concluded that 5000 or more asbestos bodies per gram of wet lung tissue were required before bodies were likely to be encountered in 10 random high power fields of iron-stained sections. Churg observed that roughly 500 asbestos bodies per gram of wet lung needed to be present before any bodies could be found in tissue sections.[66] Subsequently, Roggli and Pratt[25] reported a quantitative study relating the numbers of asbestos bodies observed in iron-stained tissue sections to asbestos body counts in lung tissue digests. The observations in this study were validated using a more rigorous mathematical model,[67] and similar results have subsequently been reported by others.[31,53]

A key factor in the calculation of the numbers of asbestos bodies per gram of wet lung tissue from the numbers observed in histologic sections is the recognition that the same asbestos body may be observed in several serial sections.[25] This is the result of the fact that the average asbestos body is considerably longer than the average section is thick. Thus, there is a finite probability that an asbestos body will be oriented in the block in such a way that it will appear on two or more adjacent sections. This concept is depicted schematically in Figure 3-11. Once the orientation of the asbestos body in the paraffin block has been accounted for, it is a simple matter to calculate asbestos bodies per gram, using a conversion factor from volume of paraffin-embedded tissue to wet weight of lung. The relevant formulas are as follows:[25]

$$N_g = \frac{N_c}{A_s t . O_c . R} \qquad (3\text{-}1)$$

where

N_g = number of asbestos bodies per gram of wet lung tissue
N_c = number of asbestos bodies counted on iron-stained tissue section
A_s = area of tissue section in mm^2
t = thickness of tissue section in mm
O_c = orientation correction factor (see Ref. 25 for details)
R = ratio of wet weight of fixed lung tissue to volume of paraffin-embedded lung tissue

Typical values for these variables in our laboratory are as follows:

t = 5 μm = 0.005 mm
O_c = 2.56 for an average asbestos body length of 35 μm
R = 2.1 g/cm^3 (includes a factor for shrinkage of lung during paraffin embedding[25])

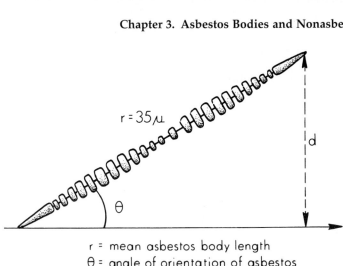

r = mean asbestos body length
θ = angle of orientation of asbestos
    body with respect to face of
    paraffin tissue block
d = r sin θ

Figure 3-11. Model for determining the orientation correction factor for counting asbestos bodies in tissue sections. Bodies are assumed to be rigid, straight structures with a mean length of 35 μm. The abscissa is parallel to the paraffin block face, θ is the angle between the asbestos body and the plane of the block face, which can range from 0–90°, and d is the projection of the asbestos body (in μm) in a direction perpendicular to the plane of the tissue section. As d increases, so does the probability that the asbestos body will be observed in two or more serial sections. (Reprinted from Ref. 25, with permission.)

Therefore,

$$N_g = \frac{N_c}{A_s} \times 37,200 \, mm^2/gm \qquad (3-2)$$

It should be noted that equation (3-2) is only applicable to sections cut at 5 μm thickness, and an average asbestos body length of 35 μm. Also, these formulas were derived using iron-stained sections examined at 200× magnification using a mechanical stage.[25] Because asbestos bodies are not necessarily distributed uniformly through tissue sections, the more sections and the more total area examined, the greater the accuracy of the estimated asbestos body concentration. Similar results can be obtained by using the regression line in Figure 3-12 (in lieu of equation 3-2) to estimate the asbestos body concentration per gram of wet lung from the numbers of asbestos bodies per mm^2 of tissue section.[25] Also, Table 3-2 shows the number of 400× microscopic fields that have to be examined on the average to find the first asbestos body for a given tissue asbestos body concentration.[67] These calculations indicate that asbestos body detection in tissue sections (i.e., one asbestos body per 4 cm^2 section area) requires 100 or more asbestos bodies per gram of wet lung tissue.[25,67]

Lung Tissue Digests

A variety of techniques have been described for the extraction of asbestos bodies from lung tissue for subsequent quantification or iden-

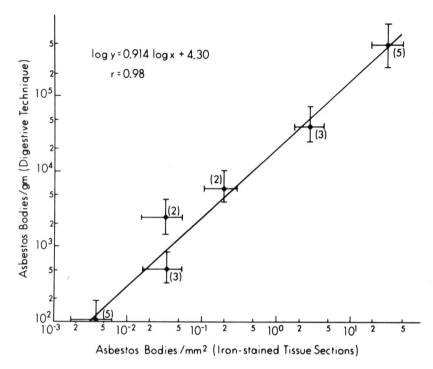

Figure 3-12. Relation (log-log scale) of the number of asbestos bodies seen in iron-stained sections (in units of bodies per mm²) to the number measured by a tissue digestion technique (in units of asbestos bodies per gram of wet, formalin-fixed lung tissue). The number of sections evaluated per case is shown in parentheses, and each data point represents the mean result for one case, with error bars indicating one standard deviation. The least squares fitted regression equation is shown at upper left, and the correlation coefficient is significant at the $P < 0.001$ level. (Reprinted from Ref. 25, with permission.)

tification.[14,20,28,45–53,68–75] Most of these techniques employ wet chemical digestion, although low temperature plasma ashing techniques have been used as well.[55,73,74] The inorganic residue remaining after digestion is then suspended in ethanol and collected on an acetate or poly-

Table 3-2. Average number (N) of 400× microscopic fields examined to find first asbestos body for a given Asbestos Body Concentration (AB/gm)[a]

N	AB/gm
1	181,000
5	36,200
10	18,100
18	10,000
25	7,240
36	5,000
50	3,620
100	1,810
181	1,000
362	500
1,810	100

[a] Modified after Ref. 67, with permission

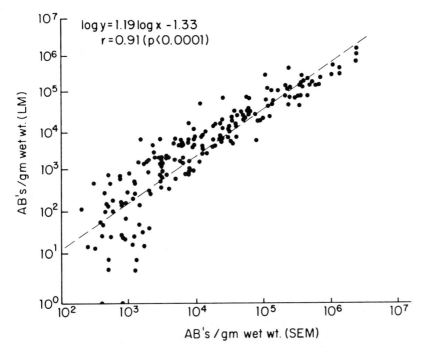

Figure 3-13. Correlation between asbestos body counts by light and scanning electron microscopy in 189 cases. Each dot represents one case. The linear regression line has a correlation coefficient of 0.91 (p < 0.0001). Note log-log scale.

carbonate filter with an appropriate pore size (0.45 µm or less). If the intent of the study is to quantify asbestos bodies alone, then the filter can be examined by light microscopy at a magnification of 200 to 400×. However, scanning electron microscopy (SEM) can be used to count asbestos bodies just as well,[41,55] and there is an excellent correlation between asbestos body concentrations determined by light microscopy and those determined by SEM (Figure 3-13). Once the number of asbestos bodies on the filter has been determined, the asbestos body concentration per gm of wet lung,[1,41,71] gm of dry lung,[20,31,69] or cm^3 of lung tissue[45,54] can be calculated. The relationship between these three ways of reporting results varies somewhat from case to case, but a useful rule of thumb for comparative purposes is

$$1 \, AB/gm \, wet \, wt. \simeq 1 \, AB/cm^3 \simeq 10 \, AB/gm \, dry \, wt. \qquad (3\text{-}3)$$

Digestion studies must be carefully performed, as there are a number of potential sources of error. Asbestos bodies (and fibers) may be lost during the extraction process through adhesion to glass surfaces, and this can result in substantial underestimation of the actual tissue concentration.[74] However, Corn et al.[76] have shown that with their bleach digestion technique, the percentage error due to adherence of fibers or bodies to glass surfaces in cases with a heavy tissue asbestos burden is negligible. Whether this is true for low or moderate tissue asbestos burdens is unknown. Ashing of the specimen (especially in a muffle furnace at 400–500 °C) causes tissue shrinkage resulting in fracture of long fibers, which increases the asbestos body count.[55,74] Morgan and Holmes have also reported that dicing of the tissue sample prior to bleach digestion results in a decrease in median asbestos body length and thus an apparent increase in asbestos body concentration.[62] However, this effect on asbestos body counts appears to be of the same order of magnitude as the coefficient of variation for counting different aliquots of the same sample (i.e., about 10%), and is substantially less than the five- to tenfold variation which can occur from sampling different sites in the same lung.[61,62] This serves to emphasize the importance of sampling multiple sites for digestion whenever this is feasible.

The asbestos body concentrations which have been reported on lung samples from the general population as well as from individuals with various asbestos-related diseases are discussed in Chapter 11. The range of values observed spans at least nine orders of magnitude (from 0.1 to 10^7 ABs/gm wet lung tissue). It should be noted that while there is fairly good agreement in the determination of tissue asbestos body concentrations among different laboratories employing different analytical techniques, the agreement is considerably worse for the determination of uncoated asbestos fiber concentrations.[77] However, there may be significant variation in tissue asbestos body content from one region of the country to another.[1,20,41,50,71] Therefore, it is important for laboratories engaged in such determinations to calculate their own normal range of asbestos body concentrations.

It is important to recognize that asbestos body counts in decomposed human lungs decrease over time. This was shown in a study by Mollo et al.[78] in 8 cases where asbestos bodies were measured shortly after death and again after 1 to 18 months of decomposition. This is probably the result of loss of proteins in the matrix of the ferruginous material, so that the coating becomes brittle and shatters off during the recovery process.

Lymph Nodes

Gloyne in 1933 described asbestos bodies in histologic sections of lymph nodes, and noted that when present, they are usually found in areas of the node containing pigment.[79] Godwin and Jagatic reported asbestos bodies in the regional lymph nodes of 6 of 7 patients with malignant mesothelioma.[80] Others have also mentioned the presence of asbestos bodies in histologic sections of lymph nodes.[20] Roggli and Benning reported asbestos bodies in histologic sections in 20 cases (Figure 3-14).[81] Seventeen of these patients had histologically confirmed asbestosis, and all were heavily exposed to asbestos for durations ranging from 4 to 40 years. The median asbestos body concentration in the lung parenchyma as determined by light microscopy of lung tissue digests was more than 1000 times our upper limit of normal.[81] In four cases, lymph node tissue was also available for digestion, and the asbestos body concentration in the lymph nodes ranged from 3000 to more than 300,000 asbestos bodies per gram wet weight of lymph node. Asbestos bodies were not observed in iron-stained sections of lymph

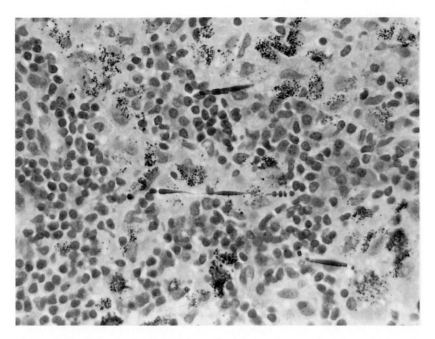

Figure 3-14. Asbestos bodies within a histologic section of a hilar lymph node from an insulator with asbestosis and squamous cell carcinoma of the right upper lobe. Hematoxylin and eosin, magnified ×520. (Reprinted from Ref. 81, with permission.)

nodes in 14 autopsied controls, all of which had lung asbestos body counts within our normal range of 0 to 20 ABs/gm. However, a few asbestos bodies were found in lymph node digests in 6 of 14 controls. The range of values for the lymph nodes was roughly the same as for normal lung parenchyma (0–17 ABs/gm of wet lymph node tissue).[81] Dodson and Huang found asbestos (ferruginous) bodies in lymph node digests from 2 of 21 nonoccupationally exposed individuals.[82]

Considerations similar to those used for the determination of asbestos body concentrations from asbestos body counts in tissue sections of lung (see above) can be used to estimate the minimum asbestos body concentration necessary in lymph node tissue for asbestos bodies to be observed in lymph node histologic sections. For an average lymph node measuring 1.0 by 0.5 cm, average asbestos body length of 35 μm, tissue section thickness of 6 μm, and lymph node density of 1 gm/cm³, the finding of one asbestos body in an iron-stained section of lymph node is equivalent to approximately 1600 asbestos bodies per gram wet weight of lymph node[81] (Figure 3-15). Several conclusions can be drawn from these observations. First, the finding of asbestos bodies in histologic sections of lymph nodes is indicative of a heavy asbestos body burden within the node and is associated with considerably elevated lung asbestos body burdens. Second, a few asbestos bodies can be found in digests of lymph nodes in many individuals with no known exposure to asbestos, indicating transport of some long fibers to the lymph nodes even at low tissue asbestos burdens. Finally, in some

Bodies in nodes of non-asb exposed

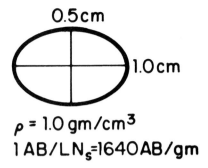

0.5 cm

1.0 cm

$\rho = 1.0 \, gm/cm^3$

$1 \, AB/LN_s = 1640 \, AB/gm$

Figure 3-15. Schematic diagram of a typical hilar lymph node section, measuring 1×0.5 cm and with approximate density (ρ) of $1.0 \, gm/cm^3$. The finding of one asbestos body in such a paraffin section is equivalent to roughly 1600 asbestos bodies per gram of wet fixed nodal tissue. (Reprinted from Ref. 81, with permission.)

cases, the asbestos body content of the hilar nodes exceeds that of the lung parenchyma at both low and high tissue asbestos burdens.

Extrapulmonary Tissues

As early as 1933, Gloyne had observed that asbestos bodies are readily transported from place to place on a scalpel or microtome blade, and can easily be carried over from one specimen jar to another.[79] It is common practice for pathologists to place portions of multiple organs in a single container of formalin. The author has recovered scores of asbestos bodies from one cc of formalin within a container in which lungs (and other organs) from an individual with a heavy pulmonary asbestos burden had been placed. In addition, asbestos bodies may adhere to glassware used in the digestion procedure, and thus potentially be carried over from one case to the next.[74,83] All of these sources of contamination would have to be considered in studies of asbestos bodies in extrapulmonary tissues, especially because the tissue concentrations would be so low that confirmation by means of histologic sections would be lacking.[25] Nevertheless, most investigators reporting asbestos bodies in extrapulmonary sites have failed to take these considerations into account. Therefore, the reader should keep these confounding factors in mind when considering the literature on this subject.

Extrapulmonary organs from which asbestos bodies have been recovered are listed in Table 3-3. Auerbach et al.[84] reported the occurrence of asbestos bodies in extrapulmonary sites in 37 cases, including 19 with asbestosis and 18 with parietal pleural plaques. These investi-

Table 3-3. Extrapulmonary tissues from which asbestos bodies have been recovered

Adrenal gland	Mesentery
Bone marrow	Omentum
Brain	Pancreas
Esophagus	Prostate
Heart	Small intestine
Kidney	Stomach
Larynx	Spleen
Liver	Thyroid
Large intestine	Urinary bladder

Source: From Refs. 84, 85, 88 and 89

gators recovered 20 mm³ of tissue from paraffin blocks deparaffinized in xylene and digested in potassium hydroxide, with the residue collected on an ashless paper filter and ashed on a glass slide within a low temperature plasma asher. Asbestos bodies were recovered from the kidney, heart, liver, spleen, adrenals, pancreas, brain, prostate, and thyroid. The authors concluded that in individuals with heavy pulmonary asbestos body burdens, asbestos bodies are likely to be present in other organs as well.[84] Kobayashi et al.[85] reported a similar study of 26 cases with varying levels of pulmonary asbestos body burden. They used up to five grams of formalin-fixed tissue which was digested with potassium hydroxide and the residue collected on a membrane filter. Asbestos bodies were found in esophagus, stomach, small and large intestine, spleen, pancreas, liver, heart, kidney, urinary bladder, bone marrow, thyroid, and adrenals. These investigators also noted that the incidence and the number of asbestos bodies in extrapulmonary organs tends to increase as the pulmonary asbestos burden increases.[85] However, this observation is also consistent with contamination of formalin by pulmonary asbestos bodies.

Ehrlich et al.[86] reported a case of an asbestos insulator with asbestosis who underwent a resection for carcinoma of the colon. Asbestos bodies were recovered from digests of 3 to 5 gm of tumor, adjacent normal bowel, mesentery, and serosal fat. In contrast, Rosen et al.[87] found no asbestos bodies in digests of colonic tissue from 21 cases of colon cancer from the general population. Dodson et al.[88] studied 20 cases with mesothelioma, and found asbestos bodies in mesentery samples from five and in the omentum from two. Roggli et al.[89] recovered asbestos bodies from digests of laryngeal mucosa in two of five asbestos workers, but in none of 10 autopsy controls. The occurrence of asbestos bodies in the upper airway and the gastrointestinal tract is not unexpected, since asbestos bodies may be found in mucus from the lower respiratory tract, which is then coughed up and swallowed (see Chapter 9). Although asbestos bodies in other extrapulmonary sites may be artifactual (see above), there are some data to indicate that vascular transport of dust from the lungs can occur.[90,91] Once an asbestos fiber gains access to the intravascular compartment, hematogenous transport to any of the organs listed in Table 3-3 could theoretically occur. However, one would then expect to find the largest number of asbestos bodies in the organs which receive the greatest percentage of systemic blood flow, that is, the brain, the heart, and the kidneys. This has not been the case in the reported studies.[84,85]

Asbestos Bodies and Fiber Type

The vast majority of asbestos bodies isolated from human lungs have been found to have an amphibole asbestos core.[13,16,17,20,30,71,92-95] Asbestos workers[41,71] and men from the general population[96] generally have the commercial amphiboles, amosite or crocidolite, forming the cores of asbestos bodies within their lungs. On the other hand, women from the general population are more likely to have one of the noncommercial amphiboles, tremolite or anthophyllite, as the core to asbestos bodies found in their lungs.[96] This latter finding may be related to contamination of commercial talcum powder with tremolite and anthophyllite.[97] The predominance of amphibole asbestos body cores is somewhat curious, considering that the bulk of asbestos used commercially is chrysotile (Figure 3-16).[98] Chrysotile asbestos bodies do occur, however (Figure 3-17), and account for approximately 2% of all asbestos bodies that have been analyzed by our laboratory[41,99] and by others as well.[20,100] Moulin et al.[101] reported that chrysotile asbestos bodies accounted for 10% of bodies analyzed from asbestos-exposed workers, but only 3% of bodies from members of the Belgian urban population. They are especially likely to occur in individuals exposed to long fibers of chrysotile, such as asbestos textile workers or chrysotile miners or millers. In the latter group of workers, most asbestos bodies isolated from lung tissue have chrysotile asbestos cores.[102] Thicker chrysotile bundles are more likely to become coated than thin chrysotile fibrils.[28] The rarity of chrysotile asbestos bodies apparently results from the ready fragmentation of chrysotile into shorter fibrils, and the fact that asbestos bodies tend to form only on fibers which are 20 μm or more in length.[27,28] As a result, asbestos bodies are generally a poor indicator of the pulmonary chrysotile asbestos burden.[20,31,69,70,103] On the other hand, the pulmonary asbestos body content correlates very well with the burden of uncoated fibers 5 μm or greater in length (Figure 3-18).[41,61,62,71,104,105] Among individuals exposed occupationally to asbestos, most fibers in this size range are commercial amphiboles.[41,71] An obvious exception to this is the relatively small percentage of asbestos workers exposed exclusively to chrysotile.

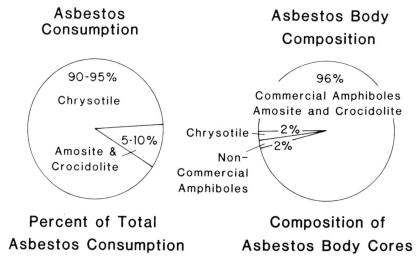

Figure 3-16. Diagram showing the proportion of the various types of asbestos fibers that are consumed commercially (*left*) versus the composition of asbestos body cores (*right*). Although chrysotile accounts for the great bulk (90%–95%) of asbestos consumed commercially, asbestos bodies infrequently (approximately 2%) have a chrysotile core. (Reprinted from Ref. 99, with permission.)

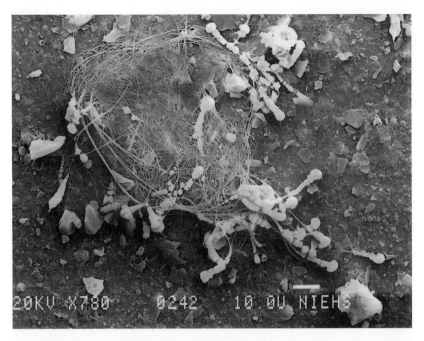

Figure 3-17. Cluster of chrysotile asbestos fibers on a Nuclepore filter isolated from the lungs of an asbestos textile worker with a pleural mesothelioma. The fiber ends appear to spin off the central mass like the arms of a spiral galaxy, and have become coated to form numerous chrysotile asbestos bodies. Scanning electron microscopy, magnified ×850. (Reprinted from Ref. 41, with permission.)

Nonasbestos Ferruginous Bodies

As noted in the section on "Historical Background," fibrous dusts other than asbestos can become coated with iron, or ferruginized, so that one must be cautious in identifying asbestos bodies by light microscopy.[14,15] Fortunately, most of the nonasbestos ferruginous bodies, or pseudoasbestos bodies, can be distinguished from true asbestos bodies at the light microscopic level.[13,17,20,106] The author has observed nonasbestos ferruginous bodies in tissue digests from 97 out of 406 cases (24%), but only rarely are they found in numbers approaching those of true asbestos bodies.[20] The morphologic features of the various types of nonasbestos ferruginous bodies are reviewed below.

Sheet Silicates

These structures may form ferruginous bodies with a distinctive broad, yellow core. Churg et al.[17] described two patterns of ferruginous body formation with sheet silicate cores: bodies with a highly irregular shape and platy structure with irregular, often sparse coating (Figure 3-19), and bodies with a rectangular shape, more uniform coating, and diameter only slightly greater than that of true asbestos bodies. The second pattern may be confused with true asbestos bodies, and when the core is particularly thin, this distinction may not be possible at the light

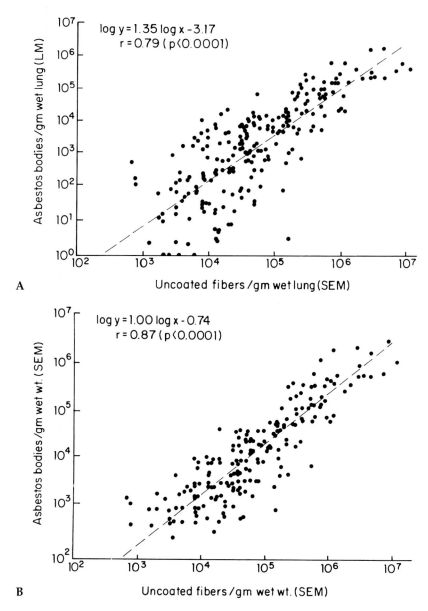

Figure 3-18. (A) Scattergram showing the relation between asbestos body counts by light microscopy and uncoated fiber counts by scanning electron microscopy, for 223 cases. The correlation coefficient for the least squares fitted linear regression line is 0.79 (p < 0.0001). **(B)** Correlation between asbestos body and uncoated fiber counts by scanning electron microscopy in 193 cases (r = 0.87, p < 0.0001). Note log-log scale.

microscopic level. Electron diffraction shows a pseudohexagonal pattern, and energy dispersive spectrometry shows that most of these bodies have cores of talc, mica, or kaolinite.[20] They are commonly found in the lungs of roofers and rubber factory workers, who are exposed to substantial amounts of talc,[20] and the author has observed them

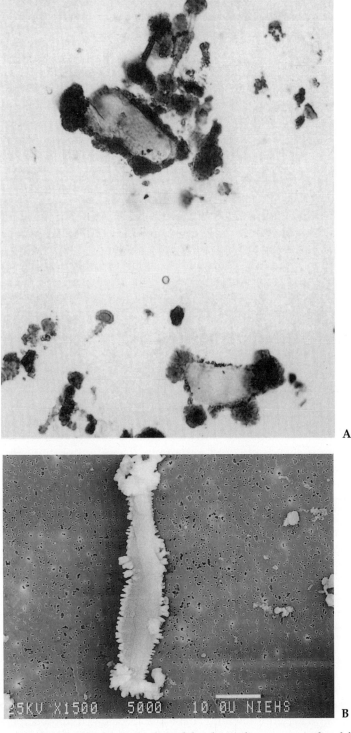

Figure 3-19. **(A)** Pseudoasbestos bodies of the sheet silicate type, isolated from the lungs of an insulator with asbestosis and small cell carcinoma of the lung, have broad yellow cores. True asbestos bodies are also present (*upper center* and *lower left*). Nuclepore filter preparation, ×520. (Reprinted from Ref. 13, with permission.) **(B)** Scanning electron micrograph of a sheet silicate pseudoasbestos body. Note the heavy coating on the ends and the serrated edges. Magnified ×1500.

commonly in the lungs of shipyard welders. In the general population, they may contribute up to 20% of the total ferruginous body burden.[17]

Carbon Fibers

Some ferruginous bodies have black cores, ranging from uniform, very thin black filaments to broader, more irregular platy forms. Gross described ferruginous bodies of this type from human lungs and suggested that they had carbon cores.[107] The coating on these bodies is also variable, and may be segmented, sheathlike, or form right angle branches.[17] Electron diffraction shows that these core fibers are amorphous, and energy dispersive spectrometry indicates that there are no elements with an atomic number greater than or equal to that of sodium ($Z = 11$).[20] These observations are consistent with the carbonaceous nature of the cores. We have observed bodies of this type in the lungs of coal miners,[108] and also in the lungs of a woman with an unusual exposure to woodstove dust (Figure 3-20).[109] In the general population, they may contribute to as much as 90% of the total ferruginous body burden in some cases,[20] and in our case with the unusual woodstove dust exposure, they accounted for 100% of the ferruginous bodies that were analyzed.[109]

Metal Oxides

Fibrous forms of a variety of metal oxides can form ferruginous bodies with dark brown to black cores.[13] These structures usually have a core with a uniform diameter and segmented coating which, except for the color of the core, otherwise resemble typical asbestos bodies (Figure 3-21). We have identified such ferruginous bodies with cores of titanium, iron, chromium, and aluminum. These are presumably in the form of the metal oxide. Titanium particles and fibers are commonly found in lung specimens,[41,108] and when they reach a certain critical length,[27] may then become coated to form a ferruginous body. Dodson et al.[110] described ferruginous bodies with iron-rich core fibers isolated from the lungs of a worker at an iron reclamation and manufacturing facility. We have observed ferruginous bodies with iron-rich cores and rarely with aluminum-rich cores from the lungs of shipyard welders. These individuals have large numbers of non-fibrous iron and aluminum oxide particles in their lungs. Finally, a unique case has been reported in which chromium-rich cores were identified in ferruginous bodies isolated from the lungs of a metal polisher.[111]

Manmade Mineral Fibers

Manufactured manmade mineral or vitreous fibers are commonly used in insulation materials and can form ferruginous bodies in experimental animals.[14] Therefore, it would not be unexpected to find such fibers at the cores of ferruginous bodies isolated from human lungs. Langer et al.[93] studied 50 ferruginous bodies isolated from the lungs of members of the general population of New York City and concluded that the cores in most were either degraded chrysotile or fibrous glass. Roggli et al.[112]

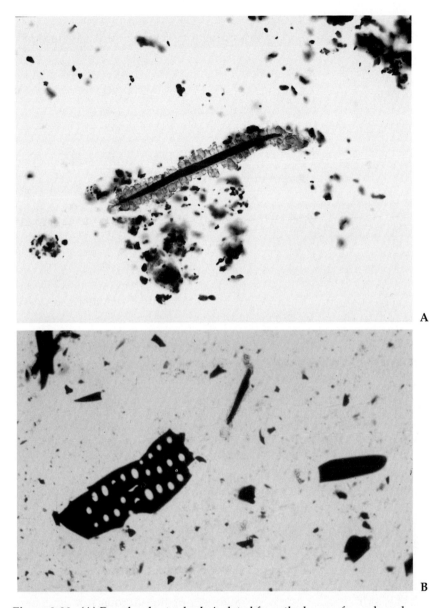

Figure 3-20. (A) Pseudoasbestos body isolated from the lungs of a coal-worker has a black carbon core which is coated with segmented ferroprotein material. Magnified ×800. (Reprinted from Ref. 108, with permission.) **(B)** Dust recovered from bronchoalveolar lavage fluid from a woman exposed to woodstove dust. Fiber in upper middle portion of field is iron coated. Note grid-like structure left of center. Nuclepore filter preparation, magnified ×330. (Reprinted from Ref. 111, with permission.)

examined 90 ferruginous bodies isolated from the lungs of six individuals with malignant pleural mesothelioma and three with asbestosis and found two with cores that had a chemical composition consistent with fibrous glass. Although fibrous glass may occasionally be found in samples of human lung tissue (Figure 3-22),[108] it is uncommonly identi-

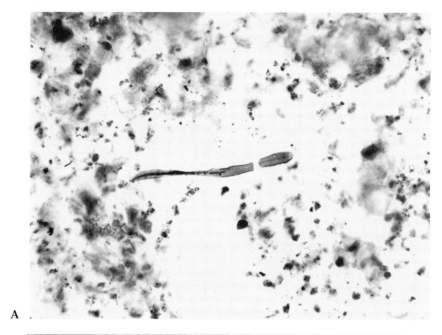

A

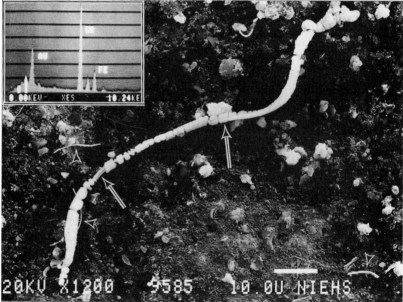

B

Figure 3-21. (A) Pseudoasbestos body with black core fiber recovered from lungs of a 76-year-old metal polisher. Magnified ×500. **(B)** Scanning electron micrograph of pseudoasbestos body, showing beaded iron coating as well as bare area revealing the core fiber (*arrows*). Additional uncoated fibers are present (*arrowheads*). Inset: EDXA spectrum from bare area of coated fiber, showing prominent peaks for chromium, and a smaller peak for iron. Au peak is due to sputter-coating. Magnified ×1200. (Reprinted from Ref. 111, with permission.)

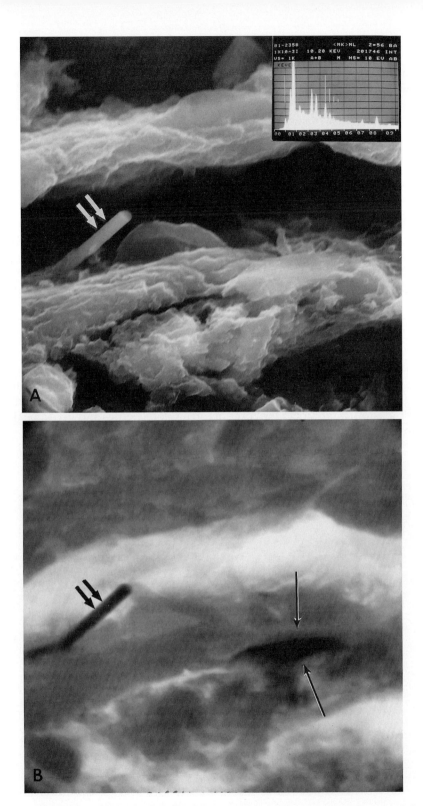

Figure 3-22. Lung tissue from a young woman with interstitial fibrosis. **(A)** Secondary electron image, showing a fiber protruding from an alveolar septum (*double arrow*). **(B)** Backscattered electron image of the same field shown in A), demonstrating the *fiber* (*double arrow*) and an additional particle of talc (magnesium-silicate) embedded in the tissue (*single arrows*). Inset: EDXA spectrum obtained from the fiber shown in (A)) and (B), indicating a chemical composition of Na-Al-Si-K-Ca-Ba. This composition is consistent with fibrous glass. (A) and (B) magnified ×3300. (Reprinted from Ref. 108, with permission.)

fied as the core of ferruginous bodies. This observation is most likely the result of the brittleness of these fibers so that they tend to break transversely producing shorter fibers[113] and to the tendency for fibrous glass to dissolve in vivo.[114] On the other hand, refractory ceramic fibers tend to be more biopersistent,[115] and thus are more likely to form ferruginous bodies. Such bodies are indistinguishable from true asbestos bodies at the light microscopic level, but have aluminum silicate cores when examined by energy dispersive spectrometry (Figure 3-23).[116]

Diatomaceous Earth

Ferruginous bodies with cores of diatomaceous earth are infrequently encountered. By light microscopy, they are large, broad, segmented, and frequently serpiginous. They do not have the clubbed ends so often observed in true asbestos bodies, and their color varies from golden-yellow to deep orange-brown.[17] In some examples, the sievelike skeletal pattern of the diatom can be observed by electron microscopy (Figure 3-24).[17,108] Because the diatom skeleton is composed of amorphous silica, the cores would be silicon-rich with energy dispersive spectrometry and show no pattern with electron diffraction. Some silica "fibers" encountered in the lung may be acicular cleavage fragments of quartz, and it is conceivable that such fragments, if of the proper dimension, might form the cores of ferruginous bodies and give a peak for silicon only with energy dispersive spectrometry.

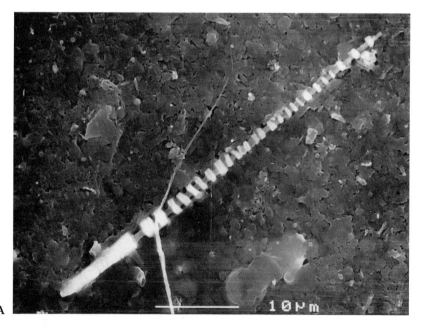

A

Figure 3-23. (A) Ferruginous body isolated from the lungs of a refractory ceramic fiber worker. Magnified ×2300. (B) EDXA spectrum from bare area of coated fiber, showing peaks for aluminum and silicon. Au peak is the result of sputter-coating.

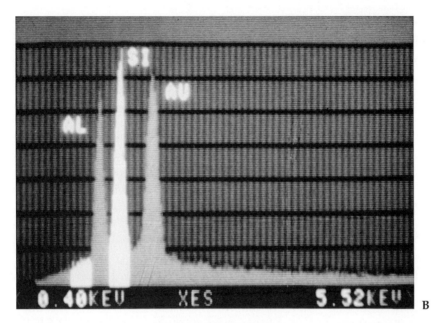

B

Figure 3-23. *Continued*

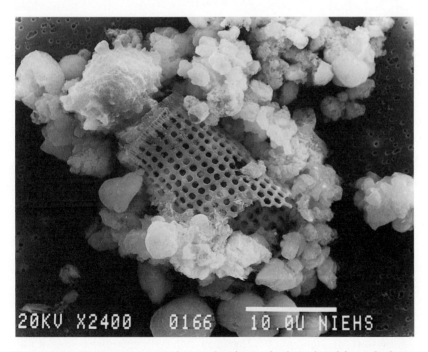

Figure 3-24. Diatomaceous earth pseudoasbestos body isolated from the lungs of an asbestos insulator in a shipyard. The diatom fragment with symmetrically aligned holes represents the silicon-containing diatom skeleton, which is surrounded by irregular granules of hemosiderin. Magnified ×2400. (Reprinted from Ref. 108, with permission.)

Zeolite Bodies

Zeolites are hydrated aluminum silicates which are naturally occurring, and some forms of zeolite, such as erionite, are fibrous. Erionite is found in volcanic tuff in Turkey, and has physical characteristics which closely resemble those of amphibole asbestos. Sebastien et al.[117] have isolated ferruginous bodies with erionite cores from the lungs of individuals from Turkish villages situated on volcanic tuff rich in erionite. By light microscopy, they are indistinguishable from typical asbestos bodies. The villagers in this region of Turkey have a high incidence of pleural mesothelioma (see Chapter 5) and pleural fibrosis and calcification (see Chapter 6). Zeolite bodies have thus far not been reported in lung tissue from individuals in North America.[13]

Others

Silicon carbide ceramic fibers can form ferruginous bodies in experimental animals,[14] and ferruginous bodies with black cores have been observed in the lung tissues of silicon carbide workers.[118-120] In addition, elastic fibers under certain conditions can undergo fragmentation and ferruginization, and hence form the cores of ferruginous bodies.[20] In consideration of the wide variety of nonasbestos mineral fibers which can be recovered from human lungs (see Chapter 11), it is likely that nonasbestos ferruginous bodies of types other than those described above will be reported in the future.

References

1. Roggli VL, Greenberg SD, Seitzman LH, McGavran MH, Hurst GA, Spivey CG, Nelson KG, Hieger LR: Pulmonary fibrosis, carcinoma, and ferruginous body counts in amosite asbestos workers: A study of six cases. *Am J Clin Pathol* 73:496–503, 1980.
2. Greenberg SD: Asbestos lung disease. *Sem Respir Med* 4:130–136, 1982.
3. Greenberg SD: Asbestos. Ch. 22 In: *Pulmonary Pathology* (Dail DH, Hammar SP, eds.), New York: Springer-Verlag, 1988, pp. 619–635.
4. Craighead JE, Abraham JL, Churg A, et al.: The pathology of asbestos-associated diseases of the lungs and pleural cavities: Diagnostic criteria and proposed grading schema (Report of the Pneumoconiosis Committee of the College of American Pathologists and the National Institute for Occupational Safety and Health). *Arch Pathol Lab Med* 106:544–596, 1982.
5. Marchand F: Ueber eigenttimliche Pigmentkristalle in den Lungen. *Verhandl d Deutsch path Gesellsch* 10:223–228, 1906.
6. Fahr T: Demonstrationen: Praparate und Microphotogrammes von einen Falle von Pneumokoniose. *Muench Med Woch* 11:625, 1914.
7. Cooke WE: Pulmonary asbestosis. *Br Med J* 2:1024–1025, 1927.
8. Stewart MJ, Haddow AC: Demonstration of the peculiar bodies of pulmonary asbestosis ("asbestosis bodies") in material obtained by lung puncture and in the sputum. *J Pathol Bact* 32:172, 1929.
9. Cooke WE: Asbestos dust and the curious bodies found in pulmonary asbestosis. *Br Med J* 2:578–580, 1929.
10. Gloyne SR: The presence of the asbestos fibre in the lesions of asbestos workers. *Tubercle* 10:404–407, 1929.

11. Craighead JE: Eyes for the epidemiologist: The pathologist's role in shaping our understanding of the asbestos-associated diseases. *Am J Clin Pathol* 89:281–287, 1988.

12. Castleman BI: *Asbestos: Medical and Legal Aspects.* New York: Harcourt, Brace, Jovanovich, 1984.

13. Roggli VL: Pathology of human asbestosis: A critical review. In: *Advances in Pathology,* (Vol. 2) (Fenoglio-Preiser CM, ed.), Chicago: Yearbook Pub Inc., 1989, pp. 31–60.

14. Gross P, de Treville RTP, Cralley LJ, Davis JMG: Pulmonary ferruginous bodies: Development in response to filamentous dusts and a method of isolation and concentration. *Arch Pathol* 85:539–546, 1968.

15. Gaensler EA, Addington WW: Asbestos or ferruginous bodies. *N Engl J Med* 280:488–492, 1969.

16. Churg A, Warnock ML: Analysis of the cores of ferruginous (asbestos) bodies from the general population. I: Patients with and without lung cancer. *Lab Invest* 37:280–286, 1977.

17. Churg A, Warnock ML, Green N: Analysis of the cores of ferruginous (asbestos) bodies from the general population. II. True asbestos bodies and pseudoasbestos bodies. *Lab Invest* 40:31–38, 1979.

18. Davis JMG: Further observations on the ultrastructure and chemistry of the formation of asbestos bodies. *Exp Mol Pathol* 13:346–358, 1970.

19. Governa M, Rosanda C: A histochemical study of the asbestos body coating. *Br J Ind Med* 29:154–159, 1972.

20. Churg AM, Warnock ML: Asbestos and other ferruginous bodies: Their formation and clinical significance. *Am J Pathol* 102:447–456, 1981.

21. Vorwald AJ, Durkan TM, Pratt PC: Experimental studies of asbestosis. *Arch Ind Hyg Occup Med* 3:1–43, 1951.

22. McLemore TL, Mace ML, Roggli V, Marshall MV, Lawrence EC, Wilson RK, Martin RR, Brinkley BR, Greenberg SD: Asbestos body phagocytosis by human free alveolar macrophages. *Cancer Letts* 9:85–93, 1980.

23. Ghio AJ, LeFurgey A, Roggli VL: In vivo accumulation of iron on crocidolite is associated with decrements in oxidant generation by the fiber. *J Toxicol Environ Health* 50:125–142, 1997.

24. Governa MM, Amati M: Role of iron in asbestos-body-induced oxidant radical generation. *J Toxicol Environ Health* 58:279–287, 1999.

25. Roggli VL, Pratt PC: Numbers of asbestos bodies on iron-stained tissue sections in relation to asbestos body counts in lung tissue digests. *Hum Pathol* 14:355–361, 1983.

26. Farley ML, Greenberg SD, Shuford EH, Jr., Hurst GA, Spivey CG, Christianson CS: Ferruginous bodies in sputa of former asbestos workers. *Acta Cytologica* 27:693–700, 1977.

27. Morgan A, Holmes A: Concentrations and dimensions of coated and uncoated asbestos fibres in the human lung. *Br J Ind Med* 37:25–32, 1980.

28. Morgan A, Holmes A: The enigmatic asbestos body: Its formation and significance in asbestos-related disease. *Environ Res* 38:283–292, 1985.

29. Dodson RF, O'Sullivan MF, Williams MG, Jr., Hurst GA: Analysis of cores of ferruginous bodies from former asbestos workers. *Environ Res* 28:171–178, 1982.

30. Dodson RF, Williams MG, O'Sullivan MF, Corn CJ, Greenberg SD, Hurst GA: A comparison of the ferruginous body and uncoated fiber content in the lungs of former asbestos workers. *Am Rev Respir Dis* 132:143–147, 1985.

31. Warnock ML, Wolery G: Asbestos bodies or fibers and the diagnosis of asbestosis. *Environ Res* 44:29–44, 1987.

32. Suzuki Y, Churg J: Structure and development of the asbestos body. *Am J Pathol* 55:79–107, 1969.
33. Koerten HK, Hazekamp J, Kroon M, Daems WTH: Asbestos body formation and iron accumulation in mouse peritoneal granulomas after the introduction of crocidolite asbestos fibers. *Am J Pathol* 136:141–157, 1990.
34. Haque AK, Kanz MF: Asbestos bodies in children's lungs: An association with sudden infant death syndrome and bronchopulmonary dysplasia. *Arch Pathol Lab Med* 112:514–518, 1988.
35. Gloyne SR: The formation of the asbestosis body in the lung. *Tubercle* 12:399–401, 1931.
36. Botham SK, Holt PF: Development of asbestos bodies on amosite, chrysotile, and crocidolite fibres in guinea-pig lungs. *J Pathol* 105:159–167, 1971.
37. Mace ML, McLemore TL, Roggli V, Brinkley BR, Greenberg SD: Scanning electron microscopic examination of human asbestos bodies. *Cancer Letts* 9:95–104, 1980.
38. Koerten HK, de Bruijn JD, Daems WTH: The formation of asbestos bodies by mouse peritoneal macrophages: An in vitro study. *Am J Pathol* 137:121–134, 1990.
39. DeVuyst P, Jedwab J, Robience Y, Yernault J-C: "Oxalate bodies", another reaction of the human lung to asbestos inhalation? *Eur J Respir Dis* 63:543–549, 1982.
40. Le Bouffant L, Bruyere S, Martin JC, Tichoux G, Normand C: Quelques observations sur les fibres d'amiante et les formations minerales diverses rencontrees dans les pulmons asbestosiques. *Rev Fr Mal Respir* 4:121–140, 1976.
41. Roggli VL: Scanning electron microscopic analysis of mineral fibers in human lungs. Ch. 5 In: *Microprobe Analysis in Medicine* (Ingram P, Shelburne JD, Roggli VL, eds.), Washington, DC Hemisphere Pub. Corp., 1989, pp. 97–110.
42. Brody AR, Hill LH: Interstitial accumulation of inhaled chrysotile asbestos fibers and consequent formation of microcalcifications. *Am J Pathol* 109:107–114, 1982.
43. Koss MN, Johnson FB, Hochholzer L: Pulmonary blue bodies. *Hum Pathol* 12:258–266, 1981.
44. Thomson JG, Kaschula ROC, MacDonald RR: Asbestos as a modern urban hazard. *S Afr Med J* 37:77–81, 1963.
45. Bignon J, Goni J, Bonnaud G, Jaurand MC, Dufour G, Pinchon MC: Incidence of pulmonary ferruginous bodies in France. *Environ Res* 3:430–442, 1970.
46. Smith MJ, Naylor B: A method of extracting ferruginous bodies from sputum and pulmonary tissues. *Am J Clin Pathol* 58:250–254, 1972.
47. Rosen P, Melamed M, Savino A: The "ferruginous body" content of lung tissue: A quantitative study of eighty-six patients. *Acta Cytologica* 16:207–211, 1972.
48. Breedin PH, Buss DH: Ferruginous (asbestos) bodies in the lungs of rural dwellers, urban dwellers and patients with pulmonary neoplasms. *South Med J* 69:401–404, 1976.
49. Bhagavan BS, Koss LG: Secular trends in presence and concentration of pulmonary asbestos bodies—1940 to 1972. *Arch Pathol* 100:539–541, 1976.
50. Churg A, Warnock ML: Correlation of quantitative asbestos body counts and occupation in urban patients. *Arch Pathol Lab Med* 101:629–634, 1977.
51. Steele RH, Thomson KJ: Asbestos bodies in the lung: Southampton (UK) and Wellington (New Zealand). *Br J Ind Med* 39:349–354, 1982.

52. Rogers AJ: Determination of mineral fibre in human lung tissue by light microscopy and transmission electron microscopy. *Ann Occup Hyg* 28:1–12, 1984.
53. Kobayashi H, Watanabe H, Zhang WM, Ohnishi Y: A quantitative and histological study on pulmonary effects of asbestos exposure in general autopsied lungs. *Acta Pathol Jpn* 36:1781–1791, 1986.
54. Dodson RF, Williams MG, Huang J, Bruce JR: Tissue burden of asbestos in nonoccupationally exposed individuals from East Texas. *Am J Ind Med* 35:281–286, 1999.
55. King JA, Wong SW: Autopsy evaluation of asbestos exposure: retrospective study of 135 cases with quantitation of ferruginous bodies in digested lung tissue. *South Med J* 89:380–385, 1996.
56. Kishimoto T: Intensity of exposure to asbestos in metropolitan Kure City as estimated by autopsied cases. *Cancer* 69:2598–2602, 1992.
57. Arenas-Huertero FJ, Salazar-Flores M, Osornio-Vargas AR: Ferruginous bodies as markers of environmental exposure to inorganic particles: experience with 270 autopsy cases in Mexico. *Environ Res* 64:10–17, 1994.
58. Monso EA, Texido A, Lopez D, Aguilar X, Fiz J, Ruiz J, Rosell A, Vaquero M, Morera J: Asbestos bodies in normal lung of western Mediterranean population with no occupational exposure to inorganic dust. *Arch Environ Health* 50:305–311, 1995.
59. Sebastien P, Fondimare A, Bignon J, Monchaux G, Desbordes J, Bonnaud G: Topographic distribution of asbestos fibres in human lung in relation to occupational and non-occupational exposure. In: *Inhaled Particles* (Vol. IV) (Walton WH, ed.), Oxford: Pergamon Press, 1977, pp. 435–446.
60. Gylseth B, Baunan R: Topographic and size distribution of asbestos bodies in exposed human lungs. *Scand J Work Environ Health* 7:190–195, 1981.
61. Morgan A, Holmes A: Distribution and characteristics of amphibole asbestos fibres, measured with the light microscope, in the left lung of an insulation worker. *Br J Ind Med* 40:45–50, 1983.
62. Morgan A, Holmes A: The distribution and characteristics of asbestos fibers in the lungs of Finnish anthophyllite mine-workers. *Environ Res* 33:62–75, 1984.
63. Pinkerton KE, Plopper CG, Mercer RR, Roggli VL, Patra AL, Brody AR, Crapo JD: Airway branching patterns influence asbestos fiber location and the extent of tissue injury in the pulmonary parenchyma. *Lab Invest* 55:688–695, 1986.
64. Um CH: Study of the secular trend in asbestos bodies in lungs in London, 1936–1966. *Br Med J* 2:248–252, 1971.
65. Selikoff IJ, Hammond EC: Asbestos bodies in the New York City population in two periods of time, Pneumoconiosis: Proceedings of the International Conference, Johannesburg, 1969 (Shapiro HA, ed.), Capetown, South Africa: Oxford University Press, 1970, pp. 99–105.
66. Churg A: Fiber counting and analysis in the diagnosis of asbestos-related disease. *Hum Pathol* 13:381–392, 1982.
67. Vollmer RT, Roggli VL: Asbestos body concentrations in human lung: Predictions from asbestos body counts in tissue sections with a mathematical model. *Hum Pathol* 16:713–718, 1985.
68. Williams MG Jr., Dodson RF, Corn C, Hurst GA: A procedure for the isolation of amosite asbestos and ferruginous bodies from lung tissue and sputum. *J Toxicol Environ Health* 10:627–638, 1982.
69. Warnock ML, Prescott BT, Kuwahara TJ: Correlation of asbestos bodies and fibers in lungs of subjects with and without asbestosis. *Scanning Electron Microsc* 11:845–857, 1982.

70. Warnock ML, Kuwahara TJ, Wolery G: The relation of asbestos burden to asbestosis and lung cancer. *Pathol Annu* 18(2):109–145, 1983.
71. Roggli VL, Pratt PC, Brody AR: Asbestos content of lung tissue in asbestos associated diseases: A study of 110 cases. *Br J Ind Med* 43:18–28, 1986.
72. Ehrlich A, Suzuki Y: A rapid and simple method of extracting asbestos bodies from lung tissue by cytocentrifugation. *Am J Ind Med* 11:109–116, 1987.
73. Manke J, Rodelsperger K, Brückel B, Woitowitz H-J: Evaluation and application of a plasma ashing method for STEM fiber analysis in human lung tissue. *Am Ind Hyg Assoc J* 48:730–738, 1987.
74. Gylseth B, Baunan RH, Overaae L: Analysis of fibres in human lung tissue. *Br J Ind Med* 39:191–195, 1982.
75. Castro-Cordoba F, Arenas-Huertero F, Salazar-Flores M, Osornio-Vargas A: Modification of the Smith and Naylor technique for the identification of ferruginous bodies. *Arch Med Res* 24:199–201, 1993.
76. Corn CJ, Williams MG Jr, Dodson RF: Electron microscopic analysis of residual asbestos remaining in preparative vials following bleach digestion. *J Electron Microsc Tech* 6:1–6, 1987.
77. Gylseth B, Churg A, Davis JMG, Johnson N, Morgan A, Mowe G, Rogers A, Roggli V: Analysis of asbestos fibers and asbestos bodies in tissue samples from human lung: An international interlaboratory trial. *Scand J Work Environ Health* 11:107–110, 1985.
78. Mollo F, Cravello M, Andreozzi A, Burlo P, Bo P, Attanasio A, De Giuli P: Asbestos body burden in decomposed human lungs. *Am J Forens Med Pathol* 21:148–150, 2000.
79. Gloyne SR: The morbid anatomy and histology of asbestosis. *Tubercle* 14:550–558, 1933.
80. Godwin MC, Jagatic J: Asbestos and mesotheliomas. *Environ Res* 3:391–416, 1970.
81. Roggli VL, Benning TL: Asbestos bodies in pulmonary hilar lymph nodes. *Mod Pathol* 3:513–517, 1990.
82. Dodson RF, Huang J, Bruce JR: Asbestos content in the lymph nodes of nonoccupationally exposed individuals. *Am J Ind Med* 37:169–174, 2000.
83. Roggli VL, Piantadosi CA, Bell DY: Asbestos bodies in bronchoalveolar lavage fluid: A study of 20 asbestos-exposed individuals and comparison to patients with other chronic interstitial lung diseases. *Acta Cytologica* 30:470–476, 1986.
84. Auerbach O, Conston AS, Garfinkel L, Parks VR, Kaslow HD, Hammond EC: Presence of asbestos bodies in organs other than the lung. *Chest* 77:133–137, 1980.
85. Kobayashi H, Ming ZW, Watanabe H, Ohnishi Y: A quantitative study on the distribution of asbestos bodies in extrapulmonary organs. *Acta Pathol Jpn* 37:375–383, 1987.
86. Ehrlich A, Rohl AN, Holstein EC: Asbestos bodies in carcinoma of colon in an insulation worker with asbestosis. *JAMA* 254:2932–2933, 1985.
87. Rosen P, Savino A, Melamed M: Ferruginous (asbestos) bodies and primary cancer of the colon. *Am J Clin Pathol* 61:135–138, 1974.
88. Dodson RF, O'Sullivan MF, Huang J, Holiday DB, Hammar SP: Asbestos in extrapulmonary sites: omentum and mesentery. *Chest* 117:486–493, 2000.
89. Roggli VL, Greenberg SD, McLarty JL, Hurst GA, Spivey CG, Hieger LR: Asbestos body content of the larynx in asbestos workers. *Arch Otolaryngol* 106:553–555, 1980.

90. Holt PF: Transport of inhaled dust to extrapulmonary sites. *J Pathol* 133:123–129, 1981.
91. Lee KP, Barras CE, Griffith FD, Waritz RS, Lapin CA: Comparative pulmonary responses to inhaled inorganic fibers with asbestos and fiberglass. *Environ Res* 24:167–191, 1981.
92. Pooley FD: Asbestos bodies, their formation, composition and character. *Environ Res* 5:363–379, 1972.
93. Langer AM, Rubin IB, Selikoff IJ: Chemical characterization of asbestos body cores by electron microprobe analysis. *J Histochem Cytochem* 20:723–734, 1972.
94. Murai Y, Kitagawa M, Hiraoka T: Asbestos body formation in the human lung: distinctions, by type and size. *Arch Environ Health* 50:19–25, 1995.
95. Dodson RF, O'Sullivan M, Corn CJ: Relationships between ferruginous bodies and uncoated asbestos fibers in lung tissue. *Arch Environ Health* 51:462–466, 1996.
96. Churg AM, Warnock ML: Analysis of the cores of ferruginous (asbestos) bodies from the general population: III. Patients with environmental exposure. *Lab Invest* 40:622–626, 1979.
97. Miller A, Teirstein AS, Bader MD, Bader RA, Selikoff IJ: Talc pneumoconiosis: Significance of sublight microscopic mineral particles. *Am J Med* 50:395–402, 1971.
98. Craighead JE, Mossman BT: Pathogenesis of asbestos-associated diseases. *N Engl J Med* 306:1446–1455, 1982.
99. Roggli VL, Brody AR: Imaging techniques for application to lung toxicology, In: *Toxicology of the Lung* (Gardner DE, Crapo JD, Massaro EJ, eds.), New York: Raven Press, 1988, pp. 117–145.
100. Woitowitz H-J, Manke J, Brückel B, Rödelsperger K: Ferruginous bodies as evidence of occupational endangering by chrysotile asbestos? *Zbl Arbeitsmed Bd* 36:354–364, 1986.
101. Moulin E, Yourassowsky N, Dumortier P, De Vuyst P, Yernault JC: Electron microscopic analysis of asbestos body cores from the Belgian urban population. *Eur Respir J* 1:818–822, 1988.
102. Holden J, Churg A: Asbestos bodies and the diagnosis of asbestosis in chrysotile workers. *Environ Res* 39:232–236, 1986.
103. Case B: Biological indicators of chrysotile exposure. *Ann Occup Hyg* 38:503–518, 1994.
104. De Klerk NH, Musk AW, Williams V, Filion PR, Whitaker D, Shilkin KB: Comparison of measures of exposure to asbestos in former crocidolite workers from Wittenoom Gorge, W. Australia. *Am J Ind Med* 30:579–587, 1996.
105. Karjalainen A, Nurminen M, Vanhala E, Vainio H, Anttila S: Pulmonary asbestos bodies and asbestos fibers as indicators of exposure. *Scand J Work Environ Health* 22:34–38, 1996.
106. Crouch E, Churg A: Ferruginous bodies and the histologic evaluation of dust exposure. *Am J Surg Pathol* 8:109–116, 1984.
107. Gross P, Tuma J, deTreville RTP: Unusual ferruginous bodies: Their formation from non-fibrous particulates and from carbonaceous fibrous particles. *Arch Environ Health* 22:534–537, 1971.
108. Roggli VL, Mastin JP, Shelburne JD, Roe MS, Brody AR: Inorganic particulates in human lung. Relationship to the inflammatory response. In: *Inflammatory Cells and Lung Disease* (Lynn WS, ed.), Boca Raton, FL: CRC Press, Inc., 1983, pp. 29–62.
109. Ramage JE, Roggli VL, Bell DY, Piantadosi CA: Interstitial pneumonitis and fibrosis associated with domestic wood burning. *Am Rev Respir Dis* 137:1229–1232, 1988.

110. Dodson RF, O'Sullivan MF, Corn CJ, Williams MG Jr., Hurst GA: Ferruginous body formation on a nonasbestos mineral. *Arch Pathol Lab Med* 109:849–852, 1985.

111. Roggli VL: Analytical scanning electron microscopy in the investigation of unusual exposures. In: *MICROBEAM ANALYSIS—1986* (Romig AD, Jr., Chambers WF, eds.), San Francisco: San Francisco Press, Inc., 1986, pp. 586–588.

112. Roggli VL, McGavran MH, Subach JA, Sybers HD, Greenberg SD: Pulmonary asbestos body counts and electron probe analysis of asbestos body cores in patients with mesothelioma: A study of 25 cases. *Cancer* 50:2423–2432, 1982.

113. Wright GW, Kuschner M: The influence of varying lengths of glass and asbestos fibres on tissue response in guinea pigs. In: *Inhaled Particles IV* (Walton WH, ed.), Oxford: Pergamon Press, 1977, pp. 455–474.

114. Morgan A, Holmes A, Davison W: Clearance of sized glass fibres from the rat lung and their solubility in vivo. *Ann Occup Hyg* 25:317–331, 1982.

115. Mast RW, McConnell EE, Anderson R, Chevalier J, Kotin P, Bernstein DM, Thevenaz P, Glass LR, Miller WC, Hesterberg TW: Studies on the chronic toxicity (inhalation) of four types of refractory ceramic fiber in male Fischer 344 rats. *Inhal Toxicol* 7:425–467, 1995.

116. Dumortier P, Broucke I, De Vuyst P: Pseudoasbestos bodies and fibers in bronchoalveolar lavage of refractory ceramic fiber users. *Am J Respir Crit Care Med* 164:499–503, 2001.

117. Sebastien P, Gaudichet A, Bignon J, Baris YI: Zeolite bodies in human lungs from Turkey. *Lab Invest* 44:420–425, 1981.

118. Hayashi H, Kajita A: Silicon carbide in lung tissue of a worker in the abrasive industry. *Am J Ind Med* 14:145–155, 1988.

119. Funahashi A, Schlueter DP, Pintar K, Siegesmund KA, Mandel GS, Mandel NS: Pneumoconiosis in workers exposed to silicon carbide. *Am Rev Respir Dis* 129:635–640, 1984.

120. Dufresne A, Loosereewanich P, Armstrong B, Infante-Rivard C, Perrault G, Dion C, Masse S, Begin R: Pulmonary retention of ceramic fibers in silicon carbide (SiC) workers. *Am Ind Hyg Assoc J* 56:490–498, 1995.

4

Asbestosis

Thomas A. Sporn and Victor L. Roggli

Introduction

The term *pneumoconiosis* dates to Zenkers' 1866 description of pulmonary disease processes related to the inhalation of dusts.[1] As some dust (asbestos fibers included) may be found in the lungs of virtually all adults from the general population, pneumoconiosis now refers to the accumulation of excessive amounts of dust in the parenchyma of the lung, and the pathologic response to its presence there.[2] Asbestosis, the form of pneumoconiosis related to excessive amounts of asbestos fibers in the substance of the lung, is the prototype of diseases caused by inhalation of mineral fibers. Much has been learned from experimental models about the pathogenesis of asbestos-induced lung injury, which is reviewed in some detail in Chapter 10. The reader is directed to Chapter 3 for a discussion of asbestos bodies, the hallmark of asbestos exposure, and an important component of the histologic diagnosis of asbestosis. Chapter 11 discusses the methodology and results of quantitative tissue analysis for asbestosis, other asbestos-related diseases, and normal and disease control populations. The present chapter describes the morphologic features of asbestosis and relates them to the clinical and radiographic features of the disease.

Historical Background

Asbestos usage and observations regarding its attendant health hazards date to antiquity. Pliny the Younger described sickness in slaves who worked with asbestos, but these descriptions received little attention.[3] With the widespread usage of asbestos after the Industrial Revolution, the number of individuals exposed to asbestos increased dramatically. Dr. H. Montague Murray is credited with the first description of asbestos-related pulmonary disease, which occurred in a 33-year-old man who had been working for 14 years in the carding section of an asbestos textile plant. This case was not published, but was reported to a British parliamentary committee in 1906.[3,4] Eight years later the German pathologist Fahr described diffuse interstitial fibrosis in the lungs of a 35-year-old asbestos worker, which he attributed to the patient's exposure to asbestos. Fahr also called attention to crystals in the lung parenchyma.[4,5] An additional report of pulmonary fibrosis in an asbestos worker was recorded by Cooke in 1924, who subsequently coined the term *asbestosis*.[6,7] Numerous cases of asbestosis have since been reported, including workers exposed to asbestos through the processes of mining and milling asbestos-containing ores, the manufacture of asbestos-containing products, or through the utilization of such products.[4,8]

The term asbestosis is best defined as diffuse and bilateral pulmonary interstitial fibrosis caused by inhalation of asbestos. The incorporation of the asbestos-related pleural diseases under the heading of asbestosis is to be avoided, as this unnecessarily groups together diseases with different epidemiologic and pathophysiologic features, as well as different clinical features and outcomes.[9,10] Historically, asbestosis has been defined in pathologic terms by a number of investigators, but pathologists have not applied these uniformly.[11–13] The most comprehensive description of the pathologic characteristics of human asbestosis is that reported by the Pneumoconiosis Committee of the College of American Pathologists and the National Institute for Occupational Safety and Health.[14] This document sets forth the *minimal histologic* criteria for the diagnosis of asbestosis. *Histologic criteria* are those that permit the definitive diagnosis without the requirement of clinical and radiographic data, or exposure history. Such criteria have included "the demonstration of discrete foci of fibrosis in the walls of respiratory bronchioles associated with accumulations of asbestos bodies."

The definition's phraseology is somewhat vague with regard to the number of asbestos bodies requisite for the diagnosis, perhaps intentionally so. The term "asbestos bodies" implies that a minimum of two must be unequivocally identified. However, some investigators have suggested that the demonstration of one asbestos body is sufficient for the diagnosis, whereas others have recommended the demonstration of clusters of three or more asbestos bodies as necessary for the histologic diagnosis.[15,16] These studies specify neither the number of slides to be examined, nor the magnification, nor the preferred staining methodology (hematoxylin-eosin vs. iron stains).[8] Nonetheless, the identification of asbestos bodies within tissue sections remains the diagnostic *sine qua non* in view of the nonspecificity of interstitial fibrosis as a response to diffuse lung injury, and the large number of disorders that may cause scarring in the lung.[17–19]

Epidemiology

Asbestosis occurs in individuals exposed to large amounts of asbestos over long periods of time,[20,21] with threshold asbestos fiber dosage of between 25 to 100 fibers per cubic centimeter/year.[9] Moreover, there is a direct relationship between intensity and duration of asbestos exposure and the prevalence of asbestosis.[22] Workers likely to sustain such high levels have historically included spray insulators and asbestos miners and millers. Brief, but intense, exposures to asbestos may be sufficient to attain threshold fiber burdens. The development of asbestosis following a less than three-year exposure to asbestos in the case of an insulator has been reported, and asbestosis has been reported in a worker exposed to crocidolite for nine months in the dusty process of manufacturing certain cigarette filters.[20,23] The outcome of short-term exposure has also included the demonstration of 20% prevalence of parenchymal opacities on radiographic studies in a cohort of amosite asbestos factory workers after as little as one month's employment.[24] While there is a direct relationship between intensity and duration of exposure to asbestos and the prevalence of asbestosis,[22] it is interesting to note that not all those suffering high level exposure to asbestos will develop asbestosis. Asbestosis may result from exposure to any of the commercial forms of asbestos (chrysotile, amosite or crocidolite) as well as the noncommercial amphibole anthophyllite.[23]

The incidence appears to be higher in cigarette smokers than non-smokers with similar levels of asbestos exposure.[25-30] This may be the result of retention of larger amounts of asbestos in the lungs of smokers because of the inhibitory effect on pulmonary clearance mechanisms and direct enhancement of asbestos penetration into respiratory epithelium by cigarette smoking.[31] Experimental models have shown that cigarette smoke increases the degree of asbestos-induced pulmonary fibrosis, with increased asbestos fiber retention and rate of fiber penetration.[32-35] Schwartz has posited a role for cigarette smoking in the causation of asbestosis, attributing the increased inflammatory cell counts in lavage fluid to the effects of cigarette smoke.[36] Comparison of lavage cell counts in patients with asbestosis and asbestos-related pleural fibrosis showed that smoking strongly influenced lavage fluid cellularity, in particular the constituency of alveolar macrophages and eosinophils, independent of the effects of asbestos alone. Such changes are believed to play a role in the fibrogenesis seen in asbestosis.[37]

Radiographic studies have also shown a relationship between cigarette smoking and the prevalence of small irregular opacities on chest x-rays among asbestos workers.[25-30] However, a case-control study of South African asbestos miners undergoing autopsy showed no positive association between smoking and histopathologic evidence of asbestosis.[38] These findings suggest that the increased prevalence of small irregular opacities on chest films of asbestos workers who smoke might be due to some effect of cigarette smoke on the lung other than enhancing the severity of asbestosis (see below).

In addition to smoking habits, individual variance in fiber retention likely plays a role in the development of asbestosis. The interval of time between exposure to asbestos and the development of clinical disease is referred to as the latency period. The latency period for asbestosis is typically measured in decades. Latency periods are generally inversely proportional to exposure intensity, with shorter latency periods following heavy exposure, and are rarely less than 15 years from the time of initial exposure.[39] Asbestos fibers trapped within the pulmonary interstitium have a prolonged residence time in the lung. Consequently, asbestosis may continue to progress many years after exposure has ceased.[24]

Clinical Features

The clinical features of asbestosis are not unique to this entity, and are similar to those of other chronic pulmonary parenchymal fibrosing disorders. Dyspnea and dry cough are accompanied by basilar rales, and digital clubbing may be present in earlier as well as advanced disease. Late stage disease is often indicated by the presence of constitutional symptoms and signs of cor pulmonale. In general, asbestosis differs from idiopathic pulmonary fibrosis in that clinical manifestations are less severe and physiologic derangements milder. The rate of disease progression in asbestosis is generally slower paced than that seen with idiopathic pulmonary fibrosis. Such physiologic derangements on pulmonary function studies are not specific to asbestosis, and are those of restrictive ventilatory defects, with reduction in lung volumes, decreased diffusion capacity and arterial hypoxemia. The reduction in forced vital capacity appears proportional to the profusion of irregular opacities on chest radiographs, which may be further exaggerated by the presence of diffuse pleural thickening.[40]

Obstructive ventilatory defects, characterized by reduction in the FEV_1/FVC ratio, are usually the result of cigarette smoking. Some data suggest that exposure to mineral dusts can contribute to the development of airflow obstruction, likely related to peribronchiolar fibrosis. A study of 17 nonsmoking asbestos workers demonstrated reduced airflow at low lung volumes consistent with obstruction at the level of the small airways.[41] Another study contrasting the physiologic derangements in workers exposed to silica, asbestos, and coal dust found lower FEV_1/FVC ratios in the cohort of coal workers, suggesting exposure to coal dust is responsible for the development of obstructive ventilatory defects independent of the degree of any underlying coal worker's pneumoconiosis. Restrictive ventilatory defects were observed in the cohort of asbestos workers, accompanied by increases in FEV_1/FVC ratios as a function of progression of fibrosis and adjustment for smoking status. The authors suggest that this effect is due to the salutary effects of fibrosis upon peripheral airflow conductance and lung recoil.[42] It remains controversial whether peribronchiolar fibrosis related to asbestos causes clinically significant airflow obstruction in the absence of cigarette smoking. In the presence of smoking, the additive contribution of asbestos exposure to airflow obstruction is likely negligible.[43,44] There is no evidence that asbestos exposure alone contributes to clinically significant emphysema.[8,9]

Asbestosis is uncommonly associated with systemic manifestations. Kobayashi et al. described a case of asbestosis in which interstitial fibrosis was also observed in the liver, kidney, myocardium and thyroid gland.[45] Asbestos fibers were also identified in each of these sites using electron microscopy. Such an occurrence is analogous to the phenomenon of extrapulmonary silicotic nodules, which may be found in the liver, spleen, bone marrow and abdominal lymph nodes in those patients with heavy exposure and advanced silicosis.[46] Experimental studies clearly showing the transport of asbestos fibers in sufficient quantity to cause fibrosis have not to our knowledge been reported. Kobayashi's case more likely represents coincident asbestosis and progressive systemic sclerosis (scleroderma). Scleroderma is an uncommon, poorly understood, but well-recognized complication of exposure to crystalline silica, and it is possible that the development of systemic sclerosis in asbestosis shares a similar pathophysiology.[47]

Asbestos exposure is known to produce immunologic alterations in the host that affect both humoral and cell-mediated immunity.[48,49] However, it is unclear what clinical manifestations may result from these derangements. Maguire et al. reported a case of immunoblastic lymphadenopathy in a 71-year-old man with asbestosis.[50] Cooke et al. described another patient with lymphomatoid granulomatosis and proliferative glomerulonephritis in which asbestos fibers were observed in the renal mesangial matrix.[51] Immunoblastic lymphadenopathy and lymphoma have all been reported in association with asbestosis.[52,53]

Historically, deaths in asbestosis have been the result of the development of intractable respiratory failure. The prognosis associated with asbestosis is variable, but in general is associated with decreased life expectancy in proportion to disease severity.[54-56] In cases of heavy exposure, progressive disease generally occurs and is resistant to medical therapy. It is not clear whether such progression of fibrosis is inevitable in all cases. Studies from the United Kingdom and Finland document considerable and excessive mortality from carcinoma of the lung in workers with asbestosis.[54,57] A review of 525 autopsy cases of asbestosis from Japan between the years 1958 and 1996 noted an incidence of malignancy in approximately 60% of the entire autopsied series, represented chiefly by carcinomas of the lung and malignant mesothelioma. The highest rate of malignancy was observed in the cohort dying between 1990 and 1996, in which the rate of malignancy was 65%, compared to a rate of 43% observed in the cohort dying between 1958 and 1979.[58]

Pathogenesis

In brief, the mechanisms of asbestos-related fibrosis center on the development of a protracted cycle of inflammation in the setting of epithelial cell injury, apoptosis, and fibroblast proliferation, following upregulation of certain oncogenes and macrophage expression of cytokines and growth factors. The inhalation of fibrogenic dust thus results in a complex cascade of interactions between injured and dying epithelial cells, inflammatory effector cells, and reactive oxygen and nitrogen species, leading to fibroblast proliferation and the deposition of collagen culminating in the clinical entity termed asbestosis.[59,60] A detailed discussion of these pathways and the cellular and molecular basis for tissue injury related to inhalation of asbestos is to be found in Chapter 10.

Diagnosis

Radiographic Features

The radiographic features of asbestosis are those of lower lung zone reticulonodular infiltrates and small irregular opacities detectable on plain chest roentgenograms. The identification of pleural thickening or calcification helps to raise the index of suspicion for asbestosis, as such changes are not typical of the other forms and causes of pulmonary interstitial fibrosis.[17,19] An upper or mid-zone distribution of infiltrates argues against the diagnosis of asbestosis.[61] Profusion of these opacities increases with the severity of disease. Typical findings include fine lower lung zone reticulation likely resultant from early interstitial fibrosis, prominent interstitial and pleural changes with partial obliteration of the cardiac border (the "shaggy heart" sign), and finally late stage changes where reticulation becomes prominent in the mid and upper lung zones and the cardiac and diaphragmatic silhouettes become yet more obscured (Figure 4-1). Large opacities (>1 cm) are uncommon in asbestosis, and in some cases may be related to concomitant inhalation of quartz dust.

The International Labor Office (ILO) has developed a classification scheme for the radiographic assessment of pneumoconiosis based on the size and profusion of radiographically detected opacities. The availability of standard films representing the various degrees of severity is necessary to enhance the reproducibility of the classification scheme.[20] Such radiographic findings are integral to an acceptable clinical diagnosis of asbestosis. The American Thoracic Society has proposed the criteria of ILO category 1/1 reticulonodular opacities accompanied by FVC and DL_{CO} reduction to less than the lower limit predicted in the setting of appropriate exposure to asbestos. Although chest roentgenography is a useful screening tool and an important aid in epidemiologic surveys, limitations of this diagnostic technique exist. Standard chest x-rays may be negative in some individuals with histologically proven asbestosis.[62–64] Therefore, a negative film does *not* exclude the presence of disease. Also, some investigators have reported an excess of small irregular opacities in chest x-rays from individuals without a dust exposure history.[28,30,65] Some have found an increased prevalence of small irregular opacities in cigarette smokers.[28,30] Other studies have failed to confirm this observation.[26]

Because standard chest x-rays may produce both false-positive and false-negative results, it is of interest that computed tomography (CT) has been shown to enhance sensitivity and specificity for the recognition of asbestosis.[66] Furthermore, CT provides finer resolution of anatomic detail of the lesions of interstitial lung disease than can be achieved with routine chest roentgenograms (Figure 4-2).[67,68] In addi-

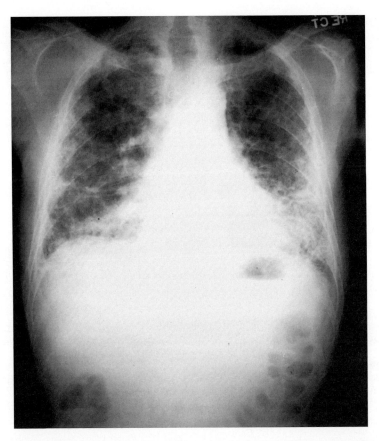

Figure 4-1. Posteroanterior chest radiograph from an insulator with asbestosis, showing small lung volumes and bilateral reticulonodular infiltrates most prominent in the lung bases. (Courtesy of Dr. Colleen Bergin, Department of Radiology, Duke University Medical Center. Reprinted from Ref. 8, with permission.)

tion, CT is a useful adjunct to conventional chest radiography in assessing the presence of emphysema, which is often present in asbestos workers who smoke cigarettes.[69–71] While the advent of high-resolution computed tomography has certainly increased the sensitivity for detection of early asbestos-related parenchymal lesions,[72–74] the plain chest roentgenogram remains the radiographic gold standard. The clinical diagnosis of asbestosis in the setting of heavy asbestos exposure and the above-described radiographic and/or physiologic derangements seldom requires biopsy for histologic confirmation. The demonstration of asbestos bodies in sputum or bronchoalveolar lavage fluid correlates both with heavy exposure and asbestosis[75] (see Chapter 9), but their presence in cytologic specimens is in and of itself insufficient for the diagnosis of asbestosis. Since those exposed to asbestos are not immune to other and potentially treatable forms of interstitial fibrosis, biopsy is recommended in instances where exposure history is not compelling and uncertainty exists on the basis of radiographic and/or clinical grounds.[76–78]

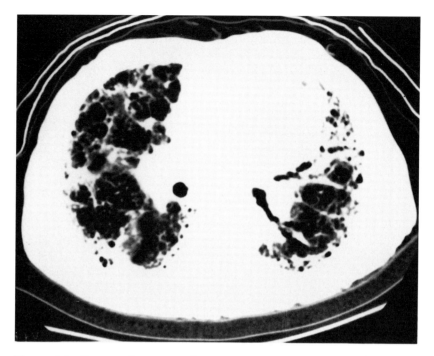

Figure 4-2. Computed tomography of the thorax from an insulator with asbestosis (same case as Fig. 4-1), showing prominent interstitial markings with honeycomb changes and peripheral accentuation. (Courtesy of Dr. Colleen Bergin, Department of Radiology, Duke University Medical Center. Reprinted from Ref. 8, with permission.)

Pathologic Features

Gross Morphology

For optimal visualization of fibrosis and concomitant pathologic processes such as emphysema, we recommend prosection of surgical or autopsy material following formalin inflation and distension, with adequate tissue fixation of at least two days duration.[14,79] In the earliest stages of asbestosis, the lungs may appear normal on gross examination. It is important not to misinterpret accompanying visceral pleural fibrosis as asbestosis, and the diagnosis must include the description of diffuse parenchymal fibrosis. As the disease progresses, gray streaks of fibrous tissue become visible at the lung bases, accentuated at the periphery, with sparing of the central lung zones.[14] This pattern may be followed by coarse linear scarring with loss of lung volume (Figure 4-3). Such areas are the pathologic counterpart to the reticular markings and small irregular opacities seen on plain chest films, and provide the anatomic basis for the physiologic derangements observed in asbestosis. The excessive collagen deposition results in increased lung weight and consistency. Honeycomb changes are identified in advanced disease, most conspicuously in the subpleural areas of the lower lung zones. The honeycomb foci consist of cystic spaces, which measure up to 1.0 cm in areas of dense fibrosis (Figure 4-4). In exceptional cases, and for uncertain reasons, the interstitial fibrosis may be most severe in the upper lung zones.[80] Progressive massive fibrosis has also been described in rare instances and is likely attributable to exposure to asbestos and silica. There are no typical asbestos-associated lesions in the airways, although traction bronchiectasis may develop in areas of dense scarring. Regional lymph nodes are generally unremarkable on gross inspection.

The changes described above are not specific for asbestosis and may be observed in a wide variety of chronic interstitial diseases and fibrosing disorders. A useful feature that may aid in the distinction of asbestosis from other fibrosing diseases is the frequent association of

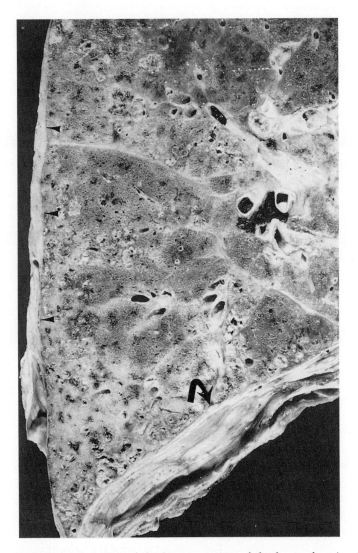

Figure 4-3. Coronal section of the lower portion of the lung of an insulator with asbestosis. There is pale gray, linear interstitial fibrosis especially prominent in the lower lobe. Note the visceral pleural thickening laterally (*arrowheads*) and adhesion of the diaphragm to the undersurface of the lung (*curved arrow*).

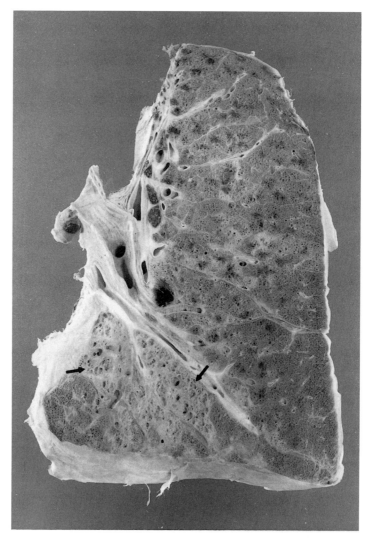

Figure 4-4. Coronal section of the left lung of an insulator with asbestosis and cavitary squamous cell carcinoma of the right lower lobe. Note the honeycomb changes in the medial portion of the lower lobe (*arrows*). (Reprinted from Ref. 8, with permission.)

pleural abnormalities with the former (see Chapter 6). Diffuse thickening of the visceral pleura is often present (Figure 4-3), whereas fibrous pleuropulmonary adhesions are variable. A finding yet more characteristic of asbestos exposure is the parietal pleural plaque, circumscribed areas of ivory-colored pleural thickening over the domes of the diaphragm or on the posterolateral chest wall running along the direction of the ribs.[81,82] Pleural plaques may be smooth or nodular (the so-called candle wax dripping appearance) when viewed grossly, and have a cartilaginous consistency. They are often calcified. The demonstration of such pleural abnormalities does not indicate a diagnosis of asbestosis, but rather alerts the pathologist to the possible presence of asbestos-related interstitial fibrosis and advises a search for asbestos bodies. Not all patients with asbestosis have pleural plaques, and certainly not all patients with pleural plaques have the interstitial fibrosis requisite for the diagnosis of asbestosis. Some have argued that there is no need to distinguish the clinically and epidemiologically disparate entities of pleural and parenchymal fibrosis as they both are causally related to asbestos exposure.[83] The weakness of this argument is apparent when one considers that asbestos exposure may result in asbestosis, malignant mesothelioma, or both. Certainly there is no rationale for including malignant mesothelioma under the rubric of asbestosis, and there is no reason to include benign pleural fibrosis under that rubric either.

Because of the prevalence of cigarette smoking among asbestos workers, this group often exhibits parenchymal changes in the lung related to exposure to tobacco smoke. The pathologist must therefore take care to distinguish abnormalities resultant from the two different types of exposure. Centrilobular emphysema is frequently observed in the lungs of cigarette smokers,[79] and may be of such a severe degree as to overshadow the fibrosis of asbestosis (Figure 4-5). Emphysema must be distinguished from the honeycomb changes observed in advanced asbestosis. The gross distribution of the lesions is helpful in this regard, with emphysema tending to be most severe in the upper lobes, and the honeycomb changes most severe in the lower lung zones. The cystic changes of honeycomb lung are usually of uniform size (approximately 0.5 cm), with thickened fibrotic walls. The emphysematous spaces by contrast are of variable size, from barely visible to several centimeters in diameter. Representing areas of destroyed lung tissue, they have no "walls" and are not accompanied by visible fibrosis.[79] Another helpful gross feature is the presence of thin, delicate tissue strands that traverse the emphysematous spaces. These represent vascular remnants that persist following destruction of alveolar tissue. The presence of a significant amount of emphysema (i.e., involvement of 25% or more of the lung parenchyma) is generally accompanied by obstructive ventilatory defects on pulmonary function studies.[79]

Cytologic Features/Bronchoalveolar Lavage

Clinical evaluation of patients with diffuse interstitial lung disease often begins with analysis of exfoliative cytologic preparations obtained by fiberoptic bronchoscopy. Demonstration of asbestos bodies using this methodology may alert to the presence of asbestos-related pathology, but the diagnosis of asbestosis is not possible based solely on cytologic grounds. Bronchoalveolar lavage is a useful technique to diagnose diseases involving the peripheral alveoli in the most distal anatomic regions of the lung.[84] The technique involves the instillation of aliquots of sterile saline via a peripherally placed fiberoptic bronchoscope. The bronchoalveolar lavage fluid (BALF) is subsequently retrieved via the bronchoscope suction port and submitted for cytologic analysis.

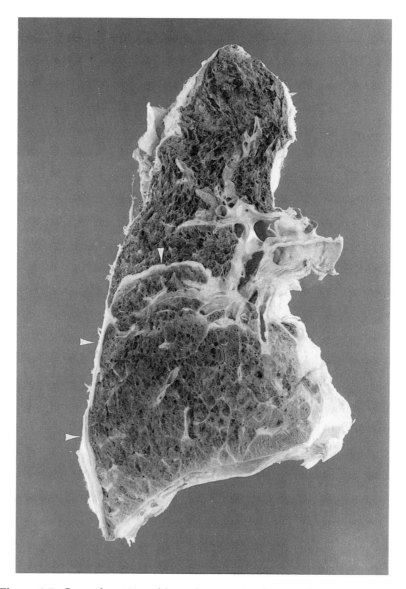

Figure 4-5. Coronal section of lung from an insulator and cigarette smoker showing moderate asbestosis and severe centrilobular emphysema (compare with honeycomb changes in Fig. 4-4). Notice the visceral pleural thickening enveloping the lung and extending into the interlobar fissure (*arrowheads*). (Reprinted from Ref. 8, with permission.)

Asbestos bodies can be found in BALF in more than 95% of patients with asbestosis, and have been considered markers of exposure rather than disease.[75,85] Some studies have shown a direct relationship between concentration of asbestos bodies in BALF and the degree of exposure and lung tissue asbestos burden.[75] However, Schwartz studied the BALF asbestos body counts in a cohort of American construction workers and determined that in at least this cohort, predominantly exposed to chrysotile, the concentration of BALF asbestos bodies was not a valid measure either of asbestos exposure or of asbestos-related lung disease.[86] It seems reasonable to treat the presence of asbestos bodies in BALF as a reproducible indicator of exposure to asbestos and to use this piece of information as a single point in the patient's clinical database. A negative BALF examination for asbestos bodies does not exclude the possibility of asbestos-related pulmonary pathology. The examination of BALF to derive inflammatory cell counts and profiles remains a research technique, and conclusions regarding the limited clinical utility of BALF appear substantiated.

Histopathology

The *sine qua non* for the histologic diagnosis of asbestosis is the demonstration of diffuse interstitial fibrosis *and* asbestos bodies in routine 5 μm sections.[14] Observations of lung tissue obtained at autopsy from asbestos workers, as well as experimental models, have demonstrated that the earliest microscopic abnormality is the presence of increased collagen in the walls of respiratory bronchioles.[14,87] With more advanced disease, fibrosis extends into the terminal bronchioles proximal to the respiratory bronchioles, as well as into distal alveolar ducts. Ultimately, the fibrotic process extends to involve the alveolar septa surrounding these structures (Figure 4-6). The most extensive involvement is typically in the subpleural tiers of alveoli and in those alveoli in closest proximity to the bronchioles.

In advanced cases, large zones of lung parenchyma consist of fibrotic alveolar walls, and honeycomb change may be present. The honeycomb areas consist of cystic spaces generally 1 to 15 mm in diameter, and are lined by cuboidal to low columnar epithelium. These spaces frequently contain mucus and inflammatory debris. A lymphoplasmocellular infiltrate may be observed within the fibrotic interstitium. The secondary interlobular septa may also be markedly thickened by fibrous tissue, and diffuse visceral pleural fibrosis may be observed as well. The fibrotic process may be patchy in the early stages, requiring the examination of multiple sections to find the diagnostic features.[14,88] Masson's trichrome stains can facilitate the assessment of the extent and distribution of the interstitial fibrosis.

The second component required for the histologic diagnosis of asbestosis is the identification of asbestos bodies in paraffin sections. Asbestos bodies may be found lying free within alveolar spaces, or embedded within the fibrotic pulmonary interstitum[8,14,88] (see Figure 4-6). (The morphologic appearance of asbestos bodies and their distinction from other ferruginous bodies are described in detail in Chapter 3.) Occasionally, asbestos bodies are observed within foreign-body giant cells. The authors have also observed asbestos bodies within hilar or mediastinal lymph nodes, often associated with fibrosis of the lymph node parenchyma. This curious observation is largely confined to patients with a heavy pulmonary parenchymal fiber burden, and is likely related to overloading of the clearance mechanisms.[89] Among 20 patients with asbestos bodies observed in thoracic lymph nodes, 17 had histologically confirmed asbestosis.[90]

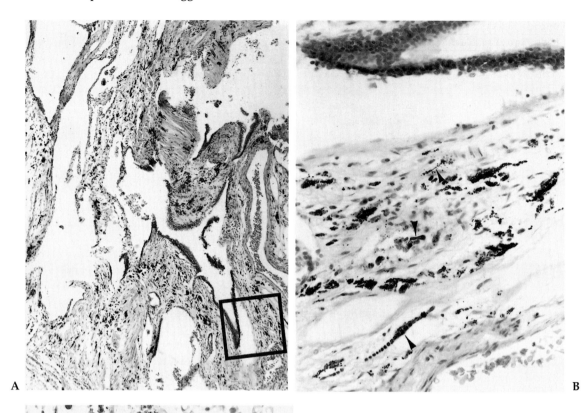

A

B

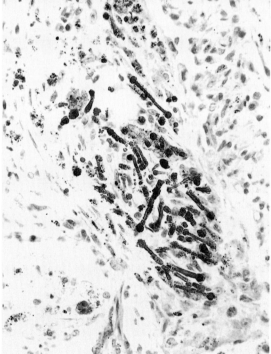

C

Figure 4-6. (A) Low power photomicrograph of a bronchiole from an insulator with asbestosis. There is peribronchiolar fibrosis with distortion of the bronchiole. The fibrosis extends to involve adjacent alveoli. **(B)** Higher magnification of the rectangular area marked in part (A) shows asbestos bodies embedded within fibrotic peribronchiolar connective tissue (*arrowheads*). **(C)** Elsewhere, clusters of asbestos bodies are embedded within fibrotic pulmonary interstitium. Hematoxylin and eosin, magnification (A) ×52; (B) ×250; (C) ×325. (Reprinted from Ref. 8, with permission.)

Table 4-1. Histological findings in 100 cases of asbestosis

Histological feature	Percent
Always Present	
Asbestos bodies	100%
Peribronchiolar fibrosis	100%
Often Present	
Alveolar septal fibrosis	82%
Occasionally Present	
Honeycomb changes	15%
Foreign-body giant cells	15%
Bronchiolar metaplasia	10%
Cytoplasmic hyaline	7%
Desquamative interstitial pneumonitis-like areas	6%
Rarely Present	
Osseous metaplasia (dendriform pulmonary ossification)	2%
Pulmonary blue bodies	1%

Source: Reproduced from Ref. 8, with permission

Other less frequent histologic changes have been observed in asbestosis (Table 4-1). These include the presence of foreign-body-type giant cells within alveoli, or less commonly the fibrotic interstitium, in some 15% of cases. Scarring and distortion of bronchioles with necrosis and disruption of the transitional zone from the respiratory bronchiole to the alveolar duct occasionally results in the lining of adjacent alveoli by cuboidal bronchiolar epithelium (Figure 4-7). This process occurs in some 10% of cases, and has sometimes been termed "pulmonary adenomatosis," but is more properly referred to as bronchiolar metaplasia. Hyperplastic Type II alveolar pneumocytes may also line the fibrotic alveolar septa in asbestosis. These cells may, in approximately 7% of cases, contain deposits of waxy, deeply eosinophilic material (Figure 4-8). This so-called cytoplasmic hyaline has tinctorial and ultrastructural characteristics identical to those observed in Mallory's hyaline of alcoholic hepatitis.[91] This unusual phenomenon is not specific for asbestosis, as once believed, and likely represents a nonspecific reaction to injury.[14,92] Alveolar macrophages are present in increased numbers in asbestosis, and in a minority of cases may so densely pack the alveoli as to mimic the pattern of desquamative interstitial pneumonia (Figure 4-9).[8,14,18]

Dendriform pulmonary ossification is another unusual phenomenon, observed in 2% of cases in the authors' series.[93] This process is characterized by branching spicules of bone, often containing marrow elements, embedded within the pulmonary interstitium (Figure 4-10). It is thought that this process represents osteoblastic metaplasia involving interstitial fibroblasts.[94] An additional unusual process observed in asbestosis is the occurrence of pulmonary blue bodies. These basophilic laminated concretions consist primarily of calcium carbonate and are present within alveolar spaces in some 1% of cases (see Table 4-1). They are not visualized with polarizing microscopy using hematoxylin-eosin stained sections, but are brightly birefringent in unstained paraffin-embedded sections, or in filter preparations of

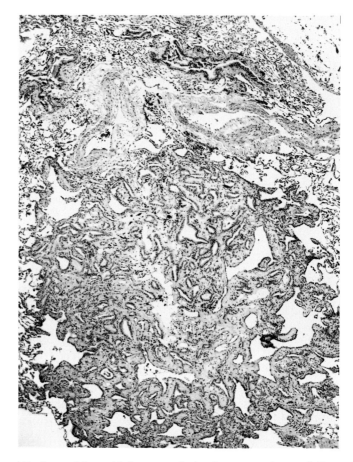

Figure 4-7. Area of bronchiolar metaplasia shows scarring and distortion of bronchiole with lining of adjacent fibrotic alveolar septa by cuboidal bronchiolar epithelium. Hematoxylin and eosin, magnification ×40.

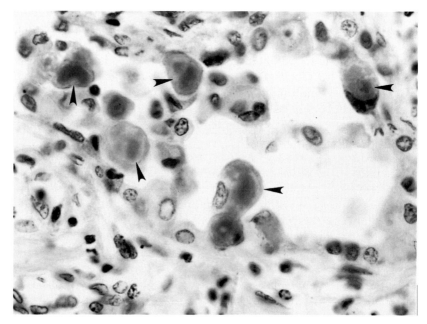

Figure 4-8. Photomicrograph of lung parenchyma in patient with asbestosis, showing hyperplastic alveolar type II pneumocytes. Many of these cells contain cytoplasmic hyalin (*arrowheads*), which has the same tinctorial characteristics as the hyalin found within hepatocytes in patients with alcoholic hepatitis. Hematoxylin and eosin, magnification ×680. (Reprinted from Ref. 8, with permission.)

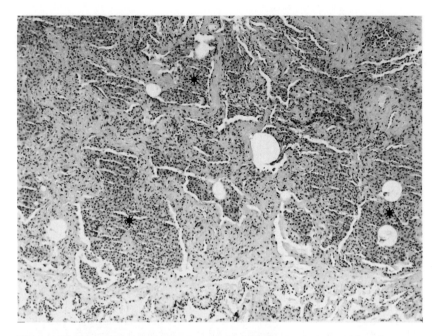

Figure 4-9. Low power photomicrograph of lung in patient with asbestosis, showing alveoli packed with sheets of alveolar macrophages (*asterisks*). This pattern resembles that seen in desquamative interstitial pneumonia. Hematoxylin and eosin, magnification ×68. (Reprinted from Ref. 8, with permission.)

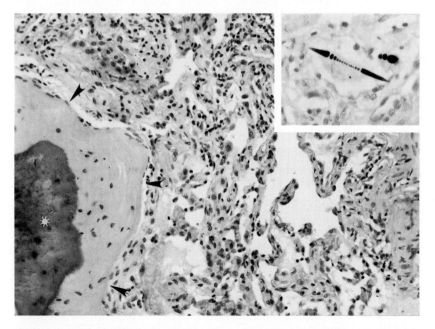

Figure 4-10. Pulmonary ossification in a patient with asbestosis, showing spicule of bone (*arrowheads*) with central calcification (*asterisk*) embedded within fibrotic interstitium. Inset shows asbestos bodies found elsewhere in the same section. Hematoxylin and eosin, magnification ×175; inset, Prussian blue, magnification ×325. (Reprinted from Ref. 93, with permission.)

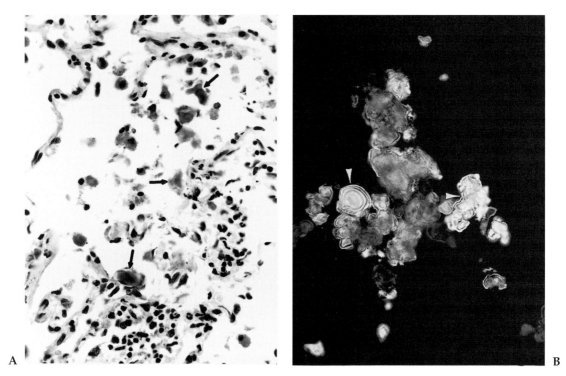

Figure 4-11. (A) Intraalveolar pulmonary blue bodies exhibit a somewhat laminated appearance (*arrows*) and consist primarily of calcium carbonate. Hematoxylin and eosin. **(B)** Nuclepore filter preparation of lung tissue digested in sodium hypochlorite [same case as illustrated in part (A)] shows brightly birefringent "blue bodies" with clearly visible laminations (*arrowheads*). Unstained filter, polarizing microscopy. Magnification (A) ×400; (B) ×325. (Courtesy of Dr. Fred Askin, Department of Pathology, Johns Hopkins Hospital, Baltimore, MD. Reprinted from Ref. 8, with permission.)

tissue digests[8,95] (Figure 4-11). The mechanism of formation of blue bodies is unknown, but calcium salts have been observed to accumulate in the pulmonary interstitium of experimental animals exposed to aerosolized asbestos fibers (see Chapter 10).[96] Pulmonary blue bodies are not specific for asbestos exposure and similar to cytoplasmic hyaline likely represent an unusual but nonspecific reaction to injury. These uncommon histologic abnormalities are generally observed in the more advanced cases of asbestosis.

Infection with aspergillus species is uncommonly associated with asbestosis, perhaps related to suppression of local cell mediated immunity by asbestos.[97] Hillerdal and Hecksher reported four cases of this unusual association and suggested the infection may be related to anatomical alterations of the bronchial tree or lung parenchyma resultant from asbestos exposure.[98] One of the authors (VLR) has also observed five additional cases[99] (and unpublished observations) (Figure 4-12), one of which was diagnosed by fine needle aspiration. No other opportunistic fungal infections associated with asbestosis have been reported or observed by the authors, and the reason for the specificity for aspergillus remains obscure.

Ultrastructural Findings

Few ultrastructural studies of the lung have been reported in patients with asbestosis. Shelburne et al.[100] observed that transmission electron microscopy (TEM) is an inefficient way to detect asbestos bodies, even in patients with heavy asbestos tissue burdens, due to the minute volume of tissue examined using this technique. Corrin et al. studied eight cases of asbestosis using TEM and observed a number of ultra-structural abnormalities, especially within the interstitium of the lung. Within the alveolar spaces, excess numbers of alveolar macrophages were observed. There was patchy loss of Type I alveolar epithelium, and the thickened alveolar septa demonstrated interstitial edema and collagen deposition.[101] Changes were also observed in the capillary compartment, consisting of endothelial swelling with basement membrane thickening and reduplication. The changes observed were similar to those seen in seventeen cases of idiopathic pulmonary fibrosis, except for a paucity of interstitial inflammatory cells and the presence of asbestos fibers in the patients with asbestosis.[101] There was no ultrastructural evidence of immune complex deposition. From this work, it appears that the parenchymal fibrosis and hallmarks of epithelial and endothelial cell injury noted in asbestosis share common ultrastructural attributes with the family of idiopathic fibrosing interstitial pneumonitides.

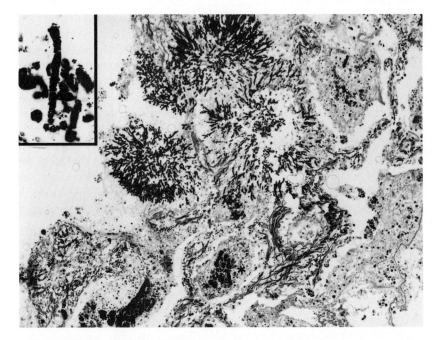

Figure 4-12. Numerous acutely branching, septate hyphae are present within the lung parenchyma. A clump of asbestos bodies can be seen in a nearby alveolus (*asterisk*). Grocott's methenamine silver technique, ×100. *Inset:* detailed view of clump of asbestos bodies. Hematoxylin and eosin, magnification ×250. (Reprinted from Ref. 99, with permission.)

Differential Diagnosis

Asbestosis must be distinguished from the group of idiopathic fibrosing interstitial pneumonitides, and also from the pulmonary injury resultant from inhalation of other dusts. Shipyard workers constitute a group of asbestos workers who may be exposed in the course of their occupation to substantial amounts of silica, talc or welding fumes in addition to asbestos.[8] Crystalline silica is used in sandblasting, and also constitutes one component of the lining of steam boilers in ships. Individuals engaged in sandblasting, boiler scaling, or even working in the vicinity of these operations often exhibit silicotic nodules within the hilar lymph nodes or parenchyma of the lung, especially the upper lobes. Silicosis may be readily distinguished from asbestosis, as it results in a circumscribed nodular pattern of fibrosis, as opposed to the irregular linear fibrosis of asbestosis. The changes of silicosis are most severe in the upper lobes, whereas asbestosis typically involves the lower lobes. Furthermore, silicotic nodules are invariably present in the hilar lymph nodes and pleural involvement, when present, consists of subpleural nodules up to several millimeters in size.[102]

Similarly, shipyard welders are invariably exposed to some asbestos, so that the pathologist must take care to distinguish asbestosis from welders' pneumoconiosis. This is characterized by interstitial deposits of iron oxides, which appear as dark brown to black spherical particles, often featuring golden-brown rims. Pseudoasbestos bodies with broad yellow or black cores are frequently seen (see Chapter 3). Welder's pneumoconiosis generally results in little collagen deposition, and the presence of substantial amounts of interstitial fibrosis in a shipyard welder should alert the pathologist to the possibility of concomitant asbestosis. Among 76 cases of welder's pneumoconiosis from the consultation files of one of the authors (VLR), only 22 cases contained peribronchiolar fibrosis and true asbestos bodies requisite for the diagnosis of asbestosis. In extreme examples, isolated instances of asbestosis, talcosis, silicosis and berylliosis have been reported in a single individual,[103] and diffuse interstitial fibrosis can follow exposure to a variety of inorganic particulates. In such cases of fibrosis due to dusts other than asbestos, analysis of lung mineral content is invaluable (see Chapter 11). Another useful feature to raise the index of suspicion for asbestosis is the frequent occurrence of visceral pleural fibrosis and parietal plaques.

In the earliest stages of the disease, the diagnosis of asbestosis may be subtle and the distinction must be made from other causes of peribronchiolar fibrosis. Inhalation of mineral dusts such as silica, iron or aluminum oxides, as well as cigarette smoke[104] has been associated with peribronchiolar fibrosis. These types of exposure generally result in a less conspicuous pattern of peribronchiolar fibrosis than that observed with asbestos exposure.[104,105] The distinction is made by the demonstration of asbestos bodies in tissue sections. The small airway lesions in cigarette smokers are most often characterized by goblet cell metaplasia, mucous plugging and peribronchiolar chronic inflammation. Many asbestos workers are also smokers, and the peribronchiolar

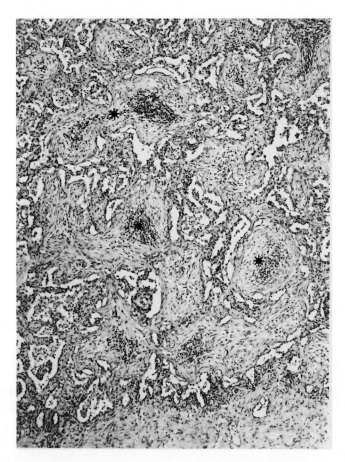

Figure 4-13. Photomicrograph of area of organizing pneumonia in a patient with asbestosis. The patient had undergone resection of a lobe for a mass suspected to be carcinoma. Note the plugs of young, edematous connective tissue filling alveolar ducts and adjacent alveolar spaces (*asterisks*). Hematoxylin and eosin magnification ×52.

fibrosis of asbestosis and the small airway lesions of smoking are often coexistent in the same patient.

Asbestosis must also be distinguished from cryptogenic organizing pneumonia (COP), formerly known as bronchiolitis obliterans organizing pneumonia (BOOP). COP may present as discrete pulmonary masses or infiltrates on chest radiographs, and thereby mimics carcinoma.[106] COP is characterized by serpiginous plugs of loose young edematous connective tissue within distal bronchioles, filling the alveolar ducts and sacs (Figure 4-13). These plugs often incorporate clusters of chronic inflammatory cells. Pathologists may encounter this entity in asbestos workers, in view of the increased surveillance given this group related to its increased risk of lung cancer (see Chapter 7), or perhaps an increased predisposition toward the development of organizing pneumonia in this group. A useful diagnostic feature is the tendency for COP to occur as a localized process, whereas asbestosis is by definition bilateral and diffuse. COP is often associated with some degree of fibrotic thickening of alveolar septa and may be accompanied by alveolar Type II pneumocyte hyperplasia, so that the diagnostic features of asbestosis may be overshadowed or obscured by super-imposed COP.

Asbestosis must also be distinguished from iatrogenic pulmonary disease related to the treatment of pulmonary and nonpulmonary malignancies. External beam radiation and cytotoxic chemotherapy may both result in pulmonary interstitial fibrosis. Radiation pneumonitis is usually, but not invariably, confined to irradiated lung, and may be suspected on the basis of its distribution in any given case.[107] Radiation pneumonitis may feature prominent changes in the vasculature, including thickening and fibrosis of vessel walls and endothelial vacuolization. Pathologic changes related to cytotoxic chemotherapeutic agents are generally more diffuse than is asbestosis, and often show atypical alveolar Type II pneumocyte hyperplasia as a prominent feature. When pulmonary fibrosis due to the administration of such chemotherapeutic agents is superimposed on asbestosis, it may be necessary to refer to pretreatment radiographs to confirm the diagnosis of asbestosis.

Perhaps the most difficult differential diagnosis is the separation of asbestosis from idiopathic pulmonary fibrosis in a patient with a history of asbestos exposure. There are gross and microscopic findings common to both entities, particularly in late stage disease. If the exposure history is not compelling and diagnostic material shows interstitial fibrosis but no asbestos bodies, then a diagnosis of idiopathic pulmonary fibrosis is more likely. Criteria for the diagnosis of the various patterns of idiopathic pulmonary fibrosis, including usual interstitial pneumonia (UIP), acute interstitial pneumonia (AIP), desquamative interstitial pneumonia (DIP), and nonspecific interstitial pneumonia (NSIP) are well established.[108] In the absence of asbestos bodies in histological sections, these patterns should not be attributed to asbestos.

Some investigators have suggested that transbronchial biopsy may be useful in the diagnosis of asbestosis.[109,110] In general, transbronchial biopsies share the same profound limitations and inadequacies in the diagnosis of asbestosis as they do in cases of idiopathic pulmonary fibrosis. Rare transbronchial biopsies have demonstrated interstitial fibrosis and asbestos bodies, allowing the diagnosis to be made in concert with a review of radiographic findings. However, transbronchial biopsy is inadequate diagnostically in the majority of cases,[9,14] and generous sampling of open or thoracoscopically obtained lung tissue is normally required to make the subtle and intricate histologic distinctions as outlined above.

Assessment of Diagnostic Criteria

The histological diagnosis of asbestosis is of considerable importance, as it provides confirmation of the presence, or absence, of a fibrosing interstitial lung disease related to the inhalation of asbestos-containing dust. The histological diagnosis of asbestosis rests upon the demon-stration of peribronchiolar fibrosis and asbestos bodies in tissue sec-tions, with or without alveolar septal fibrosis.[8,14] As other insults may result in some peribronchiolar fibrosis,[104,105] it is recommended that in the absence of alveolar septal fibrosis, a histologic diagnosis of asbesto-sis should be made only when a majority of the bronchioles show excessive amounts of connective tissue in their walls. The detection of fibrosis can be difficult when there is atelectasis, vascular congestion or consolidation with pneumonia, and care should be taken not to over-interpret such sections as showing interstitial fibrosis.[111] Examination of Masson's trichrome-stained sections is indicated to evaluate the presence and extent of fibrosis in those cases where its presence is not straightforward on routine sections.

Ferruginous bodies in histologic sections should be examined care-fully so that pseudoasbestos bodies are not mistaken for true asbestos bodies. The former will contain broad yellow or black cores and are discussed in further detail in Chapter 3. In those cases where asbesto-sis is suspected, but asbestos bodies are not readily detected on routine sections, it is recommended that iron-stained sections be prepared and examined systematically and in their entirety at 200× magnification using a mechanical stage.[112,113] Using this approach, several asbestos bodies should be observed in most 2 × 2 cm sections of lung parenchyma in cases of *bona fide* asbestosis[8] (see Chapter 11). Since asbestos bodies are not always evenly distributed in histologic sec-tions,[14,113] more than one iron-stained section should be examined when asbestos bodies are sparse.

Fibrosis was confined to the walls of bronchioles in 18% of our cases (see Table 4-1), and some investigators have challenged the inclusion of such cases in the definition of asbestosis, preferring the term asbestos airway disease.[114] The reasons given for excluding such cases include the observation that inhalation of dusts other than asbestos can result in peribronchiolar fibrosis, and a lack of direct evidence that such lesions may progress to alveolar septal fibrosis.[104,105] Inhalation of other dusts may also produce alveolar septal fibrosis,[2] but in such cases, the detection of asbestos bodies provides evidence that the fibrosis results from asbestos exposure.[8,15] Restriction of the definition of asbestosis to those cases in which the majority of the bronchioles are involved greatly reduces the chances of diagnosing such lesions as being asbestos-related. Furthermore, experimental animal studies have demonstrated that the peribronchiolar region is an early site of asbestos-induced fibrosis.[87] The most compelling argument for includ-ing isolated peribronchiolar fibrosis (accompanied by the observation of asbestos bodies) within the scope of the definition of asbestosis is that asbestos exposure can produce increased fibrous tissue deposition within all portions of the pulmonary interstitium, which includes the interstitial space of the alveolar septa, the subpleural connective tissue matrix, the secondary interlobular septa, and the connective tissue sheaths surrounding the broncho- and bronchiolovascular bundles. The preponderance of evidence warrants the inclusion of isolated peri-bronchiolar fibrosis under the diagnostic heading of asbestosis.

The identification of asbestos bodies in histologic sections as a diagnostic prerequisite for asbestosis has not gone unchallenged. Arguments against such a requirement have included the observation that chrysotile forms asbestos bodies poorly in contrast to the amphiboles, and many asbestos workers are primarily exposed to chrysotile.[115] Second, there is great individual variability with regard to the efficiency in which inhaled fibers are coated to make asbestos bodies, with some individuals poorly capable of doing so.[116,117] Holden and Churg have shown, however, that in chrysotile miners and millers, individuals with asbestosis do have asbestos bodies in histologic sections, and these bodies contain chrysotile cores.[118] Furthermore, as the number of cases with overt asbestosis decreases due to diminishing numbers of survivors of the heavy asbestos exposures of the past, there will be a concomitant and necessary increase in the proportion of cases with idiopathic pulmonary fibrosis. Therefore, loosening the requirement for asbestos bodies in histological sections in order to diagnose asbestosis would greatly reduce the specificity of the histological criteria. Furthermore, it has been our observation that those patients lacking asbestos bodies in histological sections invariably have uncoated fiber levels well below those observed in cases with *bona fide* asbestosis[77] (see Chapter 11). Similar observations have been reported by Gaensler et al.[76] In the absence of asbestos bodies on histologic sections, the detection of tissue levels of asbestos typical of asbestosis is unlikely. The analysis presented in Chapter 11 indicates that *clinically significant* interstitial fibrosis is unlikely to be the result of asbestos exposure when there are fewer than one million fibers 5μm or greater in length per gram of dry lung tissue. The fibrogenicity of fibers in this size range is well established,[119-122] whereas that of fibers less than 5μm remains unproven (see Chapter 10).[123] Therefore, no tissue level of fibers in the latter range can be used at present for a diagnosis of asbestosis.[8]

Grading Scheme

It is generally sufficient for pathologists to incorporate gross and microscopic features to estimate the extent of fibrosing or destructive processes within the lung, and to term such extent as mild, moderate or severe. It is possible using proposed histologic grading systems to assess the extent of asbestosis in a semiquantitative manner and augment the qualitative descriptors.[124-127] One such system is that proposed by the College of American Pathologists (CAP) and the National Institute for Occupational Safety and Health (NIOSH) in 1982.[14] The inter- and intraobserver variability for pathologists using this scheme was assessed, and the application of the criteria to a set of cases was found to be reasonably reproducible. Universal application of such a scheme would be highly desirable for epidemiologic studies, as well as for comparison with established radiologic schemes for classification of pneumoconiosis[128] (see earlier section on Radiographic Features). It should be noted that the diagnosis of asbestosis must be established using the criteria outlined in the previous section prior to any attempt at grading the disease.

Accurate histological grading depends on adequate tissue sampling, preferably the examination of sections obtained from the central and peripheral regions from each lobe of both lungs.[14] The limitations of sampling should be recognized; that is, grading should be possible on thoracoscopically obtained lung tissue, whereas a transbronchial biopsy specimen is not sufficient. The grading scheme of CAP-NIOSH includes scores for both severity and extent of disease.[14] A score for each of these parameters is determined for each slide examined, the two values multiplied to give a single value for each slide, and the individual values obtained for each slide averaged to give an average histological grade for each case. Grading of severity is as follows:

Grade 0 = No peribronchiolar fibrosis
Grade 1 = Fibrosis confined to the walls of respiratory bronchioles and the first adjacent tier of alveoli
Grade 2 = Fibrosis extending to involve alveolar ducts, or two or more tiers of alveoli adjacent to the bronchiole, with sparing of some alveoli between adjacent bronchioles
Grade 3 = Fibrotic thickening of the walls of all alveoli between at least two adjacent respiratory bronchioles
Grade 4 = Honeycomb changes (see earlier section on "Histopathology")

Grading of the extent of disease is classified according to the percentage of bronchioles showing excessive peribronchiolar connective tissue:

Grade A = Only occasional bronchioles involved
Grade B = More than occasional involvement, but less than half
Grade C = More than half of all bronchioles involved by fibrosing process

This scheme allows 12 possible grades for each slide. However, practical application of this scheme by the authors indicates that certain combinations occur rarely, or not at all. Virtually all cases with Grade 3 or 4 severity show grade C profusion on the same slide, as do most cases with Grade 2 severity. Furthermore, if one restricts the diagnosis in cases with Grade 1 severity to those in which most of the bronchioles are involved (see earlier section on Assessment of Diagnostic Criteria), then one is left with only four grades of severity to consider. We recommend the adoption of this simplified version of the CAP-NIOSH grading scheme,[14] summarized in Table 4-2 and illustrated in Figure 4-14. Others have proposed a similar scheme and applied it to experimental models of asbestosis.[129] In view of reasonable inter- and intraobserver concordance obtained with the more extensive scheme,[14] similar if not better concordance is expected with the modified and simpler version.

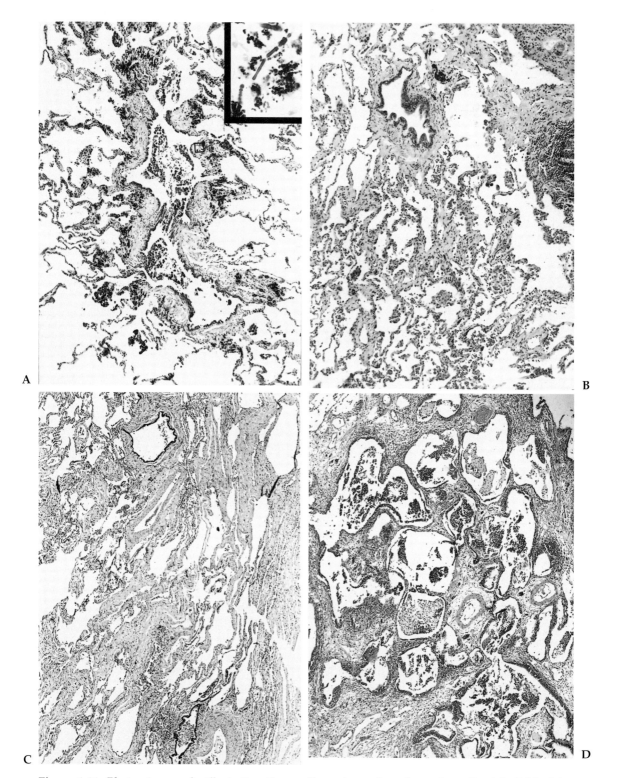

Figure 4-14. Photomicrographs illustrating the grading scheme for asbestosis outlined in Table 4-2. Each of the cases satisfied the histologic criteria for the diagnosis of asbestosis outlined in the text. **(A)** *Grade 1:* Fibrosis is confined to the walls of respiratory bronchioles. *Inset:* Higher magnification shows several asbestos bodies embedded in fibrous tissue of bronchiolar wall. **(B)** *Grade 2:* Fibrosis extends to involve alveolar ducts and two or more tiers of adjacent alveoli. **(C)** *Grade 3:* All alveoli between adjacent bronchioles show fibrotic thickening. **(D)** *Grade 4:* Honeycomb changes, consisting of cystic spaces lined by bronchiolar-type epithelium and with fibrotic walls. Hematoxylin and eosin, magnification (A) ×52, inset ×520; (B) ×62; (C) ×32; (D) ×40.

Table 4-2. Histological grading scheme for asbestosis*

Grade 0	No appreciable peribronchiolar fibrosis, or less than half of bronchioles involved
Grade 1	Fibrosis confined to the walls of respiratory bronchioles and the first tier of adjacent alveoli, with involvement of more than half of all bronchioles on a slide
Grade 2	Extension of fibrosis to involve alveolar ducts and/or two or more tiers of alveoli adjacent to the respiratory bronchiole, with sparing of at least some alveoli between adjacent bronchioles
Grade 3	Fibrotic thickening of the walls of all alveoli between at least two adjacent respiratory bronchioles
Grade 4	Honeycomb changes

Source: Modified from the scheme presented in Ref. 14

*An average score is obtained for an individual case by adding the scores for each slide (0 to 4), then dividing by the number of slides examined

References

1. Zenker FA: Staubinhalations Krankheiten der Lungen, 1866.
2. Roggli VL, Shelburne JD: Pneumoconioses, mineral and vegetable. Ch. 27 In: *Pulmonary Pathology*, 2nd ed. (Dail DH, Hammar SP, eds.), New York: Springer-Verlag, 1994, pp. 867–900.
3. Lee DHK, Selikoff IJ: Historical background to the asbestos problem. *Environ Res* 18:300–314, 1979.
4. Castleman BI: *Asbestos: Medical and Legal Aspects*. New York: Harcourt Brace Jovanovich, 1984.
5. Craighead JE: Eyes for the epidemiologist: The pathologist's role in shaping our understanding of the asbestos-associated diseases. *Am J Clin Pathol* 89:281–287, 1988.
6. Cooke WE: Fibrosis of the lungs due to the inhalation of asbestos dust. *Br Med J* II:147, 1924.
7. Cooke WE: Pulmonary asbestosis. *Br Med J* II:1024–1025, 1927.
8. Roggli VL: Pathology of human asbestosis: A critical review. In: *Advances in Pathology* (Vol. 2) (Fenoglio-Preiser CM, ed.), Chicago: Year Book Med. Pub., 1989, pp. 31–60.
9. Churg A: Nonneoplastic diseases caused by asbestos. Ch. 9 In: *Pathology of Occupational Lung Disease*, 2nd ed. (Churg A, Green FHY, eds.), Baltimore: Williams & Wilkins, 1998, pp. 277–339.
10. Murphy RL, Becklake MR, Brooks SM, et al.: The diagnosis of non-malignant diseases related to asbestos. *Am Rev Respir Dis* 134:363–368, 1986.
11. McCullough SF, Aresini G, Browne K, et al.: Criteria for the diagnosis of asbestosis and considerations in the attribution of lung cancer and mesothelioma to asbestos exposure. *Int Arch Occup Environ Health* 49:357–361, 1982.
12. Kannerstein M, Churg J: *Pathology of Asbestos Associated Diseases*. Washington, DC: Armed Forces Institute of Pathology, 1979.
13. Hinson KFW, Otto H, Webster I, et al.: Criteria for the diagnosis and grading of asbestosis. In: *Biologic Effects of Asbestosis* (Bogovski P, ed.), Lyon, France: World Health Organization, 1973.
14. Craighead JE, Abraham JL, Churg A, et al.: The pathology of asbestos-associated diseases of the lungs and pleural cavities: Diagnostic criteria

and proposed grading schema. (Report of the Pneumoconiosis Committee of the College of American Pathologists and the National Institute for Occupational Safety and Health) *Arch Pathol Lab Med* 106:544–596, 1982.

15. Churg A: Analysis of asbestos fibers from lung tissue: Research and diagnostic uses. *Sem Respir Med* 7:281–288, 1986.

16. Warnock ML, Prescott BT, Kuwahara TJ: Correlation of asbestos bodies and fibers in lungs of subjects with and without asbestosis. *Scanning Electron Microsc* II:845–857, 1982.

17. Hasleton PS: *Spencer's Pathology of the Lung*, 5th ed. New York: McGraw-Hill, 1996.

18. Katzenstein A-LA, Askin FB: *Surgical Pathology of Non-Neoplastic Lung Disease* 3rd ed. Philadelphia: W.B. Saunders Co., 1997, pp. 112–137.

19. Dail DH, Hammar SP, eds.: *Pulmonary Pathology*, 2nd ed. New York: Springer-Verlag, 1994, pp. 901–983.

20. Seaton A: Asbestos-related diseases. Ch. 13 In: *Occupational Lung Diseases*, 2nd ed. (Morgan WKC, Seaton A, eds.), Philadelphia: Saunders, 1984, pp. 323–376.

21. Beljan JR, Cooper T, Dolan WD, et al.: A physician's guide to asbestos-related diseases: Council on scientific affairs. *JAMA* 252:2593–2597, 1984.

22. Segarra F, Monte MB, Ibanez LP, Nicolas JP: Asbestosis in a Barcelona fibrocement factory. *Environ Res* 23:292–300, 1980.

23. Goff AM, Gaensler EA: Asbestosis following brief exposure in cigarette filter manufacter. *Respiration* 29:83–93, 1972.

24. Selikoff IJ, Lee DHK: *Asbestos and Disease*. New York: Academic Press, 1978.

25. McMillan GHG, Pethybridge RJ, Sheers G: Effect of smoking on attack rates of pulmonary and pleural lesions related to exposure to asbestos dust. *Br J Ind Med* 37:268–272, 1980.

26. Kilburn KH, Lilis R, Anderson HA, Miller A, Warshaw RH: Interaction of asbestos, age and cigarette smoking in producing radiographic evidence of diffuse pulmonary fibrosis. *Am J Med* 80:377–381, 1986.

27. Finkelstein MM, Virgilis JJ: Radiographic abnormalities among asbestos-cement workers: An exposure-response study. *Am Rev Respir Dis* 129:17–22, 1984.

28. Ducatman AM, Withers BF, Yang WN: Smoking and roentgenographic opacities in US Navy asbestos workers. *Chest* 97:810–813, 1990.

29. Barnhart S, Thornquist M, Omenn GS, Goodman G, Feigl P, Rosenstock L: The degree of roentgenographic parenchymal opacities attributable to smoking among asbestos-exposed subjects. *Am Rev Respir Dis* 141:1102–1106, 1990.

30. Weiss W: Cigarette smoke, asbestos, and small irregular opacities. *Am Rev Respir Dis* 130:293–301, 1984.

31. Hobson J, Gilks B, Wright J, Churg A: Direct enhancement by cigarette smoke of asbestos fiber penetration and asbestos-induced epithelial proliferation in rat tracheal explants. *J Natl Cancer Inst* 80:518–521, 1988.

32. Tron V, Wright JL, Harrison N, et al.: Cigarette smoke makes airway and early parenchymal asbestosis worse in the guinea pig. *Am Rev Respir Dis* 136:271–275, 1987.

33. Churg A: The uptake of mineral particles by pulmonary epithelial cells. *Am J Respir Crit Care Med* 154:1124–1140, 1996.

34. McFadden D, Wright J, Wiggs B, Churg A: Smoking increases the penetration of asbestos fibers into airway walls. *Am J Pathol* 123:95–99, 1986.

35. Churg A, Stevens B: Enhanced retention of asbestos fibers in the airways of human smokers. *Am J Respir Crit Care Med* 151:1409–1413, 1995.

36. Schwartz DA, Galvin JR, Merchant RK: Influence of cigarette smoking on bronchoalveolar lavage cellularity in asbestos-induced lung disease. *Am Rev Respir Dis* 145:400–405, 1992.

37. Schwartz DA, Galvin JR, Yagla SJ: Restrictive lung function and asbestos-induced pleural fibrosis. *J Clin Invest* 91:2685–2692, 1993.

38. Hnizdo E, Sluis-Cremer GK: Effect of tobacco smoking on the presence of asbestosis at postmortem and on the reading of irregular opacities on roentgenograms in asbestos-exposed workers. *Am Rev Respir Dis* 138:1207–1212, 1988.

39. Selikoff IJ, Hammond EC, Seidman H: Latency of asbestos disease among insulation workers in the United States and Canada. *Cancer* 46:2736–2740, 1980.

40. Miller A, Lilis R, Godbold J, Chan E, Selikoff IJ: Relationship of pulmonary function to radiographic interstitial fibrosis in 2611 long term asbestos insulators. *Am Rev Respir Dis* 145:263–270, 1992.

41. Begin R, Cantin A, Berthiaume Y, Boileau R, Peloquin S, Masse S: Airway function in lifetime non-smoking older asbestos workers. *Am J Med* 75:631–638, 1983.

42. Wang XR, Christiani DC: Respiratory symptoms and functional status in workers exposed to silica, asbestos and coal mine dust. *J Occup Environ Med* 42:1076–1084, 2000.

43. Kilburn KH, Warshaw R, Thornton JC: Asbestosis, pulmonary symptoms and functional impairment in shipyard workers. *Chest* 88:254–259, 1985.

44. Sue DY, Oren A, Hansen JE, Wasserman K: Lung function and exercise performance in smoking and non-smoking asbestos-exposed workers. *Am Rev Respir Dis* 132:612–618, 1985.

45. Kobayashi H, Okamura A, Ohnishi Y, et al.: Generalized fibrosis associated with pulmonary asbestosis. *Acta Pathol Jpn* 33:1223–1231, 1983.

46. Slavin RE, Swedo D, Gonzales-Vitale JC, Osornio-Vargas A: Extrapulmonary silicosis: A clinical, morphologic and ultrastructural study. *Hum Pathol* 16:393–412, 1985.

47. Cowie RL: Silica-dust exposed mine workers with scleroderma (systemic sclerosis). *Chest* 92:260–262, 1987.

48. Kagan E, Solomon A, Cochrane JC, Beissner EI, Gluckman J, Rocks PH, Webster I: Immunological studies of patients with asbestosis I. Studies of cell mediated immunity. *Clin Exp Immunol* 28:261–267, 1977.

49. Kagan E, Solomon A, Cochrane JC, Kuba P, Rocks PH, Webster I: Immunological studies of patients with asbestosis. II. Studies of circulating lymphoid cell numbers and humoral immunity. *Clin Exp Immunol* 28:268–275, 1977.

50. Maguire FW, Mills RC, Parker FP: Immunoblastic lymphadenopathy and asbestosis. *Cancer* 47:179–197, 1981.

51. Cooke CT, Matz LR, Armstrong JA, Pinerua RF: Asbestos-related interstitial pneumonitis associated with glomerulonephritis and lymphomatoid granulomatosis. *Pathology* 18:352–356, 1986.

52. Colby TV, Carrington CB: Pulmonary lymphomas simulating lymphomatoid granulomatosis. *Am J Surg Pathol* 6:19–32, 1982.

53. Churg A: Pulmonary angiitis and granulomatosis revisited. *Hum Pathol* 14:868–883, 1983.

54. Huuskonen MS: Clinical features mortality and survival of patients with asbestosis. *Scand J Work Environ Health* 4:265–274, 1978.

55. Courts II, Turner-Warwick M: Factors predicting outcome in intrapulmonary fibrosis associated with asbestos exposure (asbestosis). In: *Occu-*

pational Lung Disease (Gee JBL, Morgan WKC, eds.), New York: Raven Press, 1984, pp. 208–209.

56. Oksa P, Klockars M, Karjalainen A, Huuskonen MS, Vattulainen K, Pukkala E, Nordman H: Progression of asbestosis predicts lung cancer. *Chest* 113:1517–1521, 1998.

57. Berry G: Mortality of workers certified by pneumoconiosis reference panels as having asbestosis. *Br J Ind Med* 38:130–137, 1981.

58. Murai Y, Kitagawa M: Autopsy cases of asbestosis in Japan: A statistical analysis on registered cases. *Arch Environ Health* 55:447–452, 2000.

59. Kamp DW, Weitzman SA: The molecular basis of asbestos-induced lung injury. *Thorax* 54:638–650, 1999.

60. Mossman BT, Churg A: Mechanisms in the pathogenesis of asbestosis and silicosis. *Am J Respir Crit Care Med* 157:1666–1680, 1998.

61. Weiss W: Asbestosis: A marker for increased risk of lung cancer among workers exposed to asbestos. *Chest* 115:536–549, 1999.

62. Rockoff SD, Schwartz A: Roentgenographic underestimation of early asbestosis by International Labor Organization Classification: Analysis of data and probabilities. *Chest* 93:1088–1091, 1988.

63. Epler GR, McLoud TC, Gaensler EA, Mikus JB, Carrington CB: Normal chest roentgenograms in chronic diffuse infiltrative lung disease. *N Engl J Med* 298:934–939, 1978.

64. Kipen HM, Lilis R, Suzuki Y, Valciukas JA, Selikoff IJ: Pulmonary fibrosis in asbestos insulation workers with lung cancer: A radiological and histopathological evaluation. *Br J Ind Med* 44:96–100, 1987.

65. Meyer JD, Islam SS, Ducatman AM, McCunney RJ: Prevalence of small lung opacities in populations unexposed to dusts: A literature analysis. *Chest* 111:404–410, 1997.

66. Friedman AC, Fiel SB, Fisher MS, Radecki PD, Lev-Toaf A-S, Caroline DF: Asbestos-related pleural disease and asbestosis: A comparison of CT and chest radiography. *Am J Roentgenol* 150:269–275, 1988.

67. Bergin CJ, Mueller NL: CT in the diagnosis of interstitial lung disease. *Am J Roentgenol* 145:505–510, 1985.

68. Aberle DR, Gamsu G, Ray CS: High resolution CT of benign asbestos-related diseases: Clinical and radiographic correlation. *Am J Roentgenol* 151:883–891, 1988.

69. Pratt PC: Role of conventional chest radiography in diagnosis and exclusion of emphysema. *Am J Med* 82:998–1006, 1987.

70. Foster WL, Pratt PC, Roggli VL, Godwin JD, Halvorsen RA, Putman CE: Centrilobular emphysema: CT-Pathologic correlation. *Radiology* 159:27–32, 1986.

71. Bergin C, Muller N, Nichols DM, Lillington G, Hogg JC, Mullen B, Grymalsoki MR, Osborne S, Pare PD: The diagnosis of emphysema: A computed tomographic pathologic correlation. *Am Rev Respir Dis* 133:541–546, 1986.

72. Gamsu G, Salmon CJ, Warnock ML, Blanc PD: CT quantification of interstitial fibrosis in patients with asbestosis: a comparison of two methods. *Am J Roentgenol* 164:63–68, 1995.

73. Lynch DA, Gamsu G, Aberle DR: Conventional and high resolution computed tomography in the diagnosis of asbestos-related diseases. *Radiographics* 9:523–551, 1989.

74. Staples CA, Gamsu G, Ray CS, Webb NR: High resolution computed tomography and lung function in asbestos-exposed workers with normal chest radiographs. *Am Rev Respir Dis* 139:1502–1508, 1989.

75. De Vuyst P, Dumortier P, Moulin E, Yourassowsky N, Yernault JC: Diagnostic value of asbestos bodies in bronchoalveolar lavage fluid. *Am Rev Respir Dis* 134:363–368, 1987.
76. Gaensler EA, Jederlinic PJ, Churg A: Idiopathic pulmonary fibrosis in asbestos-exposed workers. *Am Rev Respir Dis* 144:689–696, 1991.
77. Roggli VL: Scanning electron microscopic analysis of mineral fiber content of lung tissue in the evaluation of diffuse pulmonary fibrosis. *Scanning Microsc* 5:71–83, 1991.
78. Parkes WR: An approach to the differential diagnosis of asbestosis and non-occupational diffuse interstitial pulmonary fibrosis. In: *Occupational Lung Disorders*, 3rd ed. (Parkes WR III, ed.), London: Butterworths, 1994, pp. 505–535.
79. Pratt PC: Emphysema and chronic airways disease. Ch. 26 In: *Pulmonary Pathology*, 2nd ed (Dail DH, Hammar SP, eds.), New York: Springer-Verlag, 1994, pp. 847–866.
80. Hillerdal G: Asbestos exposure and upper lobe involvement. *Am J Roentgenol* 139: 1163–1166, 1982.
81. Hillerdal G: Pleural plaques: Occurrence, exposure to asbestos, and clinical importance. *Acta Univ Upsaliensis* 363:1–227, 1980.
82. Wain SL, Roggli VL, Foster WL: Parietal pleural plaques, asbestos bodies and neoplasia: A clinical, pathologic and roentgenographic correlation of 25 consecutive cases. *Chest* 86:707–713, 1984.
83. Franzblau A, Lilis R: The diagnosis of non-malignant diseases related to asbestos. *Am Rev Respir Dis* 136:790–791, 1987.
84. Hunninghake GW, Gadek JE, Kawanami O, Ferrans VJ, Crystal RG: Inflammatory and immune processes in the human lung in health and disease: Evaluation by bronchoalveolar lavage fluid. *Am J Pathol* 97: 149–205, 1979.
85. Teschler H, Friedrichs KH, Hoheisel GB, et al.: Asbestos fibers in bronchoalveolar lavage and lung tissue of former asbestos workers. *Am J Respir Crit Care Med* 149:641–645, 1994.
86. Schwartz DA, Galvin JR, Burmeister LF, et al.: The clinical utility and reliability of asbestos bodies in bronchoalveolar fluid. *Am Rev Respir Dis* 144:684–688, 1991.
87. Vorwald AJ, Durkan TM, Pratt PC: Experimental studies of asbestosis. *Arch Ind Hyg Occup Med* 3:1–43, 1951.
88. Hammar SP, Dodson RF: Asbestos. Ch. 28 In: *Pulmonary Pathology*, 2nd ed. (Hammar SP, Dail DH, eds.), New York: Springer-Verlag, 1994, pp. 901–984.
89. Vincent JH, Jones AD, Johnston AM, McMillan C, Bolton RE, Cowie H: Accumulation of inhaled mineral dust in the lung and associated lymph nodes: Implications for exposure and dose in occupational lung disease. *Ann Occup Hyg* 31:375–393, 1987.
90. Roggli VL, Benning TL: Asbestos bodies in pulmonary hilar lymph nodes. *Mod Pathol* 3:513–517, 1990.
91. Kuhn C, Kuo T-T: Cytoplasmic hyaline in asbestosis: A reaction of injured alveolar epithelium. *Arch Pathol* 95:190–194, 1973.
92. Warnock ML, Press M, Churg A: Further observations on cytoplasmic hyaline in the lung. *Hum Pathol* 11:59–66, 1980.
93. Joines RA, Roggli VL: Dendriform pulmonary ossification: report of two cases with unique findings. *Am J Clin Pathol* 91:398–402, 1989.
94. Ndimbie OK, Williams CR, Lee MW: Dendriform pulmonary ossification. *Arch Pathol Lab Med* 111:1062–1064, 1987.

95. Koss MN, Johnson FB, Hochholzer L: Pulmonary blue bodies. *Hum Pathol* 12:258–266, 1981.
96. Brody AR, Hill LH: Interstitial accumulation of inhaled chrysotile asbestos and consequent formation of microcalcifications. *Am J Pathol* 109:107–114, 1982.
97. Kagan E: Current perspectives in asbestosis. *Ann Allergy* 54:464–474, 1985.
98. Hillerdal G, Hecksher T: Asbestos exposure and aspergillus infection. *Eur J Respir Dis* 63:420–424, 1982.
99. Roggli VL, Johnston WW, Kaminsky DB: Asbestos bodies in fine needle aspirates of the lung. *Acta Cytol* 28:493–498, 1984.
100. Shelburne JD, Wisseman CL, Broda KR, Roggli VL, Ingram P: Lung: Nonneoplastic conditions. In: *Diagnostic Electron Microscopy* (Vol. 4) (Trump BF, Jones RJ, eds.), New York: Wiley, 1983, pp 475–538.
101. Corrin B, Dewar A, Rodriguez–Roisin R, Turner-Warwick M: Fine structural changes in cryptogenic fibrosing alveolitis and asbestosis. *J Pathol* 147:107–119, 1985.
102. Craighead JE, Kleinerman J, Abraham JL, et al.: Diseases associated with exposure to silica and nonfibrous silicate minerals. *Arch Pathol Lab Med* 112:673–720, 1988.
103. Mark GJ, Monroe CB, Kazemi H: Mixed pneumoconiosis: silicosis, asbestosis, talcosis and berylliosis. *Chest* 75:726–728, 1979.
104. Wright JL, Churg A: Morphology of small airways lesions in patients with asbestos exposure. *Hum Pathol* 15:68–74, 1984.
105. Churg A, Wright JL: Small airway lesions in patients exposed to non-asbestos mineral dusts. *Hum Pathol* 14:688–693, 1983.
106. Ackerman LV, Elliott GV, Alanis M: Localized organizing pneumonia: Its resemblance to carcinoma: A review of its clinical, roentgenographic and pathologic features. *Am J Roentgenol Radium Ther Nucl Med* 71:988–996, 1954.
107. Schmidt RA: Iatrogenic Injury: Radiation and Drug Effects. Ch. 23 In: *Pulmonary Pathology*, 2nd ed. (Hammar SP, Dail DH, eds.), New York: Springer-Verlag, 1994, pp. 779–806.
108. Katzenstein A-LA, Myers JL: Idiopathic pulmonary fibrosis: Clinical relevance of pathologic classification. *Am J Respir Crit Care Med* 157: 1301–1315, 1998.
109. Kane PB, Goldman SL, Pillai BH, Bergofsky EH: Diagnosis of asbestosis by transbronchial biopsy: A method to facilitate demonstration of ferruginous bodies. *Am Rev Respir Dis* 115:689–694, 1977.
110. Dodson RF, Hurst GA, Williams MG, Corn C, Greenberg SD: Comparison of light and electron microscopy for defining occupational asbestos exposure in transbronchial lung biopsies. *Chest* 94:366–370, 1988.
111. Churg A: An inflation procedure for open lung biopsies. *Am J Surg Pathol* 7:69–71, 1983.
112. Roggli VL, Pratt PC: Numbers of asbestos bodies on iron-stained tissue sections in relation to asbestos body counts in lung tissue digests. *Hum Pathol* 14:355–361, 1983.
113. Vollmer RT, Roggli VL: Asbestos body concentrations in human lung: predictions from asbestos body counts in tissue sections with a mathematical model. *Hum Pathol* 16:713–718, 1985.
114. Wright JL, Cagle P, Churg A, et al.: State of the art: diseases of the small airways. *Am Rev Respir Dis* 246:240–262, 1992.
115. Becklake MR: Asbestosis criteria. *Arch Pathol Lab Med* 108:93, 1984.
116. Dodson RF, Williams MG, O'Sullivan MF, Corn CJ, Greenberg SD, Hurst GA: A comparison of the ferruginous body and uncoated fiber content in the lungs of former asbestos workers. *Am Rev Respir Dis* 132:143–147, 1985.

117. Warnock ML, Wolery G: Asbestos bodies or fibers and the diagnosis of asbestosis. *Environ Res* 44:29–44, 1987.
118. Holden J, Churg A: Asbestos bodies and the diagnosis of asbestosis in chrysotile workers. *Environ Res* 39:232–236, 1986.
119. Wright GW, Kuschner M: The influence of varying lengths of glass and asbestos fibers on tissue response in guinea pigs. In: *Inhaled Particles IV* (Walton WH, ed.), Oxford: Pergamon Press, 1977, pp. 455–474.
120. Davis JMG, Beckett ST, Bolton RE, Collins P, Middleton AP: Mass and number of fibres in the pathogenesis of asbestos-related lung disease in rats. *Br J Cancer* 37:673–688, 1978.
121. Crapo JD, Barry BE, Brody AR, O'Neil JJ: Morphological, morphometric, and X-ray microanalytical studies on lung tissue of rats exposed to chrysotile asbestos in inhalation chambers. In: *Biological Effects of Mineral Fibers* (Vol. 1) (Wagner JC, ed.), IARC Scientific Publications No. 30: Lyon, 1980, pp. 273–280.
122. Lee KP, Barras CE, Griffith FD, Waritz RS, Lapin CA: Comparative pulmonary responses to inhaled inorganic fibers with asbestos and fiberglass. *Environ Res* 24:167–191, 1981.
123. Gross P: Is short-fibered asbestos a biological hazard? *Arch Environ Health* 29:115–117, 1974.
124. Report and recommendations of the working group on asbestosis and cancer. *Br J Ind Med* 22:165–171, 1965.
125. Warnock ML, Kuwahara TJ, Wolery G: The relationship of asbestos burden to asbestosis and lung cancer. *Pathol Annu* 18:109–145, 1983.
126. Wagner JC, Moncrief CB, Coles R, et al.: Correlation between fibre content of the lungs and disease in naval dockyard workers. *Br J Ind Med* 43:391–395, 1986.
127. Davis JMG: The pathology of asbestos-related disease. *Thorax* 39:801–808, 1984.
128. International Labor Organization: International Classification of Radiographs of the Pneumoconioses. *Occupational Safety and Health Series*, No. 22 (Rev) Geneva: ILO, 1980.
129. Smith CM, Batcher S, Catazano A, Abraham JL, Phalen R: Sequence of bronchoalveolar lavage and histopathologic findings in rat lungs early in inhalation asbestos exposure. *J Toxicol Environ Health* 20:147–161, 1987.

5

Mesothelioma

Thomas A. Sporn and Victor L. Roggli

Introduction

Mesothelioma, literally "tumor of the mesothelium," is a term often used synonymously with *malignant* (diffuse) *mesothelioma*, the malignant neoplasm arising from the serosal linings of the pleural, pericardial, or peritoneal cavities. These major body cavities are lined by a single layer of flattened to cuboidal cells of mesodermal origin that constitute the mesothelium proper.[1] This serosal membranous lining includes not only the mesothelium, but also the underlying basement membrane, a matrix of elastic fibroconnective tissue containing lymphatic and vascular channels, and scattered mesenchymal cells as well. Mesothelial cells possess a complex cytoskeletal network of intermediate filaments, produce hyaluronic acid, and have distinctive ultrastructural features including numerous pinocytotic vesicles and long surface microvilli that project into the serous cavities (Figure 5-1).[2,3] It remains uncertain whether mesothelioma results from the malignant transformation of the differentiated mesothelial cell or from more primitive progenitor cells such as the submesothelial mesenchymal cell, or from both.[4]

Malignant (diffuse) mesotheliomas are rare neoplasms, with estimated incidence in North America of 15 to 20 cases per million persons per year for men, with a much lower incidence in women.[5–10] Its rarity combined with its strong association with asbestos exposure make it a signal malignancy, that is, an epidemiologic marker for exposure to asbestos.[7] The mechanism whereby asbestos induces mesothelioma is not completely understood. This mechanism is reviewed in detail in Chapter 10, and the results of quantitative tissue analysis for asbestos content in cases with malignant mesotheliomas compared with those of other asbestos-related disorders and with normal controls in Chapter 11. The present chapter reviews the pathologic features of malignant mesothelioma, the means to distinguish mesothelioma from other conditions with which it may be confused, and the agents implicated in its etiology. A certain amount of confusion exists with regard to benign tumors of the serosal membranes, which have also been variously termed fibrous mesothelioma, localized fibrous tumor, and solitary

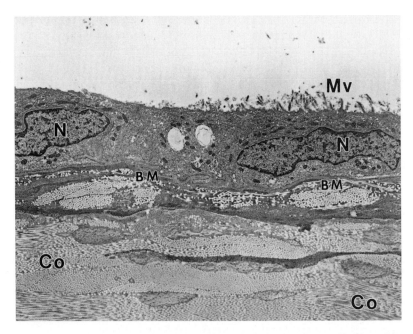

Figure 5-1. Transmission electron micrograph of normal mesothelium. Note flattened mesothelial cells, one of which has long surface microvilli (Mv). BM = basement membrane, N = nucleus, Co = collagen. Magnified ×3430. (Reprinted from Ref. 2, with permission.)

fibrous tumor. These rare tumors have not been convincingly shown to be asbestos related and are reviewed elsewhere.[2,11]

Historical Background

Mesotheliomas are uncommon tumors, accounting for fewer than 1% of cancer deaths worldwide,[12] with few descriptions in the literature until this century. In 1767, Lieutand described two pleural tumors in a series of 3000 autopsies that may have been mesotheliomas.[13] Wagner's detailed descriptions published in 1870[14] leave little doubt that he was describing what we now recognize as malignant pleural mesothelioma.[15,16] In 1924, Robertson reviewed earlier reports in the literature and concluded that only sarcomatous tumors could be regarded as primary pleural malignancies, and that tumors with epithelial morphology represented metastases from other, and possibly occult sites.[17] Klemperer and Rabin described in 1931 a series of five pleural tumors, four of which were localized and one diffuse.[18] These investigators separated the localized tumors of the pleura from the diffuse pleural malignancies and used the term *mesothelioma* to refer to the entire histologic spectrum of epithelial and spindle-cell primary malignancies that diffusely involve the pleura.[15,16] By the 1950s, growing numbers of diffuse primary peritoneal tumors were recognized, and malignant mesothelioma became generally accepted as a distinct clinicopathologic entity.[19]

The British pathologist Gloyne is credited with the first description in 1933 of pleural malignancy in an individual occupationally exposed to asbestos.[20] This report referred to a case of "squamous carcinoma of the pleura," which the author did not believe was related to the patient's asbestosis.[21] Reports from Germany in 1943 by Wedler[22] and from the United States in 1947 by Mallory[23] describing further cases of pleural malignancy associated with asbestos exposure followed subsequently. Additional reports appeared in the 1940s and 1950s,[20,24] and by 1960 Keal had described the association between peritoneal mesotheliomas and asbestos exposure.[25] Any remaining doubt concerning the association between asbestos exposure was dispelled by Wagner in 1960.[26] This classic study described 33 cases of diffuse pleural mesothelioma occurring in the Northwestern Cape Province of South Africa, in which 32 cases had a documented exposure to asbestos. In some instances, the patient's only exposure was living in proximity to an asbestos mine. Since 1960, numerous studies have appeared in the literature confirming the association between asbestos exposure and malignant mesothelioma of the pleura, peritoneum, and pericardium.[2]

Etiologic Considerations and Epidemiology

Asbestos

The association between mesothelioma and asbestos exposure is undisputed. Following Wagner's study of mesothelioma subsequent to environmental and occupational exposure to crocidolite,[26] epidemiologic and case-control studies from many industrialized nations have documented rising rates of malignant mesothelioma following the heavy commercial use of asbestos.[27–44] A large proportion of cases in these studies have derived from shipyard workers[27,33] and insulators,[45,46] where large numbers of workers had heavy exposures. Other occupational exposures to asbestos including those sustained by miners and millers,[26,34,47] railroad machinists and steam locomotive repair workers,[48,49] and workers in asbestos factories have resulted in appreciable numbers of cases.[50]

The authors have undertaken a study of 1445 cases of mesothelioma with known exposure histories, and 268 with tissue asbestos fiber burden analyses.[51] We found that these cases were classifiable into 23 predominant occupational or exposure categories and that 94% of cases had exposures in one or more of twelve different industries, six occupational categories, or one nonoccupational exposure. The industry with the largest number of cases was shipbuilding, followed by service in the U.S. Navy, the construction industry, and the insulation industry. The occupation with the largest number of cases was pipefitter (including welders), followed by boiler workers, maintenance workers, machinists, and electricians. As many individuals worked at more than one type of job, an exposure in some additional occupational setting was observed in 26% of our cases. The nonoccupational group with the largest number of cases in our study was household contacts of asbestos workers. Household contacts are believed to sustain exposure by contact with contaminated clothing or personal effects of the asbestos worker.[5,52,53] Environmental or neighborhood exposures have also been described, sustained by those living in the vicinity of asbestos factories or mines.[26] Some unusual exposures to asbestos associated with the development of mesothelioma have been documented, including the manufacture of asbestos-containing cigarette filters[54] or the preparation of silver jewelry and ceremonial clothing by members of a Native American pueblo.[55] Mesothelioma has been reported among individuals exposed as children, whose diapers were made from cotton sacks previously used to transport asbestos insulation.[56]

Mesothelioma is overwhelmingly a disease affecting men, reflecting the predominance of men in those occupations and industries most commonly associated with asbestos exposure. While the rates of mesothelioma have increased over the past decades, the rates in women have remained relatively constant.[6-10] A geographical influence is also noted in North America, with the coastal areas housing the shipbuilding industries of the World War II era having the highest rates.[57]

A prolonged *latent interval*, that period of time between initial exposure and the manifestation of disease, is typical of most asbestos-associated illnesses, and mesothelioma is not an exception. The latent interval for mesothelioma is measured in decades, peaks at 30 to 40 years post-exposure and may extend to 70 years after exposure.[45,58,59] The latent interval is virtually never less than 15 years,[9] and when claimed in any particular case, merits the search for evidence of more remote exposure.[60] Mesothelioma tends to be a disease of those in the seventh or eighth decades of life in keeping with the long latent interval. An inverse relationship between dose or level of exposure and latent interval is suggested, as we have observed the development of mesothelioma at a significantly younger age in insulators as compared to other asbestos workers.[51]

The risk for the development of mesothelioma appears to increase dramatically with time from initial exposure. Peto et al. have examined this relationship mathematically and found that the available data are best explained by a model in which the mesothelioma risk increases with the third or fourth power of time from first exposure. These investigators also concluded that there is a linear dose-response relationship between the amount of asbestos to which an individual is exposed and the risk of developing mesothelioma.[61] A threshold level of exposure below which mesothelioma will not occur has not yet been identified.[62] Peritoneal mesotheliomas, historically comprising some 30% of all cases, have fallen in proportion to approximately 10% of cases as the incidence of pleural mesotheliomas has risen. Peritoneal mesotheliomas are associated on average with heavier and/or more prolonged exposure to asbestos,[2,45,63] as evidenced by their frequency in the cohort of insulators[45,51,64,65] who tend to have the highest tissue fiber burdens. However, a similar latency period for both pleural and peritoneal forms is observed.[61] The association between peritoneal mesothelioma and higher degrees of exposure is supported by the observation of the clinical diagnosis of asbestosis in 50% of male patients with peritoneal mesotheliomas, but in only 20% of patients with pleural mesothelioma.

There are marked differences in the potential for various types of asbestos fibers to produce mesothelioma. While amosite is the most common fiber type associated with mesothelioma among U.S. workers,[51,66] crocidolite appears to pose the greatest risk among the commercially available species, followed by amosite.[67–72] Whereas the epidemiological association between exposure to commercial amphibole asbestos is indisputable, the mesotheliogenic potential of chrysotile has been much debated. The controversy surrounding chrysotile is multifaceted, influenced by the decreased biopersistence of the mineral in lung tissue and the frequent presence of its natural contaminant, the noncommercial amphibole form of asbestos tremolite.[73–75]

It is sometimes difficult to gauge the degree and type of asbestos exposure for any given worker, and indeed mesotheliomas have developed in workers in some plants believed to utilize only chrysotile asbestos, who upon analysis have been shown to contain amphibole fibers in their lungs.[76–78] Furthermore, individuals with mesothelioma who are exposed to chrysotile through the milling and mining of asbestos have more tremolite than chrysotile in their lung tissue, even though the contaminant accounts for only a fraction of a percent of the chrysotile ore.[74,79] This observation has led some investigators to suggest that it is the contaminating tremolite that is responsible for the increased risk of mesothelioma in miners and millers of chrysotile. Several studies have shown that environmental exposure to tremolite asbestos can result in an increased risk for developing mesothelioma, particularly in instances where the tremolite fibers have a high aspect ratio (i.e., ratio of length to diameter of fiber). In this regard, it is of interest to note that another noncommercial form of asbestos, anthophyllite, featuring broad fibers with low aspect ratio, has only rarely been implicated in the causation of human mesothelioma.[53,80] Finally, it is clear that sufficient exposure to chrysotile may result in the development of mesothelioma, but in contrast to the commercial amphiboles, low level exposures are not likely to increase such risk.

Mesothelioma is thought to originate in the parietal pleura. Asbestos fibers may reach the pleural surface via direct penetration following inhalational deposition in the respiratory bronchioles, or via the lymphatics. Asbestos is a powerful mesothelial carcinogen, capable of inducing DNA damage alone, or in concert with reactive oxygen species produced by inflammatory cells. Nonetheless, only a small fraction (10% or less) of asbestos workers will develop mesothelioma.[45,52,81] In our own studies, approximately 11% of mesotheliomas have a lung asbestos content indistinguishable from background, and perhaps 10 to 20% of cases are not the result of asbestos exposure. The size of the exposed population at risk for mesothelioma and the relative rarity of the disorder suggest variable individual susceptibilities, possibly genetically mediated. The observation that a substantial proportion of patients with malignant mesothelioma have no identifiable exposure to asbestos has led investigators to look for other potential etiologic or predisposing factors. These are reviewed in the following sections.

Zeolites

The discovery of an epidemic of malignant pleural mesothelioma in two villages in the Cappadocian region of Turkey[82] has prompted the current interest in the pathologic effects of zeolites.[2] The small villages of Karain and Tuzkoy are situated in a region whose caves and volcanic tuffs are rich in fibrous erionite, a hydrated aluminum silicate belonging to the family of zeolite minerals, and provide stones for dwellings there. In this area of Turkey where asbestos is ordinarily found in the volcanic terrain and construction materials containing tremolite asbestos are widely used, malignant mesothelioma attributable to environmental exposure to tremolite asbestos has been well documented.[83,84] However, the high incidence of mesothelioma in these two villages could not be explained by environmental asbestos alone. The excess incidence of mesothelioma in these villages is believed to be attributable to erionite,[85] whose fibers have been recovered from the lungs from some of the cases of mesothelioma in this area,[86] although some asbestos fibers have been identified as well.[87] Erionite has physical characteristics and dimensions closely resembling amphiboles, and in experimental animal studies, a high rate of mesothelioma has been induced following intrapleural or intraperitoneal injection.[88,89] Other studies have shown lower rates of mesothelioma induction following administration of erionite in a rodent model.[90] These variances are possibly attributable to different geographic sources of erionite used in the experimental studies. It is of interest that in the villages of Karain and Tuzkoy, a significant proportion of the villagers do not develop mesothelioma, and no other association with malignancy in this population has been demonstrated. A genetic predisposition toward the development of mesothelioma in families of these villages has been posited.[91] No cases of human mesothelioma due to erionite exposure have been reported to date in North America.

Radiation

There have been a number of case reports of the development of mesothelioma following thoracic or abdominal radiotherapy.[92,93] Radiation in these cases has been both internal and external beam, sometimes following the administration of intravascular thorium dioxide (Thorotrast).[94] The latent interval following radiotherapy to the clinical development of mesothelioma is generally prolonged, ranging from 7 to 50 years following exposure.[92] Several cases have been reported of young adults developing mesothelioma following intensive chemoradiotherapy for Wilms' tumor,[95–97] with radiation ports including the lower thorax. Lung tissue analysis yielded values within the expected range for a reference population in the single case in which it was performed.[97] Neugut et al. performed a retrospective review of 251,750 women registered with breast carcinoma, 24.8% of whom had received radiation therapy, and 13,743 patients with Hodgkins' disease, of which 50.6% had received radiation therapy. Six cases of mesothelioma were discovered, all in the cohort of breast carcinoma patients. Four of the six had not received radiotherapy, thereby finding no association in a large controlled study with thoracic radiation and the development of mesothelioma.[98] Experimental animal studies support a role for radiation in the causation of mesothelioma.[88,89,99] While it remains likely that intensive radiotherapy can cause mesothelioma in humans, the risk appears minimal. There is no evidence that whole body external radiation causes or contributes to the development of mesothelioma. Reports of mesothelioma developing following chemotherapy do not allow for the frequently unrecognized exposure to asbestos.[100]

SV 40

Following the report by Carbone et al.,[101] there has been much interest and ongoing research into the role of simian virus 40 (SV40), a DNA tumor virus, as carcinogen or cocarcinogen with asbestos in the induction of mesothelioma.[81,102,103] SV40 is capable of causing mesothelioma in animal models following intrapleural or intrapericardial injection[104] and may result in the transformation of human cell lines in tissue culture. Human exposure to SV40 is believed to have occurred following administration of contaminated live and attenuated polio virus vaccines, prepared from infected monkey kidney tissue culture cell lines.[105,106] It is estimated that between 1954 and 1963, 96 million adults and children in the United States were potentially inoculated with contaminated vaccine, and some 32 million people may have been exposed to infectious SV 40.[106–108] Hundreds of millions of people worldwide were likely exposed to SV40 in this fashion.

The SV40 viral genome encodes several oncogenic proteins, most notably large T-antigen (Tag). Tag is a potent carcinogen and mutagen and also serves to inhibit cellular tumor suppressor activity through inactivating p53 and p-retinoblastoma family proteins.[109–111] It has been demonstrated that human mesothelial cells are particularly susceptible to SV40 infection and malignant transformation, much more so than other cell types, with synergy toward malignant transformation provided by asbestos.[112] Using polymerase chain reaction (PCR) methodology, studies from multiple institutions in the USA have demonstrated the presence of SV40 Tag in some 50% of mesotheliomas.[81,113–115] The presence of SV40 sequences has been associated with a poor prognosis in nonepithelial mesothelioma. Studies have also shown selective expression of SV40 by mesothelioma cells but not in adjacent stromal cells or lung carcinomas.[116,117] Studies from Finland and Belgium have not shown the association between mesothelioma and SV40, possibly because of variances in exposure to contaminated vaccines.[118–120]

The theory of SV40 as carcinogen and cocarcinogen is not without its detractors and skeptics, which stem from fundamental disputes about the infectivity of SV40 in humans and whether it is even possible to distinguish SV40 infection from infection by other viruses in humans. Furthermore, there have been inconsistencies in the ability of different laboratories to detect SV40 sequences in the same specimens.[121] Finally, epidemiological studies have failed to document an increased risk for malignancy in those likely exposed to polio vaccine contaminated with SV40.[122] The role of SV40 as a contributor to the development of mesothelioma in humans remains to be determined.

Other Factors

Additional factors implicated as contributing causes to the development of malignant mesothelioma are uncommon, but have included chronic empyema, peritonitis and scarring of the serosa, or following the creation of therapeutic pneumothorax with intrapleural administration of leucite spheres for the treatment of pulmonary tuberculosis.[123–125] Malignant mesothelioma in such cases arises after several decades. The identification of malignant mesothelioma in oil refinery and petrochemical plant workers suggested a role for chemical cocarcinogens in the production of mesothelioma.[125] However, in the twenty years since this suggestion was made, no supporting evidence has been forthcoming. Anecdotal reports have described malignant mesotheliomas developing following exposure to beryllium and nickel.[126] One epidemiological study showed a slightly increased risk of malignant mesothelioma in fiberglass workers,[28] although this has not been confirmed. Mesothelioma has been reported in sugarcane workers following inhalation of noncrystalline silica fibers with fiber dimensions similar to those of amphibole asbestos.[127] In addition to the familial clustering of malignant mesothelioma in the Cappadocian region of Turkey discussed above, several reports of familial aggregations of mesothelioma indicate that host genetic factors may contribute to the development of malignant mesothelioma, although the specific genetic mechanism is not yet elucidated.[128–131] Of note is that in such familial clusterings, an asbestos exposure is present in the majority of cases.[132,133] While important in the causation of bronchogenic carcinoma in patients with asbestosis (see Chapter 7), cigarette smoking has not been implicated as a risk factor for the development of malignant mesothelioma.[52] Finally, reports of mesothelioma developing in childhood or even in utero for which none of these risk factors could be identified indicate that there are probably as yet unknown factors involved in the pathogenesis of this rare malignancy.[134,135]

Pathologic Features

Gross Morphology

Malignant mesotheliomas are characteristically comprised of confluent, thick growth over the distribution of the serosal surface, usually with an associated effusion, leading to the obliteration of the serosal cavity and extensive involvement of regional viscera, compressing and invading from without. The most common site of origin of malignant mesothelioma is the pleura. In a large series, the ratio of pleural to peritoneal locations is 10:1.[136] The earliest lesions typically begin as small macules or nodules on the parietal pleura,[137,138] whose subsequent growth leads to coalescence of these nodules and finally fusion of the parietal and visceral pleura.[139,140] Growth then follows the distribution

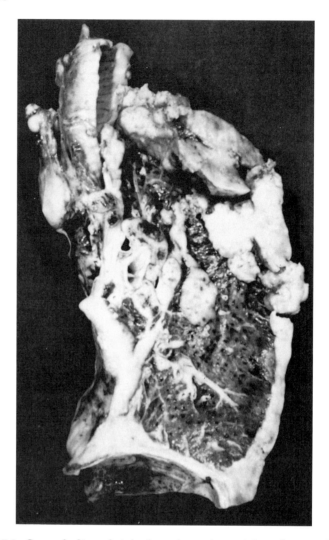

Figure 5-2. Coronal slice of right lung in patient with malignant (diffuse) pleural mesothelioma shows encasement of lung by rind of tumor. Note superficial invasion of underlying parenchyma. (Reprinted from Ref. 2, with permission.)

of the pleural surface, with extension into fissures and interlobular septa (Figure 5-2). Pleural mesotheliomas will invade mediastinal structures, chest wall, diaphragm, and in advanced cases, the contralateral pleural cavity and peritoneum. These gross features correlate well with the typical clinical symptoms of chest pain and dyspnea.

A large and often hemorrhagic pleural effusion is frequently present at the time of presentation[141] and may be responsible for some of the dyspnea observed. However, in late stage disease, obliteration of the pleural space through tumoral fusion of the pleurae may not allow for significant fluid accumulation.[2] The presence of bulky disease may be accompanied by constitutional symptoms and weight loss. Parenchymal pulmonary masses are uncommon, except in late stage disease, and dominant pulmonary masses should raise suspicions regarding the diagnosis of mesothelioma. In exceptional cases, malignant pleural mesotheliomas may present as large, localized pleural-based masses.[142–144]

The most common site of metastasis is via lymphatics to lymph nodes in the hilar areas of the lung or mediastinum, and this is commonly observed.[125,136] In rare instances extensive lymphangitic pulmonary spread may be present at the time of diagnosis.[145] The propensity for mesothelioma to grow in the subcutaneous tracks following needle biopsy or placement of ports for thoracoscopy[12] often necessitates the excision of these sites at the time of pleuropneumonectomy. Clinically evident metastatic disease outside the thorax at time of presentation is uncommon, but distant hematogenous metastases are frequently detected at autopsy, present in at least half of cases.[125,146–148]

Observations regarding gross distribution and morphologic features of the tumor are very important elements in the diagnosis of malignant mesothelioma. When this information is not available directly to the pathologist or prosector of autopsy or surgical material, it may be obtained through the observations of the surgeon at the time of thoracoscopy, thoracotomy, or pleuropneumonectomy, or from radiographic studies. Massive pleural effusions may obscure the details of tumor distribution on plain films, but additional radiographic studies may provide detailed information regarding salient gross pathologic features.[149–151] Computerized tomography (CT) can suggest the diagnosis by demonstrating effusions and nodular pleural thickening and may delineate invasion of local structures (Figure 5-3). Magnetic resonance imaging (MRI) may provide additional detailed information regarding local invasion that is of potential utility in those patients considered for pleuropneumonectomy.[148,149,151] All of the above modalities may also demonstrate evidence of other concomitant intrathoracic asbestos-related pathology such as pleural plaques.

Although the gross distribution of mesothelioma with circumferential encasement of the lung in a rind of tumor is characteristic, it is not pathognomonic of the entity. Other malignant tumors, both primary within the lung or metastatic from extrathoracic sites, may directly invade and diffusely involve the pleura. Small peripheral pulmonary adenocarcinomas may invade the pleura (Figure 5-4),[152] and so closely mimic the gross appearance of mesothelioma that some investigators have termed such tumors "pseudomesotheliomatous adenocarcinomas."[153,154] Angiosarcomas and epithelioid hemangioendotheliomas, closely related mesenchymal malignancies of vascular origin, may mimic malignant pleural mesothelioma both in terms of gross distribution and in clinical behavior.[155–158] Therefore, the differential diagnosis of mesothelioma is extensive, including chiefly peripheral primary carcinomas of the lung, metastatic carcinomas of extrathoracic sites that may be clinically occult (e.g., kidney), and primary pleural angiosarcomas. In view of this lengthy list, it is critically important to have an understanding of pertinent clinical and historical data, as well as radiographic findings, so as not to overlook primary malignancy elsewhere with secondary pleural involvement.

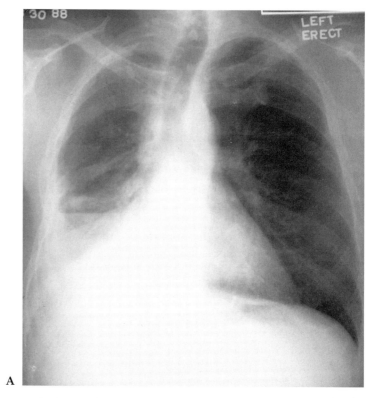

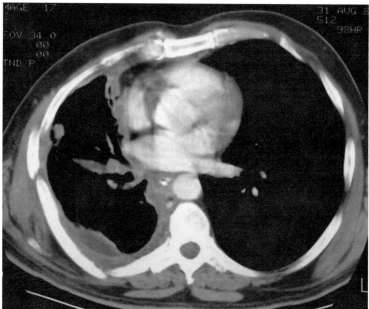

Figure 5-3. **(A)** Posteroanterior chest x-ray shows a unilateral pleural effusion. **(B)** Computed tomography of the thorax from the same patient shows irregular pleural thickening with encasement of the lung. These radiographic features are typical for malignant (diffuse) pleural mesothelioma. (Courtesy Dr. Caroline Chiles, Duke University Medical Center, Durham, NC.)

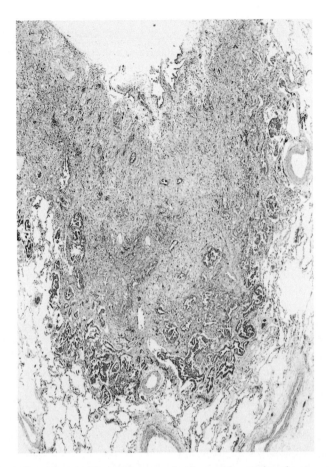

Figure 5-4. Low-power photomicrograph of a small peripheral scar carcinoma found at autopsy that measured 5 mm in maximum dimension. Multiple pleural deposits of tumor histologically identical to the adenocarcinoma at the periphery of the central scar resulted in a pattern mimicking mesothelioma. H&E ×24.

The diagnosis of malignant pleural mesothelioma depends not only on the presence of typical gross tumor distribution, but also on the identification of a histologic, histochemical, immunophenotypic, or ultrastructural pattern compatible with mesothelioma, and, moreover, exclusion of metastatic tumor. These additional and ancillary studies to complement examination of routine stained sections will be reviewed subsequently. Studies describing the cytologic features of mesothelioma in effusion cytologies and aspiration biopsies are reviewed in detail in Chapter 9. The distinction of malignant mesothelioma, reactive mesothelium, and metastatic carcinoma may be difficult or impossible on limited material. Although with the now commonplace usage of immunocytochemistry in the evaluation of cytologic material the pathologist may become highly suspicious of the diagnosis of mesothelioma, it remains our practice, and that of others,[159] to treat exfoliative and aspiration biopsy specimens as screening tests, and to rely on tissue specimens to secure the diagnosis.[2,15,139–152]

Histopathology

Malignant mesothelioma is characterized by a broad range of microscopic appearances, both across the entire spectrum of the disease entity and often within individual tumors themselves. This capability is likely a function of the potential for mesothelial cells to undergo varying pathways of differentiation. The World Health Organization recognizes four main histologic subtypes: epithelioid (epithelial) mesothelioma, sarcomatoid mesothelioma, desmoplastic mesothelioma, biphasic mesothelioma, and a separate category encompassing a variety of less common patterns, often featuring the presence of heterologous elements.[160] Epithelial, sarcomatoid, and biphasic mesotheliomas are the most common pleural forms, occurring in approximately 50, 20, and 30% of cases respectively.[2,125,139] The representation of these subtypes is different among the peritoneal mesotheliomas; Churg and Kannerstein reported in a series of 82 cases 75% epithelial mesotheliomas, 24% biphasic and 1% purely sarcomatoid.[161] Origin within the pleura or peritoneum does not confer any differences in the microscopic features of the mesothelioma subtypes themselves. The histologic classification of mesothelioma is summarized in Table 5-1.

The most common variant is the epithelial, defined as a tumor whose histologic pattern is that of tubulopapillary structures, trabeculae, acini, or sheets of atypical cells (Figure 5-5A,B). Epithelial mesotheliomas are typically heterogeneous, and may assume different combinations of the above-described patterns throughout its expanse. The tubulopapillary pattern is most commonly observed, where the tumor consists of branching tubules and papillae lined by flat to cuboidal cells. Columnar tumor cells are uncommon, and while psammoma bodies may be observed in some 5% to 10% of cases,[132] their profusion suggests papillary carcinoma, especially in peritoneal malignancies.

Table 5-1. Histological classification of malignant mesothelioma

Epithelial
  Tubulopapillary
  Solid variant
  Adenomatoid
  Small cell
  Deciduoid
  Adenoidcystic
  Pleomorphic
  Well differentiated papillary*
Sarcomatoid
  Fibrosarcomatoid
  Chondrosarcomatoid
  Osteosarcomatoid
  Malignant fibrous histiocytoma-like
  Lymphohistiocytoid
  Desmoplastic
Biphasic (mixed)

*This variant is considered to be a tumor of low grade malignant potential

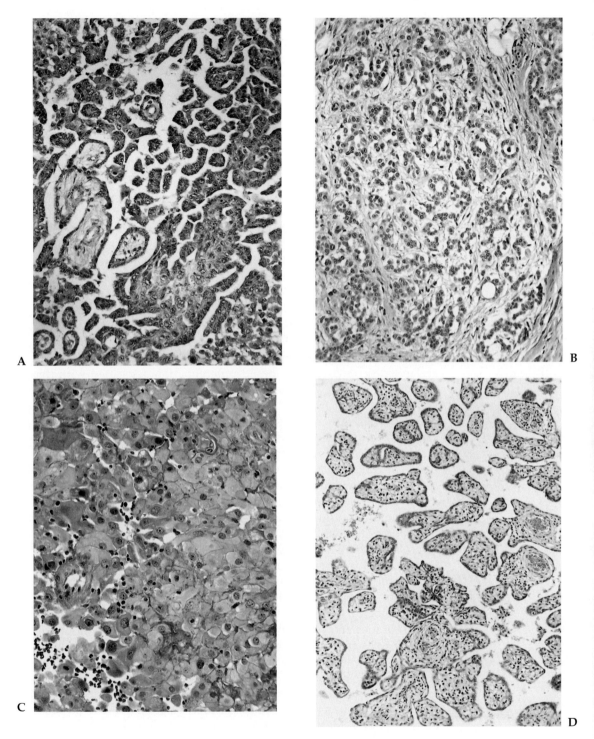

Figure 5-5. Histologic patterns of the epithelial variant of malignant (diffuse) mesothelioma. **(A)** papillary pattern; **(B)** tubular pattern; **(C)** deciduoid pattern; **(D)** well-differentiated papillary pattern. The latter pattern in pure form tends to have an indolent clinical behavior. H&E, (A), (B) and (D) ×170; (C) ×400; (D). (Reprinted from Ref. 2, with permission.)

Epithelioid cytologic features include cuboidal or polygonal shape, moderate to abundant cytoplasm, and paracentric nuclei, often with prominent nucleoli. Multinucleate forms and occasional mitoses may be observed, but anaplastic forms, extreme pleomorphism and high-grade cytologic atypia are not common features of epithelial mesotheliomas. Atypical mitoses are distinctly uncommon.[2,162] The epithelial variant is most likely to be confused with adenocarcinoma, and this distinction becomes more difficult as the epithelial tumor cells become more anaplastic.[2] A useful cytologic feature reported to be characteristic of the tumor cells of epithelial mesothelioma is a constant nuclear to cytoplasmic ratio.

Several histologic subtypes or patterns of epithelial mesothelioma are recognized. The *adenomatoid* subtype forms a microglandular pattern with lumina containing hyaluronic acid, mimicking adenomatoid tumors.[132] While typically comprised of large epithelial tumor cells, the *small cell* subtype demonstrates a diffuse growth of small tumor cells that may sometimes be confused with small cell carcinoma.[132,163] *Deciduoid* mesothelioma, originally described in young women as aggressive peritoneal tumors arising independent of exposure to asbestos,[164] features sheets of large, round to polygonal cells with typically a single nucleolus and abundant eosinophilic cytoplasm, resembling cells of the decidual reaction (Figure 5-5C). Puttagunta et al. have described focal rhabdoid differentiation associated with this tumor type as well.[165] These tumors have also been described in men and may occur in the pleura and pericardium as well as the peritoneum.[166–169] A history of asbestos exposure has been reported in a few cases.[166,168,170] Other unusual variants of epithelial mesothelioma include the *adenoid cystic* type, resembling tumors of salivary gland origin, and the *pleomorphic* variant, with a histological resemblance to pleomorphic carcinoma of the lung.[171]

Well-differentiated papillary mesothelioma (WDPM) is an uncommon tumor tending to involve the peritoneal cavity of women in the third and fourth decades of life, but rarely reported to involve the other serosal membranes. Unlike typical pleural and peritoneal mesotheliomas, a history of asbestos exposure is not present in most cases.[172,173] In a recent review, Butnor et al. described 14 cases of WDPM, including seven pleural tumors and one from the tunica vaginalis testis.[174] The histological features of tumors in the pleural, pericardial and peritoneal cavities and tunica vaginalis are similar, demonstrating prominent fibrovascular cores lined by a single layer of relatively uniform cuboidal cells with minimal nuclear atypia and no mitotic activity (Figure 5-5D). Psammoma bodies were present in one of the cases reported by Butnor et al., and focal stromal invasion was identified in two cases. An asbestos exposure history may be present in some cases.[174,175] WDPM typically has a good prognosis characterized by indolent clinical behavior, but may pursue an aggressive course with death following the development of diffuse disease.[174,175] Identification of invasion signals a poor prognosis, and such tumors should be classified as epithelial mesotheliomas.

The sarcomatoid variant is the least common of the three major histologic types. The tumor cells are elongate and spindled, and may show considerable pleomorphism and mitotic activity.[2] Architecturally complex, the broad fascicular or storiform growth pattern resembles those of typical soft tissue sarcomas, including neurogenic sarcoma, leiomyosarcoma, chondrosarcoma or osteogenic sarcoma (Figure 5-6A,B).[136,176,177] We have also observed cases in which the storiform fascicles of spindle cells contain intermixed bizarre tumor giant cells in a pattern reminiscent of malignant fibrous histiocytoma (Figure 5-6C). True heterologous elements comprised of osteosarcomatous or chondrosarcomatous foci have been noted in otherwise typical mesotheliomas.[176,177] The *lymphohistiocytoid* variant of sarcomatoid mesothelioma is an unusual form that may be misdiagnosed as an inflammatory pseudotumor or lymphoma.[178] The tumor consists of an admixture of large histiocytoid cells and dense lymphoplasma cellular infiltrate within a background of sarcomatoid tumor cells (Figure 5-7). Mesothelial differentiation in these cases has been proven using cytokeratin immunostaining and electron microscopy. The authors accept the various patterns listed above as mesothelioma, provided the gross distribution of tumor is characteristic, and there is no evidence of primary soft tissue sarcoma elsewhere in the patient.[2]

The most distinctive pattern of malignant mesothelioma is the biphasic or mixed pattern. These tumors have areas that exhibit one of the epithelial patterns described above, as well as areas with a spindle cell or sarcomatoid appearance. The transition from epithelial to sarcomatoid areas may be gradual or abrupt, with sharp demarcation between the epithelial and sarcomatoid components (Figure 5-8). Metastases from biphasic mesotheliomas may contain either component alone, or both may be present together.[2] The frequency of the biphasic pattern ranges from 25% to 50% in various series of pleural mesotheliomas, and is somewhat dependent on the thoroughness of tumor sampling.[125,137] The pathologist must be careful to differentiate a true sarcomatoid component from a cellular fibroblastic stromal response to metastatic carcinoma.

A particularly deceptive pattern of sarcomatoid malignant mesothelioma is the *desmoplastic* variant.[179,180] This uncommon form, constituting approximately 10% of all malignant mesotheliomas, is typically less cellular than its counterparts, and features largely hyalinized collagenous stroma. Desmoplastic mesothelioma mimics benign reactive processes, typically the fibrosing serositis that may occur in postoperative or postinflammatory conditions. Patients with malignant mesothelioma often have parietal pleural plaques, present in more than 70% of cases with pleural mesothelioma.[51] Plaques are a potential source of confusion as they too are generally acellular, but demonstrate hyalinized collagen with a "basket weave" pattern, never in a storiform pattern. DMM was originally described by Kannerstein and Churg in 1980.[179] Specific diagnostic criteria to more readily allow the distinction of this tumor from fibrous pleurisy have since been introduced by Mangano et al.[181] The most striking feature of this tumor is a whorled

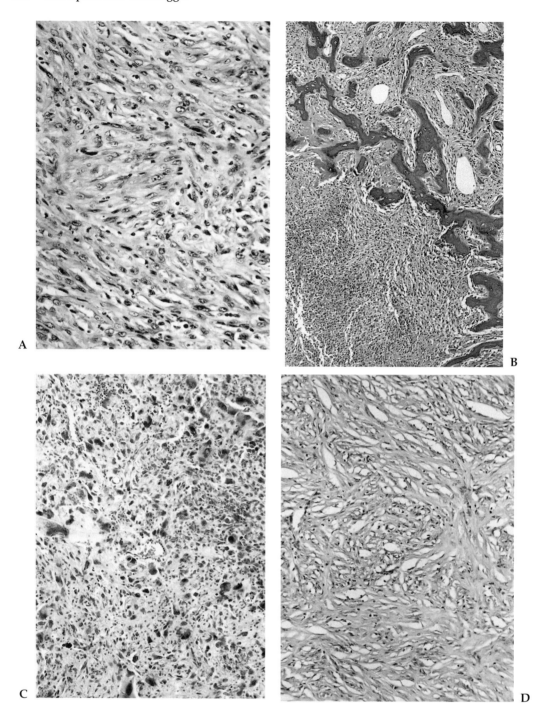

Figure 5-6. Histologic patterns of the sarcomatoid variant of malignant (diffuse) mesothelioma. **(A)** fibrosarcomatoid pattern; **(B)** osteosarcomatoid pattern. Note bony spicules surrounded by malignant spindle cells; **(C)** malignant fibrous histiocytoma-like pattern, with numerous tumor giant cells; **(D)** desmoplastic pattern, consisting of thick collagen bundles arranged in a storiform pattern with scattered inconspicuous tumor cells in spaces between the fiber bundles. H&E, (A) ×250; (B) ×70; (C) and (D) ×130. ((A) and (D) reprinted from Ref. 2; part (B) courtesy Dr. Tom Colby, Mayo Clinic, Scottsdale, AZ, and reprinted with permission from Roggli VL, Cagle PT: Pleura, Pericardium and Peritoneum, Ch 20, In: Diagnostic Surgical Pathology and Cytopathology, 4th Ed. (Silverberg SG, DeLellis RL, Frable WJ, LiVolsi VA, Wick M, eds.) Philadelphia: Elsevier 2004, with permission.)

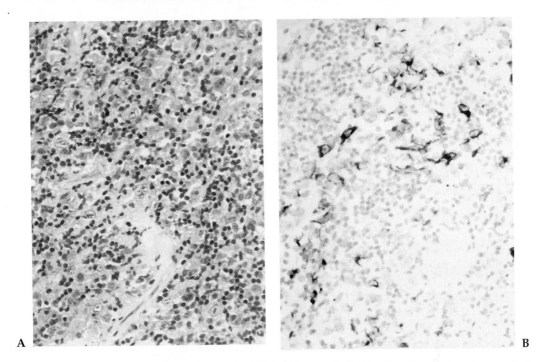

Figure 5-7. (A) Lymphohistiocytoid malignant pleural mesothelioma, showing large pale neoplastic nuclei (*arrowheads*) in a background of small lymphocytes. The pattern resembles that of a mixed small and large B-cell lymphoma. **(B)** Adjacent serial section stained for cytokeratins shows positive staining of the large neoplastic cells. H&E, (A) ×325; (B) immunoperoxidase (cytokeratins) ×325.

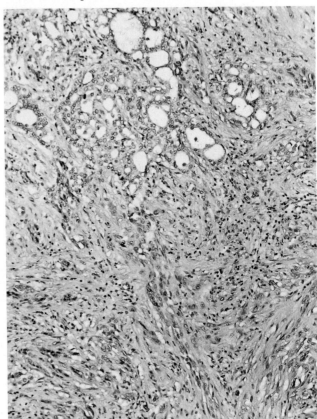

Figure 5-8. Biphasic variant of malignant (diffuse) mesothelioma showing epithelial component (*top*) with tubule formation and sarcomatoid differentiation (*bottom right*). H&E ×100. (Reprinted from Ref. 2, with permission.)

and twisting paucicellular lesion, produced by distinct broad collagen fibers in a storiform array, or in the "patternless pattern" of Stout (Figure 5-6D).[182] The storiform pattern can be focally found as a component of a large percentage of malignant mesotheliomas,[183] so the term is restricted to cases in which this pattern predominates.[179,180] Rarely, biphasic and epithelial mesotheliomas containing a predominant desmoplastic component have been described.

The diagnostic criteria for DMM include the presence of a tumor more than 50% of which consists of dense collagen bundles arranged in a storiform or patternless pattern, and at least one of the following additional findings. First is invasion of lung or chest wall by neoplastic spindle cells. This is often apparent on routine stained sections. The presence of more subtle invasion may be demonstrated with low molecular weight cytokeratin immunoperoxidase stains, showing keratin-positive spindle cells infiltrating alveolar septa or adipose tissue of the chest wall. The mere identification of cytokeratin-positive spindle cells within the lesion is not diagnostic, as keratin expression may be observed in reactive processes as well. The second criterion is the finding of bland necrosis, as evidenced by necrotic foci with minimal accompanying inflammatory infiltrate. Necrosis may be detected by subtle changes in the tinctorial quality of the fibrosis and nuclear fragmentation. The third criterion is that of frankly sarcomatoid areas, as defined by zones of transition from paucicellular fibrosis to areas of more abundant spindled cellularity. An accompanying increase in nuclear atypia may help distinguish sarcomatoid foci. Mitotic figures are not numerous in either fibrosing pleuritis or DMM. The fourth criterion is the presence of distant metastases.[181,184]

In addition to these specific criteria, other findings may also aid in distinguishing DMM from a reactive process. Churg has noted that the most cellular areas in fibrosing pleuritis are oriented toward the luminal aspect of the pleura, whereas the process closest to the chest wall is less cellular.[60] This "top heavy" cellular pattern may also feature numerous perpendicular capillaries traversing the full thickness of pleura, favoring a reactive process.[2,184] Thoracic imaging studies, particularly computed tomography or magnetic resonance imaging, are often of great value by demonstrating irregular pleural thickening, chest wall invasion or bony involvement, and may assist the pathologist in making a diagnosis of DMM in difficult cases.[151,181] Immunohistochemistry for the p53 tumor suppressor gene protein has been suggested as a useful diagnostic adjunct for distinguishing reactive pleural processes from mesothelioma and metastatic carcinoma. Mutations of this gene are more likely to result in a stable protein as compared to the wild type.[185] Staining of more than 10% of nuclei is seen more frequently in DMM than fibrosing pleuritis, but the difference is not statistically significant in the small number of cases examined.[181]

Metastases from malignant mesothelioma generally resemble the histological appearance of the primary tumor, and a review of 42 pleural mesotheliomas showed no difference in the frequency of hematogenous or lymphatic metastases among the three major histological variants,[186] despite prior reports that sarcomatoid mesothelioma has more frequent distant metastases.[187] It is interesting to note that whereas regional lymph node metastases are commonly identified,[125,136] metastases to extrathoracic lymph nodes are infrequent, occurring in eight of 77 cases of pleural mesothelioma in a single series.[188] In exceptional cases, osseous metastases have been described as the initial clinical evidence of tumor dissemination in DMM.[189] Hematogenous metastases of DMM sometimes exhibit the curious phenomenon of central hyalinization with a peripheral cellular storiform pattern.[2] Finally, rare cases have been reported in which liver metastases from a malignant pleural mesothelioma underwent dystrophic calcification and presented as hepatic calcification initially detected radiographically.

Histochemistry

The distinction of malignant mesothelioma from its mimics, and adenocarcinoma in particular, is critical in regard to decisions for treatment, prognostication, and frequently for compensation in medicolegal cases involving allegations of exposure to asbestos. In view of these crucial decision points, studies adjunctive to the examination of hematoxylin and eosin stained sections are required to secure the diagnosis of malignant mesothelioma in the vast majority of cases.

Histochemical staining for mucins and acid mucopolysaccharides provides one means for making this distinction. The histochemical basis for distinguishing malignant pleural mesothelioma from metastatic adenocarcinoma rests on the identification of hyaluronic acid production in the former instance and neutral mucin in the latter.[2] Neutral mucin may be identified by the periodic acid Schiff (PAS) stain. The specificity of the PAS stain is increased by prior digestion of the section with diastase in order to remove glycogen, which may be abundant in the cytoplasm of either mesothelioma or adenocarcinoma. The demonstration of PAS-positive, diastase-resistant droplets of neutral mucin as intraluminal secretions or cytoplasmic vacuoles within a tumor strongly supports a diagnosis of adenocarcinoma (Figure 5-9).[2,12,60,132,136,137,139,140,153] A false positive reaction with the PAS stain may occur if removal of glycogen by diastase is incomplete. Therefore, simultaneous controls should always be performed. In addition, basement membrane material, which may be prominent in epithelial mesotheliomas, will stain with the PAS reaction. Careful attention to the pattern of staining will usually prevent the confusion of residual glycogen or basement membrane material with positive staining for neutral mucin. The PAS stain is of no use for the diagnosis of sarcomatoid or desmoplastic mesotheliomas.[2] The mucicarmine stain may occasionally react with hyaluronic acid, giving a false positive result. We therefore do not recommend mucicarmine for distinguishing mesothelioma from metastatic adenocarcinoma.

Identification of hyaluronic acid as the sole or major acid mucopolysaccharide in an epithelial tumor has also been proposed as

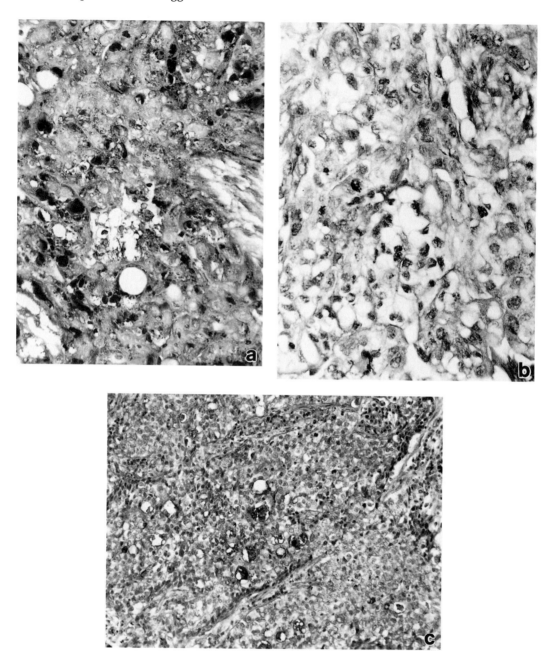

Figure 5-9. (A) In this epithelial type of mesothelioma, tumor cells contain finely granular, intracyto-plasmic PAS-positive material. **(B)** Staining reaction in an adjacent section has been abolished by prior digestion with diastase. **(C)** In this adenocarcinoma metastatic to the pleura, PAS-positive material within glandular lumens remains following digestion by diastase, indicating the presence of neutral mucin. (Reprinted from Ref. 2, with permission.)

a useful histochemical marker for the diagnosis of malignant mesothelioma.[2,12,60,132,136,137,139,140,153] Such identification may be hampered by the tendency of water-soluble hyaluronic acid to leach out of tissue sections. Acid mucopolysaccharides, including hyaluronic acid, may be identified histochemically using alcian blue or colloidal iron stains. The specificity of the reaction for hyaluronic acid is determined by digestion of a serial section with hyaluronidase prior to staining (Figure 5-10). The results seen following enzyme predigestion depend to some degree on the actual type of hyaluronidase used in the test, since *Streptomyces* hyaluronidase is specific for hyaluronic acid, whereas testicular hyaluronidase digests chondroitin sulfate as well. Only intracytoplasmic or intraluminal alcianophilia associated with epithelial cells should be considered diagnostic. Intracytoplasmic or intraluminal staining that is entirely eliminated by hyaluronidase strongly supports the diagnosis of malignant mesothelioma. Staining unaffected by hyaluronidase predigestion favors adenocarcinoma. Simultaneous controls should always be performed to ensure that the stains and enzyme are working properly.

The detection of glycosaminoglycans in pleural effusions using electrophoresis has been considered as a diagnostic adjunct,[190] as the effusions associated with malignant mesothelioma may be rich in hyaluronic acid. In patients with malignant mesothelioma, hyaluronic acid is typically the sole or predominant mucopolysaccharide (glycosaminoglycan) identified electrophoretically, whereas malignant effusions associated with adenocarcinoma generally contain a mixture of glycosaminoglycans. However, rare cases of pleural mesothelioma have been reported in which chondroitin sulfate was the predominant glycosaminoglycan, and rare instances of pleural effusions complicating metastatic pancreatic carcinoma have been shown to contain predominantly hyaluronic acid.

It should be noted that the demonstration of PAS-positive, diastase-resistant and alcian blue positive, hyaluronidase resistant intracytoplasmic vacuoles has rarely been reported in mesothelioma. MacDougall et al. reported one such case of a pleural malignancy whose ultrastructural and immunohistochemical characteristics were otherwise typical for mesothelioma.[191] Cook et al. reported a similar case involving the peritoneum that mimicked gastric adenocarcinoma.[192] Hammar et al. reported a series of ten so-called mucin-positive epithelial mesotheliomas.[193] In this study, the intensity of PAS-positivity was often eliminated or reduced following hyaluronidase treatment, suggesting that hyaluronic acid was responsible for the positive staining reaction. Ultrastructurally, the secretions had the appearance of crystalline hyaluronic acid or peptidoglycans. A diagnosis of "mucin-positive" mesothelioma should only be entertained in tumors that otherwise have clinical, gross, histologic, immunohistochemical, and ultrastructural features typical for mesothelioma.

In summary, histochemistry may be useful in discriminating between adenocarcinoma and mesothelioma. While offering generally lower cost and simpler methodology, the histochemical techniques described suffer from some limitations. A substantial proportion of

...

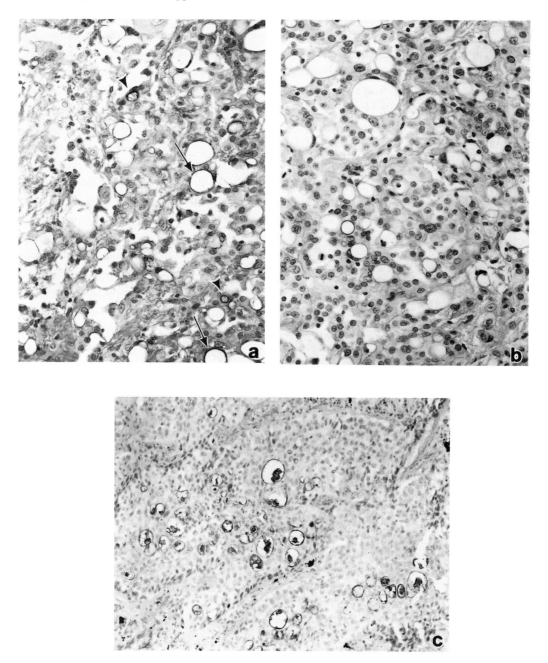

Figure 5-10. **(A)** In this epithelial pleural mesothelioma, tumor cells are forming nests with lumens that are filled with (*arrowheads*) or rimmed by (*arrows*) alcian-blue-positive material. **(B)** This material is completely removed from a serial section by prior digestion with hyaluronidase. **(C)** In this adenocarcinoma metastatic to the pleura, alcian-blue-positive material persists in the lumens following digestion with hyaluronidase. (Reprinted from Ref. 2, with permission.)

adenocarcinomas fail to produce detectable amounts of neutral mucin, and only about half of epithelial mesotheliomas produce detectable quantities of hyaluronic acid. Therefore, negative histochemical studies provide no diagnostically useful information, and in a great many cases histochemistry will not discriminate between malignant mesothelioma and metastatic adenocarcinoma. In our practice, we reserve histochemical staining for tumors that have identifiable secretions on routine hematoxylin and eosin-stained sections.

Immunohistochemistry

Among the ancillary diagnostic studies employed in the diagnosis of mesothelioma, immunohistochemical studies currently play the dominant role in separating mesothelioma from its neoplastic mimics. Following Wang's report that expression of carcinoembryonic antigen (CEA) could be used to distinguish adenocarcinoma from mesothelioma,[194] numerous different antibodies and panels of antibodies have been evaluated to strengthen this distinction. While immunohistochemistry has evolved to the point that there are arrays of immunophenotypes considered diagnostic or exclusionary of mesothelioma, several principles regarding its application remain axiomatic. First and foremost, there is no immunohistochemical marker that can distinguish per se a malignant cell, either mesothelioma or carcinoma, from a benign or hyperplastic cell with complete sensitivity and specificity. Second, there is no single marker completely sensitive and specific for the identification of mesothelial or carcinoma cells. Such limitations to the state of the art necessitate the employment of a panel of immunostains whereby one can demonstrate an immunophenotype generally considered diagnostic or exclusionary of mesothelioma. In the absence of mesothelium-specific antibodies, the major strength of immunohistochemistry in the diagnosis of mesothelioma historically has been one of exclusion. Recent advances have seen the development of antibodies with greater specificity for mesothelial differentiation, as well as markers with greater specificity for carcinoma.

Cytokeratins

Cytokeratins consist of a family of some twenty 40 to 67 kilodalton polypeptides, forming one of five intermediate filaments. They are expressed to some degree in both benign and transformed epithelial cells as well as mesothelium. Pulmonary adenocarcinomas and mesotheliomas both demonstrate simple epithelial patterns of cytokeratin immunoreactivity with expression of cytokeratins 1, 8, 18, and 19 from the Moll's catalog.[195] Typical practice in diagnostic surgical pathology often employs a "cocktail" of low and high molecular weight cytokeratins that will neither differentiate a reactive process from a neoplastic one nor reliably separate carcinoma from mesothelioma.[183,196–200] However, such staining does permit the distinction of mesothelioma from the occasional lymphoma, melanoma, or epithelioid hemangioendothelioma that may involve the pleura.

The demonstration of cytokeratin expression will in most cases allow the exclusion of localized fibrous tumors or sarcomas involving the serosal membranes. Notable exceptions to this include synovial sarcomas and epithelioid sarcomas, which often express cytokeratins, but are uncommonly encountered as primary tumors of the serosal membranes. Other mesenchymal malignancies such as some leiomyosarcomas and malignant fibrous histiocytomas may infrequently demonstrate aberrant expression of cytokeratins. Sarcomatoid mesotheliomas and the spindle cell component of biphasic mesotheliomas will generally stain positive for cytokeratins, and this remains a useful technique for distinguishing sarcomatoid mesotheliomas from other spindle cell malignancies (Figure 5-11).[201–203] Reactive fibrous pleural lesions, including parietal pleural plaques and the desmoplastic stromal response induced by metastases, will also usually show positive staining of spindle cells for cytokeratins. Therefore, this technique does not aid in distinguishing reactive from neoplastic mesothelial proliferations.[201,203] In addition, anticytokeratin antibodies will not discriminate between sarcomatoid mesotheliomas or the spindle cell component of biphasic mesotheliomas and sarcomatoid carcinomas, such as the sarcomatoid renal cell carcinoma or pleomorphic carcinoma of the lung.[204]

Recent investigation into the differential expression of the individual cytokeratins has proven useful to aid in the distinction of mesothelioma from carcinoma. Mesotheliomas selectively express cytokeratins 4, 5, 6, 14, and 17, which is not observed in adenocarcinomas (Figure 5-12A).[205] Ordonez reported immunoreactivity for cytokeratins 5/6 (CK 5/6) in each of 40 epithelial mesotheliomas but in none of 30 pulmonary adenocarcinomas. However, CK 5/6 was expressed in all 15 squamous cell carcinomas and in 3 of 5 large cell carcinomas of the lung, as well as 14 of 93 nonpulmonary adenocarcinomas.[206] Subsequent studies by Cury et al. report positive immunoreactivity for CK 5/6 in 56 of 61 epithelial mesotheliomas, compared with 9 of 63 cases of metastatic adenocarcinomas, including one case of pulmonary adenocarcinoma.[207] Mesotheliomas also stain positive for cytokeratin 7 and usually stain negative for cytokeratin 20. We have observed occasional cases with focal moderate staining for the latter marker. This pattern is similar to that observed for primary adenocarcinomas of the lung and breast, but differs from that of most adenocarcinomas of the gastrointestinal tract.[208]

Glycoproteins

Numerous antibodies to cell surface glycoproteins have been evaluated for their pattern of differential expression in adenocarcinomas and mesothelioma. The antibodies considered for discussion are those routinely employed in the practice of diagnostic surgical pathology and include CEA, Ber-EP4, Leu-M1 (CD15), B72.3, and epithelial membrane antigen (EMA). Excepting EMA, the diagnostic utility lies in that positive expression of these markers is a hallmark of most adenocarcinomas, and negative expression a feature of most mesotheliomas.

The oncofetal antigen CEA is a member of a large family of glycoproteins, and the first immunohistochemical marker proven useful in

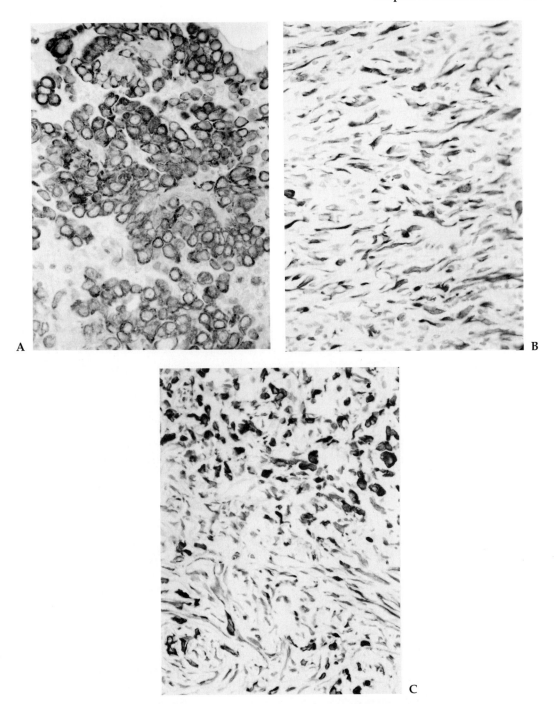

Figure 5-11. Immunohistochemical staining for cytokeratins using a cocktail of monoclonal antibodies to high- and low-molecular-weight cytokeratins. **(A)** Diffuse cytoplasmic staining in a predominately epithelial mesothelioma. **(B)** Cytoplasmic staining of spindle cells in a sarcomatoid mesothelioma. **(C)** Staining of epithelial component (*top*) and sarcomatoid component (*bottom*) of a biphasic mesothelioma.

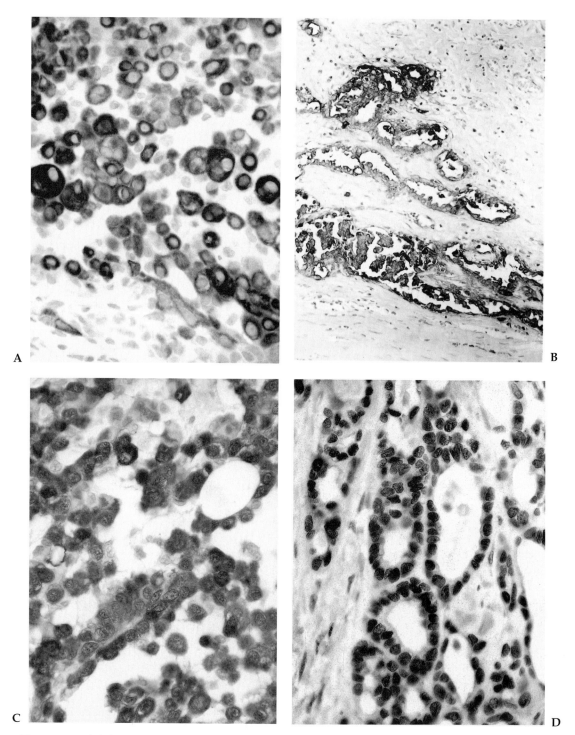

Figure 5-12. **(A)** Strong cytoplasmic staining of an epithelial mesothelioma for cytokeratins 5/6. **(B)** In this adenocarcinoma metastatic to the pleura, the tumor cells are strongly positive for carcinoembryonic antigen (CEA). (Reprinted from Ref. 2, with permission.) **(C)** Strong nuclear staining of an epithelial mesothelioma for calretinin. **(D)** Strong nuclear staining of a pulmonary adenocarcinoma for thyroid transcription factor-1 (TTF-1).

the diagnostic evaluation of mesothelioma.[194] CEA is often expressed in adenocarcinomas of pulmonary and gastrointestinal origin (Figure 5-12B), as well as those originating in the breast, liver, and pancreas.[209] Corson and Pinkus reported that some epithelial mesotheliomas may stain positively albeit weakly with CEA using polyclonal antibodies.[210] This is likely explained by the labeling of nonspecific, cross-reacting antigens and unrelated epitopes. Commercially available monoclonal CEA antibodies give cleaner backgrounds, less nonspecific cross reactivity and higher specificity for carcinoma with some reduction in sensitivity.[211] CEA is expressed in some 85% to 95% of pulmonary adenocarcinomas, and in at least 80% of carcinomas from other sites.[212–214] Staining for CEA should be interpreted with some caution, as adenocarcinomas of the kidney, thyroid, and prostate do not generally express CEA. Moreover, papillary serous carcinomas of the ovary and peritoneum are usually CEA negative, which compromises the usage of this antibody in peritoneal mesotheliomas.

Ber-EP4 is a murine monoclonal antibody prepared from mice immunized with a breast carcinoma cell line.[215] Latza et al. first demonstrated its utility in the distinction between mesothelioma and adenocarcinoma, reporting immunoreactivity to the antibody by 99% of adenocarcinomas from various sites, contrasted with no reactivity in 14 epithelial mesotheliomas.[215] Other studies indicated the potential staining for BerEP4 by some mesotheliomas. In view of the reported discrepancy, Ordonez performed a review of the collective experience with this antibody.[216] This author observed BerEP4 immunoreactivity in 18/70 mesotheliomas (26%), compared with 20/20 (100%) pulmonary adenocarcinomas and 55/59 (93%) nonpulmonary adenocarcinomas. BerEP4 staining in mesothelioma, when present, was generally weak and restricted to limited numbers of cells, whereas focal, diffuse or negative staining was observed in metastatic adenocarcinomas of unknown primary site. The primary utility of BerEP4 lies in its ability to separate adenocarcinoma of the lung from mesothelioma, with lesser ability to distinguish mesothelioma from metastatic carcinomas to the pleura originating from nonpulmonary sites.

The monoclonal antibody LeuM1 (also known as CD15) is a myelomonocytic antigen once believed to be a specific marker for Hodgkins disease, owing to its ability to decorate Reed-Sternberg cells. Immunoreactivity to this antibody has since been shown in non-Hodgkins lymphomas and leukemias, as well as some carcinomas.[217,218] Sheibani et al. were the first to report its application in the diagnosis of mesothelioma.[211,218] These authors reported LeuM1 immunoreactivity in 105/179 (59%) adenocarcinomas of various sites, in 47/50 (94%) pulmonary adenocarcinomas, and in none of 28 mesotheliomas. LeuM1 appears to be a specific but rather insensitive marker for distinguishing adenocarcinoma from mesothelioma.

B72.3 is a murine monoclonal antibody generated against a membrane-enriched fraction derived from human breast cancer cells that recognizes tumor-associated glycoproteins present in a number of pulmonary and nonpulmonary adenocarcinomas. Lefebvre et al. were the first to report its utility in the diagnosis of mesothelioma, showing immunoreactivity in 17/20 (85%) pulmonary adenocarcinomas, contrasted with weak staining in 2 of 10 mesotheliomas.[219] Subsequent studies appear in concurrence with a high degree of B72.3 expression in adenocarcinomas, especially of pulmonary origin, with up to 5% of mesotheliomas staining positive, albeit weakly and focally.[220,221]

Epithelial membrane antigens are associated with human mucins produced in a broad array of glandular and lactating epithelia, and diagnostic immunohistochemical stains have been developed using monoclonal antibodies to human milk fat globules and carcinomas. Membranous staining of tumor cells by HMFG-2 has been reported to be a feature of mesothelioma, whereas adenocarcinomas generally show cytoplasmic immunoreactivity.[222] Other studies have discounted this observation, citing difficulties in consistency and interpretation of such staining patterns.[223,224] Immunoreactivity to anti-EMA monoclonal antibodies is seen in both mesothelioma and carcinoma. However, localization and pattern of such expression have also been reported to be diagnostically useful. Similarly, it has been proposed that immunoreactivity for anti-EMA can reliably discriminate between reactive hyperplastic and neoplastic mesothelium. The authors' experience with this antibody does not support either contention, and it is concluded that immunohistochemical staining with antibodies to epithelial membrane antigens has no diagnostic value in common practice.

Calretinin
Calretinin is a 29 kilodalton protein, which belongs to a large family of cytoplasmic calcium-binding proteins that also includes S-100 protein. Calretinin differs from the majority of the commonly employed diagnostic antibodies in that positive immunoreactivity is supportive of the diagnosis of mesothelioma. Doglioni et al. described positive calretinin staining in both a nuclear and cytoplasmic distribution in 44 of 44 mesotheliomas, including sarcomatoid variants, compared to the focal staining observed in 28 of 294 adenocarcinomas (10%).[225] Subsequent studies demonstrated calretinin staining in 100% of mesotheliomas, compared with weak and focal staining in 4/34 (12%) adenocarcinomas.[226,227] Ordonez observed strong calretinin immunoreactivity in 100% of 38 mesotheliomas, as well as focal staining in 14/155 (9%) adenocarcinomas and in 11/28 squamous cell carcinomas using the Zymed monoclonal antibody.[228] Nuclear staining is far more specific than cytoplasmic staining (Figure 5-12C).[207] Staining in sarcomatoid mesotheliomas is less dependable and usually focal when present.

Thrombomodulin
Thrombomodulin is a surface glycoprotein involved in the regulation of intravascular coagulation, and may be expressed in a variety of normal and neoplastic epithelia, as well as in mesothelium and

endothelium. Collins et al. first described its expression in mesothelioma, observing immunoreactivity in all 31 cases of mesothelioma
studied, contrasted with 8% of pulmonary adenocarcinomas.[229]
Ordonez observed immunoreactivity in 75% to 80% of mesotheliomas,
contrasted with 15% of adenocarcinomas.[230] Because staining with this
antibody is primarily surface membrane in distribution and since blood
vessels also stain positive, interpretation can be difficult in some
cases.[207]

HBME-1

HBME-1 is a monoclonal antibody developed from a suspension of
cells from a well-differentiated epithelial mesothelioma, with the
immunogen originally believed present on cell surface microvilli. The
actual antigen remains unknown and this antibody is not specific for
mesothelium, with positive immunoreactivity present in a number of
adenocarcinomas. Initial experience with this antibody suggested that
differences in staining patterns observed in mesothelioma (strong
membranous staining) versus adenocarcinoma (cytoplasmic staining)
were diagnostically useful.[231,232] Subsequent studies have observed
common staining patterns shared by the two classes of tumor.[230] Some
investigators still use HBME-1 in their diagnostic armamentarium, but
only at much higher dilutions (1:5000 to 1:15,000) than that recommended by the manufacturer (1:50) (Doug Henderson, Sam Hammar,
and Hector Battifora, personal communication).

Cadherins

The cadherins constitute a family of glycoproteins involved in calcium-
dependent intercellular adhesion. E-cadherin is expressed in epithelial
cells, whereas N-cadherin is present in nerve, skeletal muscle and
mesothelium.[233] Soler et al. have reported positive immunostaining for
E-cadherin in 13/14 (93%) of pulmonary adenocarcinomas compared
with negative staining in 13 mesotheliomas.[234] Similar findings have
been reported by Leers et al. using the monoclonal antibody HECD-1,
wherein 20/21 metastatic adenocarcinomas were positive, contrasted
with 3/20 (15%) mesotheliomas.[226] Ordonez noted focal immunoreactivity for E-cadherin in 3/50 (6%) mesotheliomas, compared to diffuse
staining in 34/40 (85%) pulmonary adenocarcinomas.[235] Soler et al.
reported positive immunoreactivity for N-cadherin in 92% of mesotheliomas, contrasted with 7% of adenocarcinomas.[234] The utility of N-
cadherin is somewhat limited by its common expression in ovarian
adenocarcinomas.[236]

TTF-1

Thyroid transcription factor-1 (TTF-1) is a tissue specific transcription
factor expressed in the thyroid gland, in parts of the developing brain
and by Type II pneumocytes and Clara cells in the lung, but not in
mesothelium. Studies by Bejarano et al. and Di Loreto et al. demonstrated high rates of TTF-1 expression in pulmonary adenocarcinomas,
with no immunoreactivity observed in nonpulmonary adenocarcinomas or in epithelial mesotheliomas (Figure 5-12D).[237,238] These observa-

tions were confirmed by those of Ordonez, who detected TTF-1 immunoreactivity in 30/40 (75%) pulmonary adenocarcinomas and 10/10 thyroid carcinomas, contrasted with negative expression observed in the remainder of the adenocarcinomas from various other sites and in all 50 mesotheliomas.[235] This antibody thus may serve the dual purpose of distinguishing pulmonary adenocarcinoma from mesothelioma, and if positive, demonstrate a high degree of specificity regarding the site of tumor origin.

Ultrastructural Features

While application of the above described histochemical and immuno-histochemical studies frequently is sufficient to diagnose mesothelioma, there are cases in which those studies are not adequate or are equivocal. In such instances, the observation of characteristic ultrastructural attributes using electron microscopy may permit the diagnosis of mesothelioma. No single ultrastructural feature is unique to malignant mesothelioma. Rather, a constellation of ultrastructural features exists that is characteristic of the tumor. Such features include long surface microvilli, abundant intermediate filaments, and often prominent accumulations of intracytoplasmic glycogen.[239–244] The ultrastructural features common to mesothelioma may be demonstrated to varying degrees in individual cases, and the absence of a single feature (such as long surface microvilli) does not necessarily negate the diagnosis.[245,246]

One of the most conspicuous and useful ultrastructural feature observed in the epithelial variant of mesothelioma is the presence of long, slender, smooth surface microvilli that stand in contrast to the less abundant, shorter, blunt microvilli seen in adenocarcinomas (Figure 5-13A,B). The microvilli of adenocarcinoma may also have a fuzzy appearance, due to the presence of ample surface glycocalyx.[15,246] The microvilli of adenocarcinoma may also demonstrate glycocalyceal bodies and prominent rootlets.[15] As these differences in microvillus structure between mesothelioma and adenocarcinoma may be variable and to a degree subjective, some studies have sought to establish more objective criteria by examining the aspect (length to diameter) ratios of the microvilli in the two types of tumor cells.[242–244] Mesotheliomas have been found to have microvilli with a mean length to diameter ratio of approximately 16, compared to a value of approximately 9 for the microvilli of adenocarcinoma in most reported cases.[2,205,242–244]

Another useful finding is the presence of such microvilli in mesothelioma not only at the luminal surface, but also at the abluminal surface of the tumor cell. Dewar reported microvilli making direct contact with collagen through basal lamina defects in 10 of 12 mesotheliomas studied, compared with zero of twenty adenocarcinomas.[247] Although examination of ultrathin sections prepared from glutaraldehyde-fixed tissue is preferred, the presence of long surface microvilli can be detected using formalin-fixed, paraffin-embedded material. Jandik et al. measured the aspect ratios of microvilli in seven mesotheliomas and seven adenocarcinomas using scanning electron microscopy, with

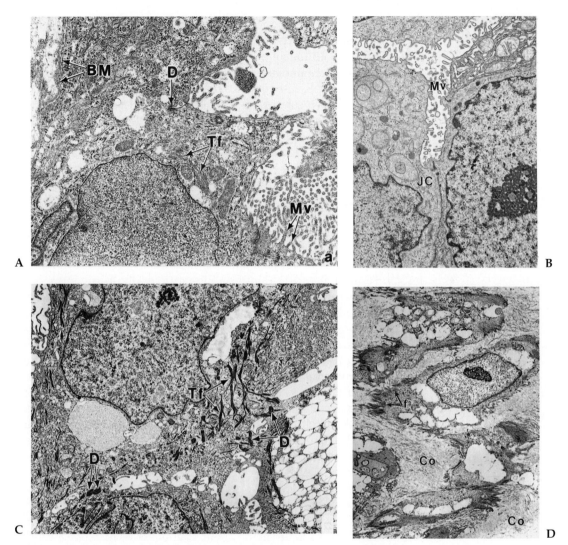

Figure 5-13. (A) This epithelial mesothelioma illustrates long, slender surface microvilli (Mv), tonofibrillar bundles (Tf), desmosomes (D), and basal lamina (BM). **(B)** Blunt surface microvilli (Mv) and a junctional complex (JC) are observed in this adenocarcinoma metastatic to the pleura. Intermediate filaments and tonofibrillar bundles are not identified. **(C)** Numerous tonofibrillar bundles (Tf) and prominent desmosomes **(D)** are present in this squamous cell carcinoma of the lung. **(D)** This sarcomatoid mesothelioma demonstrates spindle cells with cytoplasmic filaments (F) and abundant extracellular collagen (Co). Transmission electron micrographs, (A) ×10,000; (B) ×6000; (C) ×6000; (D) ×4000. ((A), (B), and (D) reprinted from Ref. 2, with permission.)

results comparable to those performed using transmission electron microscopy on the same tumors.[248]

Intercellular junctions of the macula adherens type (true desmosomes) are found with equal frequency in epithelial mesotheliomas and adenocarcinoma,[2] although some qualitative differences have been reported. Burns et al. found that "giant desmosomes" (i.e., desmosomes greater than 1 μm in length) were more frequent in mesothelioma, although mean desmosomal length was not significantly different in the two groups.[249] Ghadially found giant desmosomes in 2 of 10 epithelial mesotheliomas and in no adenocarcinomas studied.[250] Mukherjee et al. reported a freeze fracture study of intercellular junctions in two cases of pleural mesothelioma obtained by biopsy and noted that both gap and tight junctions were less well-developed and less numerous than those in exfoliated mesothelioma cells present in effusions, or in benign mesothelial cells.[251]

Mesotheliomas generally contain significantly more intermediate filaments, condensed as perinuclear tonofibrillar bundles, than do adenocarcinomas.[2,242] These tonofilaments insert into the large desmosomes connecting the cells. Whereas studies by Warhol and Roggli have shown the increased tonofilament content of mesothelioma over adenocarcinomas of lung, breast, ovary and endometrium, these may be absent in some epithelial mesotheliomas[15,242] and prominent in squamous or adenosquamous carcinomas of the lung (Figure 5-13C). Hyaluronic acid, identified ultrastructurally as medium electron-dense material, or crystalline, scroll-like structures, may be found in tumor neolumina, embedding microvilli, or in the extracellular space.[15,246]

Certain ultrastructural observations when present would tend to exclude a diagnosis of mesothelioma. These include the presence of mucous granules, dense core neuroendocrine granules, zymogen granules, and Clara cell granules. Adenocarcinomas derived from Type II pneumocytes may contain multivesicular and lamellar bodies not seen in mesothelioma cells. Similarly, the presence of pinocytotic vesicles together with Weibel-Palade bodies is pathognomonic of vascular endothelial differentiation, which would suggest a diagnosis of epithelioid hemangioendothelioma or pleural angiosarcoma.

Sarcomatoid mesotheliomas generally have ultrastructural features that resemble those of soft tissue fibrosarcomas (Figure 5-13D).[2,15,241,252] The features of these spindled tumor cells are elongate nuclei with prominent nucleoli, short cytoplasmic fragments of distended rough endoplasmic reticulum, occasionally prominent intermediate cytoplasmic filaments, and variable quantities of extracellular collagen. In some cases, the tumor cells resemble myofibroblasts, with peripherally located actin filaments, occasionally associated with dense bodies.[15,253] Cells with transitional features intermediate between epithelial and mesenchymal cells have been described. These include the presence of intercellular junctions, occasional surface microvilli, partial or incomplete basal lamina, and even a few tonofibrillar bundles.

Differential Diagnosis

Malignant mesothelioma must be distinguished from benign, reactive mesothelial proliferations on the one hand, and on the other, from various primary and secondary malignancies involving the serosal membranes. The distinction between reactive and malignant mesothelial proliferations constitutes a major difficulty in diagnostic surgical pathology, especially when dealing with small specimens such as needle biopsies. In cases of both epithelial and spindle cell proliferations, the demonstration of true stromal invasion is the most accurate hallmark of malignancy.[184] The demonstration of such invasion may not be possible in small, superficial biopsies, and caution is warranted to avoid the pitfall of overinterpreting a tangentially cut section. Additionally, benign processes and organizing effusions may result in the entrapment of reactive mesothelium in organizing fibroinflammatory and granulation tissues, mimicking stromal invasion. Linear, in situ proliferations of mesothelial cells projecting into the cavity lumen should not be diagnosed as malignant, except in the setting of unequivocal stromal invasion.

Densely packed sheets of mesothelial cells within body cavities may actually be common in reactive conditions involving the serosal membranes, but such collections within the confines of stroma favor malignancy. The demonstration of cytologic atypia may not be helpful in the distinction of benign versus malignant, as reactive mesothelial hyperplasia may be accompanied by striking atypia, and some epithelial mesotheliomas may show bland and monotonous cytologic features.[184] Necrosis is typically associated with malignant processes, but may be seen in benign conditions as well. Ordonez has shown that lesions described as nodular mesothelial hyperplasia, while not readily confused with mesothelioma, are primarily histiocytic proliferations with positive immunoreactivity for CD 68, and are cytokeratin negative.[254] In some cases, sampling may show obvious malignant mesothelioma at one site, and atypical, reactive changes at another. With generous sampling and careful attention to histologic and cytologic detail, the distinction between malignant epithelial mesothelioma and reactive mesothelial hyperplasia is generally possible in an adequate biopsy specimen.[2]

Similar difficulties may be encountered when attempting to distinguish reactive fibroblastic processes involving the serosal membranes, in particular the pleura (Figure 5-14A), and the sarcomatoid and desmoplastic variants of malignant mesothelioma. Fibrous pleurisy often features a "top heavy" zonation phenomenon, with areas of greatest cellularity and accompanying atypia at the interface with the pleural space, and increasing maturation of fibrosis with reduction in cellularity proceeding toward the chest wall. Such a graded pattern of cellularity, atypia and fibrosis is not a feature of sarcomatoid or desmoplastic tumors. The presence of elongate, vertical capillaries perpendicular to the pleural surface are typical of organizing effusions and fibrous pleurisy (Figure 5-14B), and are not a typical feature of sarcomatoid mesotheliomas. The demonstration of invasion is an important indicator of malignancy (Figure 5-14C). Immunoperoxidase stains for cytokeratins are useful in illustrating the distribution of mesothelial cells, and may reinforce the demonstration of invasion by showing cytokeratin-positive cells in subpleural soft tissues. Immunoreactivity for anticytokeratins per se is of no utility, as both benign and malignant mesothelial proliferations will display this pattern (Figure 5-14D). Patterns of immunostaining for p53, commonly positive in

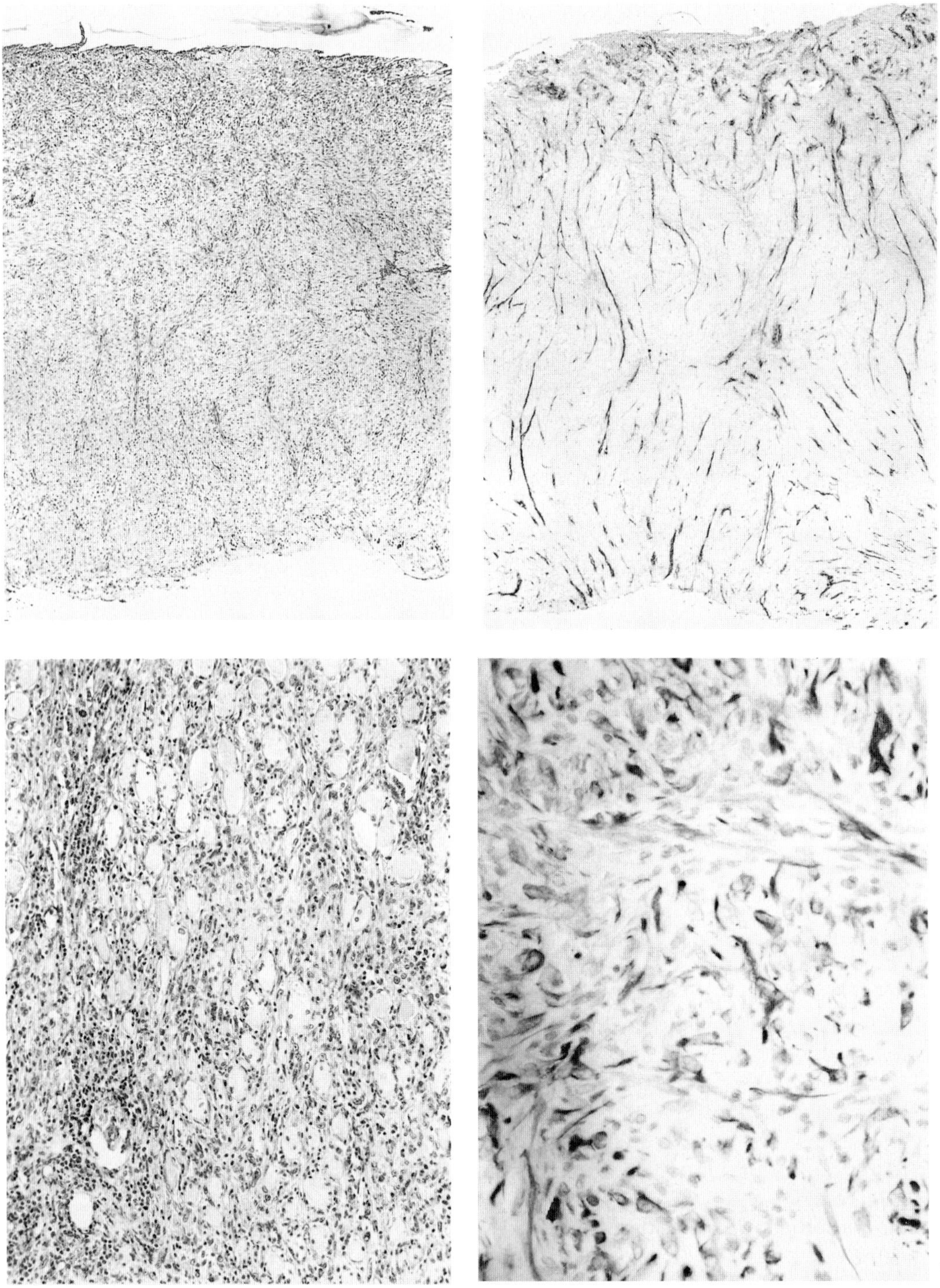

Figure 5-14. (A) Chronic organizing pleuritis shows a fibrinous surface exudate and markedly thickened parietal pleura. **(B)** Immunoperoxidase staining for Factor VIII antigen delineates capillaries oriented perpendicular to the pleural surface almost completely traversing the fibrotic, thickened pleura. **(C)** Invasion of skeletal muscle fibers of chest wall by sarcomatoid pleural mesothelioma. **(D)** Immunoperoxidase staining for cytokeratins shows positive-staining spindle cells in chronic organizing pleuritis. ((A), (B), and (D) from the same case.) (A) and (B) ×40; (C) ×130; (D) ×325.

mesothelioma, are nevertheless unreliable indicators of benign versus malignant mesothelial proliferations in individual cases.[184] In view of the gravity of the diagnosis of malignant mesothelioma, a conservative approach toward its diagnosis is favored in equivocal cases.

Distinguishing between metastatic adenocarcinoma and the epithelial variant of malignant mesothelioma is the most common diagnostic problem confronting the surgical pathologist confronted with a biopsy of an epithelioid pleural malignancy. This problem, too, is magnified in the small biopsy specimen. The diagnostic adjuncts to assist in this distinction, including histochemistry, immunohistochemistry and electron microscopy, are discussed in detail in their respective sections. In addition, the expected results of common immunohistochemical stains used to distinguish mesothelioma from adenocarcinoma are listed in Table 5-2. Renal cell carcinoma metastatic to the pleura may be especially difficult to distinguish from pleural mesothelioma, as these tumors may feature sarcomatoid foci and exhibit an overlapping immunophenotype with coexpression of cytokeratins and vimentin and negative CEA expression.[255] The authors have observed ten such cases, and believe that a diagnosis of pleural mesothelioma should not be made in a patient with a solid renal mass that has not been sampled histologically.

Other neoplasms that may involve the pleura include localized fibrous tumors as well as leukemias and lymphomas, the latter requiring distinction from the lymphohistiocytoid variant of malignant mesothelioma.[178] Localized fibrous tumors are usually distinguished by the gross distribution as a pedunculated pleural tumor displaying the cytokeratin-negative, CD 34-positive immunophenotype. Soft issue

Table 5-2. Expected immunohistochemical staining results for mesothelioma vs. adenocarcinoma

Antibody	Mesothelioma	Adenocarcinoma
Keratin cocktail	Pos.	Pos.
Cytokeratins 5/6	Pos.	Neg.[a]
Cytokeratin 7	Pos.	Pos/Neg[b]
Cytokeratin 20	Neg	Pos/Neg[b]
CEA	Neg.	Pos.
BerEP4	Neg.	Pos.
LeuM1 (CD15)	Neg.	Pos.
B72.3	Neg.	Pos.
EMA	Pos.	Pos.[c]
HMFG-2	Pos.	Pos.[c]
Calretinin	Pos. (N)	Neg.
Thrombomodulin	Pos.	Neg.
HBME-1	Pos.	Neg.
E-cadherin	Neg.	Pos.
N-cadherin	Pos.	Neg.
TTF-1	Neg.	Pos. (N)

[a] Many adenocarcinomas of extrapulmonary origin may stain positive. See Ref. 277.
[b] Varying combinations of CK7 and CK20 positivity are seen in adenocarcinomas, depending upon primary site. See Ref. 208.
[c] Distribution of staining is primarily membranous in mesothelioma, cytoplasmic in adenocarcinoma.
Pos. = positive staining; Neg. = negative staining; N = nuclear staining.

sarcomas most commonly involve the pleura via direct extension from the chest wall, or as metastatic disease with hematogenous spread to the lung and thence to the pleura. This pattern of metastatic involvement has not been observed to result in the diffuse pleural thickening seen in advanced mesothelioma.[19] Metastatic sarcomas rarely pose a diagnostic problem, which may be further simplified by observing patterns of cytokeratin expression, which should be negative in the sarcoma and positive in sarcomatoid malignant mesotheliomas. However, some soft tissue sarcomas have been reported as primary pleural tumors. Those that seem to show a predilection for this include synovial sarcoma, angiosarcoma, and epithelioid hemangioendothelioma (EHE).

Primary vascular malignancies of the pleura are uncommon. The authors have observed seven cases, with an additional 29 reported in the literature. Six of our cases and 10 of those reported in the literature were EHE. Weiss and Enzinger originally described EHE as a vascular malignancy of soft tissue with clinical behavior intermediate between hemangioma and angiosarcoma.[256] EHE has also been described in the lung, initially as intravascular bronchiolar and alveolar tumor (IVBAT),[257] subsequently recognized to be the pulmonary form of the EHE.[258] In our experience, EHE of the pleura features a gross distribution identical to that of malignant (diffuse) pleural mesothelioma, forming a thick rind of tumor encasing the lung and spreading along fissures and secondary interlobular septa. Moreover, the clinical behavior of this tumor parallels that of malignant mesothelioma, with survival measured in months. Despite an epithelioid appearance, EHE is rather easily distinguished from mesothelioma using immunohistochemistry with positive staining observed in these cases for the vascular markers CD34, CD31, and/or Factor VIII, combined with negative immunoreactivity for anticytokeratins.[155–158] Angiosarcomas of the pleura are exceedingly rare as well, and consist of pleomorphic malignant endothelial cells lining irregular and anastomosing vascular spaces. These tumors display an identical immunophenotype to that of EHE, with negative immunoreactivity to anticytokeratins and positive immunoreactivity to vascular markers. Both tumors may contain diagnostic Weibel Palade bodies ultrastructurally, although these are less common in angiosarcoma.

Synovial sarcoma (SS) may, under unusual circumstances, provide a pitfall in the diagnosis of malignant pleural mesothelioma. Typically occurring in the thorax as metastatic tumor, SS has nonetheless been reported as a primary tumor of the lung, pleura, and mediastinum.[259–262] A typically biphasic tumor with epithelial and sarcomatous components with at least focal expression of cytokeratins and EMA, SS may mimic biphasic or sarcomatoid mesotheliomas. Moreover, in a review of 103 cases of SS, Miettinen et al. found foci of calretinin expression in 29/41 (71%) biphasic SS, particularly in the spindle cell component.[259] In contrast, epithelial mesotheliomas expressed calretinin diffusely while sarcomatoid mesotheliomas showed variable expression for this marker. BerEP4 and cytokeratins 5/6 were frequently expressed by SS. Differences in expression of cytokeratins by monophasic SS compared with sarcomatoid mesotheliomas have been found to be of help in distinguishing these two tumors.[261] Finally, identification of the SYT/SSX transcript may be useful for confirming a diagnosis of SS of the pleura.[261,263]

The accurate premortem diagnosis of mesothelioma involves a multitiered approach, beginning with information regarding the gross distribution of tumor. This information is seldom directly available to the pathologist when a small biopsy specimen is received for review in the laboratory. Information about the gross distribution can be obtained from radiologic studies, such as chest roentgenograms, CT or MRI of the thorax, or observations of the surgeon at time of thoracoscopy or thoracotomy for pleural tumors, and CT or MRI of the abdomen and pelvis or observations of the surgeon at time of laparoscopy or laparotomy for peritoneal or pelvic tumors. If the gross distribution is consistent with mesothelioma, then the next tier involves histologic assessment of the tumor for one or more of the patterns listed in Table 5-1. For tumors with visible secretions on routine histology, we then employ histochemical studies including PAS following diastase predigestion and alcian blue with and without hyaluronidase. If the secretions stain with DPAS and with alcian blue both before and after hyaluronidase, then adenocarcinoma is favored. If the secretions stain with alcian blue but are negative for DPAS and for alcian blue after hyaluronidase, then mesothelioma is favored (Figures 5-9 and 5-10).

The fourth tier involves immunohistochemical studies. The panel used in our laboratory differs somewhat by tumor type and location and is summarized in Table 5-3. For epithelial or biphasic tumors involving the pleura or the peritoneum, a cocktail of anticytokeratin antibodies that includes AE1/AE3, CAM 5.2, and MNF.116 is used to exclude lymphoma, melanoma, and epithelioid hemangioendothelioma. Epithelial mesotheliomas and most carcinomas stain strongly and diffusely with this antibody cocktail. Calretinin and CK 5/6 are also employed, as these stain a high percentage of epithelial mesotheliomas but a relatively low percentage of adenocarcinomas. Nuclear staining for Zymed calretinin antibody is highly specific and sensitive for mesotheliomas. For pleural tumors, the panel is rounded out with

Table 5-3. Suggested immunohistochemical panel for mesothelioma diagnosis

| | Epithelial or Biphasic | | Sarcomatoid |
	Pleural	Peritoneal	
1st Line	Cytokeratin cocktail Calretinin Cytokeratins 5/6 CEA TTF-1	Cytokeratin cocktail Calretinin Cytokeratins 5/6 BerEP4 B72.3	Cytokeratin cocktail Vimentin
2nd Line	LeuM1 B72.3 BerEP4	LeuM1 Thrombomodulin HBME-1	

CEA = carcinoembryonic antigen; TTF-1 = thyroid transcription factor-1. See text for details.

CEA and TTF-1, which stain a high percentage of pulmonary adeno-carcinomas and a very low percentage of mesotheliomas. LeuM1, BerEP4, and B72.3 are held in reserve for cases with discordant immunohistochemical findings. For peritoneal tumors, CEA and TTF-1 are less effective at excluding adenocarcinomas, so BerEP4 and B72.3 are substituted. LeuM1, HBME-1, and thrombomodulin are second line antibodies for cases with discordant results.

Most of the antibodies that stain epithelial mesotheliomas have inconsistent or focal staining for sarcomatoid mesotheliomas. There-fore, the only antibodies we use for pure sarcomatoid malignancies involving the serosal membranes are vimentin and the cytokeratin cocktail. A high percentage of sarcomatoid mesotheliomas stain strongly and diffusely positive for low molecular weight cytokeratins, whereas most sarcomas are either negative or focally positive. Cyto-keratin stains are also useful for detecting subtle invasion in desmo-plastic mesotheliomas. Vimentin is a useful indicator of appropriate fix-ation, as a negative stain for vimentin in a sarcomatoid malignancy probably indicates poor fixation. Sarcomatoid mesotheliomas rarely are cytokeratin negative, and at least a portion of these are also vimentin negative.

The fifth tier of investigation is electron microscopy. An accurate diagnosis of mesothelioma can be made on an adequately sampled tumor in the vast majority of cases using the first four tiers of investi-gation. Therefore, we reserve ultrastructural studies for those cases in which the diagnosis remains in doubt. Examples include cases with discordant immunohistochemistry after the second line antibodies have been used, or very unusual variants such as localized malignant mesothelioma or the so-called "mucin-positive" mesothelioma.

Peritoneal Mesothelioma

The peritoneum is the second most common site of involvement by malignant (diffuse) mesothelioma, accounting for approximately 10% of cases. Peritoneal mesotheliomas demonstrate spread over the peri-toneal surface of abdominal viscera leading to encasement of the organs in a rind of tumor, a growth pattern similar to that encountered in the pleural form where growth over the visceral and parietal pleurae occurs. The tumor is typically firm and white, studding the peritoneal surface with numerous individual nodules, in a pattern indistinguish-able grossly from peritoneal carcinomatosis (Figure 5-15). Plaques of tumor or matted tumor masses may also be seen. The omentum is often thickened by infiltrating tumor, and adhesions between viscera and abdominal wall may be prominent. This gross distribution of tumor readily explains the typical clinical presenting complaints of abdomi-nal pain, weight loss, obstruction or abdominal mass. Increased abdominal girth may also be reported as a result of the accumulation of copious ascites, or peritoneal fluid. This fluid may be watery and transudative, or viscous because of the presence of hyaluronic acid, the latter feature suggestive of the diagnosis of mesothelioma but by no means specific.

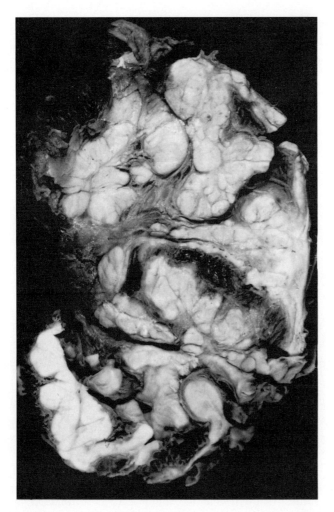

Figure 5-15. Coronal slice of abdominal viscera in patient with malignant (diffuse) peritoneal mesothelioma shows encasement and compression of bowel (dark areas) by confluent tumor nodules. (Reprinted from Ref. 2, with permission.)

As with pleural mesotheliomas, clinically evident distant metastases are seldom noted at initial presentation, although they are commonly detected at autopsy.[125,161] Extension to involve one or both pleural cavities may occur,[264] making it difficult to discern the exact site of origin.[19] At autopsy, careful inspection of the organs is necessary in order to exclude a primary malignancy with secondary peritoneal carcinomatosis, as may often occur with adenocarcinomas of the stomach, pancreas and ovaries.[2]

The diagnosis of malignant peritoneal mesothelioma depends on the findings of the typical gross features as described earlier, the identification of a histologic pattern compatible with mesothelioma, and the exclusion of metastatic disease involving the peritoneal cavity (peritoneal carcinomatosis). Information regarding the gross distribution of tumor may be obtained from computed tomographic (CT) scans of the

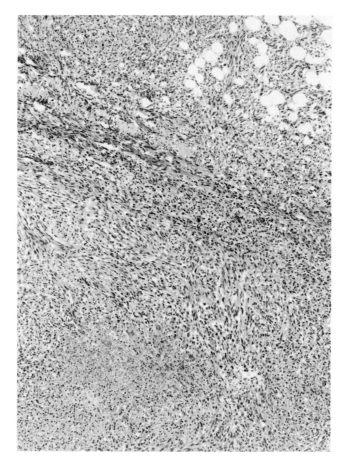

Figure 5-16. Sarcomatoid diffuse peritoneal mesothelioma shows invasion of peritoneal fat (*upper right*) and a focus of necrosis (*lower left*). Extensive sampling at autopsy showed that the tumor had a sarcomatoid appearance throughout. H&E ×68.

abdomen that may show mesenteric thickening, ascites and peritoneal studding. Some patients with advanced peritoneal mesothelioma may only have modest abnormalities on CT scans, and magnetic resonance imaging may provide additional information in this regard.[265,266] Surgical exploration may be required to inspect the abdominal viscera for the presence of primary tumors and to obtain sufficient tissue for pathologic diagnosis. The observations of the surgeon at time of laparoscopy/laparotomy are clearly useful for determining the gross distribution of tumor. In a report of eighteen cases of peritoneal mesotheliomas diagnosed by laparoscopy and peritoneal biopsy, eight diagnoses were rejected following subsequent pathologic review.[267]

Peritoneal mesotheliomas exhibit the same histologic spectrum as pleural mesotheliomas. In one of the authors' series of 185 peritoneal mesotheliomas, 127 were epithelial, 51 were biphasic, and only seven were purely sarcomatoid (Figure 5-16). Cases of diffuse peritoneal mesothelioma have also been reported in which the tumor presented as innumerable cysts involving the visceral and parietal peri-toneum.[268–270] It has been argued, however, that such cases do not rep-resent mesotheliomas at all, but are examples of nonneoplastic reactive mesothelial proliferation.[271] In this regard, we have never seen an example of so-called "peritoneal cystic mesothelioma" in over 180 peri-toneal mesotheliomas reviewed for litigation purposes. The histo-chemical, immunohistochemical, and ultrastructural features of peritoneal mesothelioma are similar to those of pleural mesothelioma, although fewer cases have been studied.[2,19,125,193,240,244,272–274]

Malignant peritoneal mesothelioma must be distinguished from other papillary peritoneal tumors in women, metastatic carcinoma with secondary involvement of the peritoneum, as well as reactive mesothe-lial hyperplasia. The peritoneal mesothelium has a remarkable capac-ity for undergoing marked hyperplastic changes, most notably in patients with cirrhosis and ascites. Florid hyperplastic changes include the formation of papillary structures, pseudoacini and squamous nests.[275] Immunoperoxidase stains will not reliably permit the separa-tion of reactive changes from neoplasia, but the demonstration of inva-sion, nuclear anaplasia, and focal necrosis may be diagnostic in this regard. Metastatic adenocarcinomas involving the peritoneum fre-quently express mucin (Figure 5-17A), which may be detected using

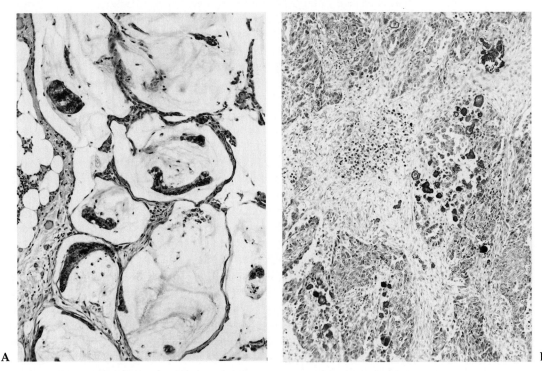

Figure 5-17. (A) Metastatic mucin-producing adenocarcinoma in the peritoneum consists of pools of mucin within spaces lined by delicate connective tissue stroma. Some of the spaces are partially lined by a layer of tall columnar tumor cells. (Reprinted from Ref. 2, with permission.) **(B)** Serous papillary adenocarcinoma of the peritoneum contains numerous psammoma bodies in this field. These tumors often have PAS-positive cytoplasmic mucin vacuoles as well. (A) and (B) ×100.

PAS stain following diastase predigestion, a histochemical finding distinctly unusual in mesothelioma.

A broad histologic spectrum of primary papillary serous tumors of the peritoneum may occur in women. These tumors may show histologic similarities to both epithelial mesothelioma as well as papillary tumors of the ovary, and presumably derive from extraovarian epithelium with Mullerian potential. Such serous papillary adenocarcinomas of the peritoneum often show considerable nuclear anaplasia and mitotic activity, and may contain numerous psammoma bodies (Figure 5-17B). Peritoneal epithelial mesotheliomas with papillary features may contain scattered psammoma bodies that are typically less prominent than those seen in papillary carcinomas.[11,19] In some serous papillary carcinomas, psammoma bodies are so prominent that the term *psammocarcinoma* has been suggested.[276] Papillary serous adenocarcinomas of the peritoneum will usually demonstrate intracytoplasmic mucin granules with the PAS stain, and display an immunophenotype typical of carcinoma. Some caution in the interpretation of negative CEA staining is warranted in peritoneal mesotheliomas, as a substantial proportion of ovarian adenocarcinomas will display this pattern. Similarly, a number of malignancies involving the peritoneal cavity will stain positive for CK 5/6, so such staining should be interpreted with caution.[277] In cases with conflicting or equivocal immunohistochemical data, examination of tumor cell ultrastructure will often demonstrate the long branching microvilli characteristic of mesothelioma[240,244,278] or the short stubby microvilli of carcinoma.[243]

Peritoneal mesotheliomas account for between 17–32% of the mesotheliomas affecting women in the United States.[5,161,279] In contrast to the generally dismal prognosis associated with pleural mesotheliomas, the prognosis for peritoneal mesotheliomas is less predictable, especially in women. Goldblum and Hart's review of 19 peritoneal mesotheliomas in women found considerable overlapping histologic features in the mesotheliomas displaying both indolent and aggressive behavior, and found survivorship to be determined largely by gross distribution, with solitary tumors conveying a good prognosis, but the opposite for diffuse tumors.[173] Kerrigan et al. reviewed a series of 25 peritoneal mesotheliomas in women that were exclusively diffuse. Controlling for age at time of diagnosis, presentation and form of treatment, these investigators found that there were no morphologic attributes that could reliably predict the behavior of any given tumor. Survivorship in this population ranged from 1 month to 15 years. The authors concluded from these observations that the spectrum of diffuse epithelial peritoneal mesotheliomas includes forms with aggressive behavior related to pleural mesotheliomas, as well as to more indolent forms, and that morphologic data alone do not appear predictive of clinical behavior in this population.[279] An indolent behavior is often observed for well-differentiated papillary mesotheliomas of the peritoneum in women (Figure 5-5D). However, when invasion is present, these tumors may behave more aggressively.[174]

Peritoneal mesotheliomas are strongly associated with asbestos exposure, especially in men. Asbestosis is present in approximately

50% of cases of peritoneal mesotheliomas, compared to approximately 20% of pleural mesotheliomas.[51] Epidemiologic studies comparing degree of asbestos exposure with occupation and ultimate site of mesothelioma development point to the peritoneal site as being associated with longer and more intense exposures to asbestos.[51,54,56] Peritoneal mesotheliomas follow exposure to commercial amphibole fibers (amosite or crocidolite), but have not convincingly been related to exposure to chrysotile asbestos.[280]

Mesothelioma of the Tunica Vaginalis Testis

The tunica vaginalis testis is formed by an outpouching of the abdominal peritoneal membrane and is lined by a layer of mesothelial cells. Thus it is an extension of the peritoneum. Infrequently, a malignant mesothelioma may originate in this location. Initially described by Barbera et al. in 1957,[281] this uncommon tumor has since been reported in single case and series form by others,[282–284] including a case reported in a 6 year old.[285] The collective experience with this tumor would indicate the reporting of fewer than 80 cases worldwide. These tumors present clinically as hydroceles or paratesticular masses, whose malignant nature may not be suspected until pathologic evaluation of surgical material. The tumor has the potential for local and regional spread, as well as distant and fatal metastases. An aggressive clinical course is typical, especially in those tumors not completely excised at the outset.

The histologic spectrum and immunophenotype are similar to that of malignant mesotheliomas from other sites, and include papillary (epithelial), sarcomatoid, and biphasic variants.[282,284] The ultrastructural features of the epithelial variants that have been examined are similar to those of epithelial mesotheliomas occurring elsewhere. A causative role for asbestos in some cases is favored. In Jones' report, the issue of asbestos exposure was specifically addressed in only 27 of 64 cases. In eleven of these cases (41%), an occupational exposure to asbestos was reported.[282] Plas' review of the literature concerning mesothelioma of the tunica vaginalis testis indicates a positive history of asbestos exposure in 34.2%.[283] The real prevalence of asbestos exposure in this patient population may be underestimated because of a lack of historical information. Causative roles for radiation, testicular trauma, or viral infection have not been convincingly demonstrated.[283]

The differential diagnosis chiefly includes carcinoma of the rete testis, which shares gross and histologic similarities with mesothelioma. Experience with the immunophenotype of rete testis carcinoma is limited, but potentially useful diagnostic information may be obtained on ultrastructural examination, as rete testis tumors tend to show microvillus features of length/width ratios more typical of carcinoma.[282,286] The differential diagnosis also includes adenomatoid tumor. This tumor often involves the epididymis, displays ultrastructural evidence of mesothelial differentiation, but is usually noninfiltrative and sharply circumscribed.[287] Carcinomas of the lung and prostate are among the tumors that may commonly metastasize to the testis, but sharp differences in histology and immunophenotype should permit the distinction.

Pericardial Mesothelioma

Primary malignant mesotheliomas of the pericardium are distinctly uncommon, with approximately 100 cases reported in the literature involving the adult and pediatric population.[2,136,288,289] These tumors invade the parietal and visceral pericardium, eventually encasing the heart in a rind of tumor (Figure 5-18). Patients typically present with pericardial effusion or mediastinal mass that may be accompanied by arrhythmias, congestive heart failure, pericardial constriction, or cardiac tamponade.[290–292] Chest roentgenograms show cardiac enlargement or a mass, and low voltage may be demonstrable in anterior precordial leads on electrocardiogram. Magnetic resonance imaging may also provide detailed information regarding location and extent of tumor.[293]

Microscopic examination of the pericardial tumors has shown a biphasic pattern in most cases, but epithelial and sarcomatoid variants have also been described.[136] Immunohistochemical and ultrastructural

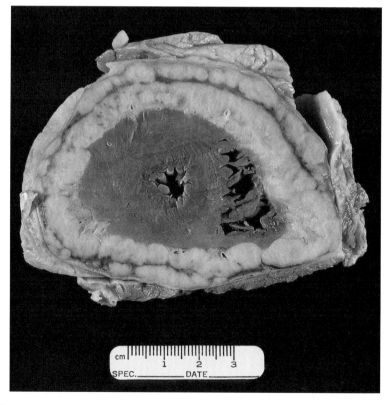

Figure 5-18. Transverse section of heart, showing complete encasement by malignant pericardial mesothelioma.

studies have only rarely been described,[290,291,294] but these tumors appear morphologically identical to their pleural and peritoneal counterparts. Pericardial mesotheliomas must be distinguished from the much more common carcinoma directly extending into or metastatic to the epicardium or pericardium.[295,296] In addition, pleural mesotheliomas may also directly extend into and invade the contiguous pericardium, further complicating the diagnosis of primary pericardial mesothelioma.[19] The so-called mesothelioma of the atrioventricular node is a benign tumor not derived from mesothelium at all, but from endoderm.[2,297–299] An exposure to asbestos has been established in several patients suffering from pericardial mesothelioma.[300–303]

Treatment and Prognosis

The prognosis of malignant (diffuse) mesothelioma is poor. In most series, a median survival between 4 and 18 months is expected for the pleural forms.[304–311] Death typically results from respiratory failure or infection, but involvement of the heart and transdiaphragmatic involvement of abdominal viscera may also contribute to mortality.[312,313] Physicians experienced in treating mesothelioma will report occasional patients with significantly greater longevity following treatment. Consequently, a limited set of prognostic factors has been derived to predict outcome and to identify those patients most likely to receive benefit from radical treatment regimens. Numerous studies evaluating clinical prognostic factors have been reported over the past 20 years, identifying the importance of age, sex, performance status, weight loss, chest pain and clinical stage.[304] Conflicting data have been reported due in part to variances in disease staging, therapies given, assessment of response, and enrollment eligibility.

The issue of clinical stage as a prognosticator is particularly problematic. Surprisingly, several studies found stage not to be an important prognostic factor.[304] This may be related to the necessity for exploratory and cytoreductive surgery to fulfill all staging descriptors. Such criteria have not been fulfilled for most patients with mesothelioma, even at centers with special expertise in treatment and management of this disease. Thus, most historical staging data are only approximate. The prognostic scoring systems of the Cancer and Leukemia Group (CALGB) and European Organization for the Research and Treatment of Cancer (EORTC) have been applied to large numbers of patients with mesothelioma.[310,311] These distinct scoring systems have identified poor prognostic indicators which include nonepithelial subtype, male gender, poor performance status, and hematologic parameters of low hemoglobin, high leukocyte and platelet counts and high serum lactic dehydrogenase (LDH).[311] In a retrospective review of 121 cases of malignant pleural mesothelioma, univariate analysis demonstrated lower rates of survival in patients with poor performance status and nonepithelial histologic subtypes, and found that any form of treatment beyond supportive care led to longer survival.[314]

Table 5-4. The Butchart staging system

Stage	Definition
I.	Tumor is confined to the capsule of the parietal pleura (i.e., involves only the ipsilateral lung, pericardium, and/or diaphragm)
II.	Tumor invades the chest wall or mediastinal structures (e.g., Esophagus, heart, and/or contraleral pleura), or Tumor involves intrathoracic lymph nodes
III.	Tumor penetrates the diaphragm to involve peritoneum, or Tumor involves the contralateral pleura, or Tumor involves extrathoracic lymph nodes
IV.	Distant blood-borne metastases

Source: From Ref. 316

Many clinicians approach patients with malignant mesothelioma with a certain amount of therapeutic nihilism, mindful that single modality therapy has failed to change the natural history of the disease in a meaningful fashion.[315] Debate continues as to the selection of patients for cytoreductive surgery and adjuvant therapeutic modalities, and the identification of patients likely to receive benefit from such an approach. This controversy is in part the result of the lack of a universally accepted staging system for pleural mesothelioma. An ideal staging system should incorporate clinical and pathologic data to stratify survival and thereby tailor a therapeutic approach to the tumor. Several such staging systems have been offered, but none are universally accepted and most do not live up to the ideal. Butchart et al. proposed their staging system in 1976, and it remained popular despite its basis on only 29 patients and failure to stratify survival (Table 5-4).[316] Other staging proposals include Sugarbaker's revised Brigham/Dana-Farber Cancer Institute system and the somewhat complex system proposed by International Mesothelioma Interest Group (IMIG) (Tables 5-5 and 5-6).[317,318] Sugarbaker's system has the advantage of simplicity and results in survival stratification, but has yet to be validated in an independent patient population. In the Brigham/Dana-Farber experience, survivals following radical pleural pneumonectomy and adjuvant chemoradiotherapy of 25, 20, and 16 months were reported for their stage I, II, and III cohorts, respectively.[317]

Table 5-5. Revised staging system proposed by Sugarbaker et al., Brigham/Dana-Farber Cancer Institute

Stage	Definition
I	Disease completely resected within the capsule of the parietal pleura without adenopathy: ipsilateral pleura, lung, pericardium, diaphragm, or chest wall disease limited to previous biopsy sites
II	All of stage I with positive resection margins and/or intrapleural adenopathy
III	Local extension into the chest wall or mediastinum; into the heart or through the diaphragm or peritoneum; or with extrapleural lymph node involvement
IV	Distant metastatic disease

Source: From Ref. 317

Table 5-6. Staging system proposed by the International Mesothelioma Interest Group (IMIG)

Tumor (T) staging

Tla Tumor limited to the ipsilateral parietal pleura, including the mediastinal and diaphragmatic pleura, without involvement of visceral pleura

Tlb Tla + scattered foci of tumor involving the visceral pleura

T2 Tumor involving each of the ipsilateral pleural surfaces (parietal, mediastinal, diaphragmatic, and visceral pleura

- Involvement of diaphragmatic muscle
- Confluent visceral pleural tumor (including the fissures) or extension of tumor from the visceral pleura into the underlying pulmonary parenchyma

T3 Locally advanced but potentially resectable tumor. The tumor involves all of the ipsilateral pleural surfaces with at least one of the following features:

- Involvement of the endothoracic fascia
- Extension into the mediastinal fat
- A solitary, completely resectable focus of tumor extending into the soft tissues of the chest wall
- Nontransmural involvement of the pericardium

T4 Locally advanced, technically unresectable tumor. The tumor involves all of the ipsilateral pleural surfaces with at least one of the following features:

- Diffuse extension or metastatic spread to the chest wall with or without rib destruction
- Direct transdiaphragmatic extension to the peritoneum
- Direct extension to the contralateral pleura
- Direct extension to any mediastinal organ
- Direct extension to the spine

Lymph node (N) staging

Nx Regional lymph nodes (LNs) cannot be assessed

N0 No regional LN metastases

N1 Involvement of ipsilateral bronchopulmonary or hilar LNs

N2 Involvement of subcarinal or ipsilateral mediastinal LNs (including the internal mammary LNs)

N3 Involvement of the contralateral mediastinal or internal mammary LNs or any supraclavicular LNs

Metastases (M) staging

Mx Presence of distant metastases cannot be assessed

M0 No distant metastases

M1 Distant metastases present

Overall staging

Stage I		
	Ia	TIa N0M0
	Ib	T1b N0 M0
Stage II		T2 N0 M0
Stage III		Any T3 M0
		Any N2 M0
Stage IV		Any T4
		Any N3
		Any MI

Source: From Ref. 318

Unimodality therapy employing radiation appears infeasible because of the requirements of a large field imposed by diffuse tumor, and the potential for injury to vital thoracic structures by large doses of radiation. Low response rates, at the expense of radiation toxicity, limit the efficacy of this modality.[317] The surgical therapies for malignant pleural mesothelioma include pleurodesis, decortication and pleurectomy, and radical extrapleural pneumonectomy. To date, no randomized studies comparing the efficacy of these three procedures exist. Talc pleurodesis to palliate symptoms caused by pleural effusion has been shown to result in median survival similar to that of untreated patients. Decortication and pleurectomy and radical extrapleural pneumonectomy effect cytoreduction with curative intent. Neither results in significant prolongation of survival when offered as single modality treatment.

The largest studies of radical extrapleural pneumonectomy followed by chemoradiotherapy have been undertaken at Brigham and Women's hospital. In a series of 183 patients undergoing this surgery, there were seven perioperative deaths. The remaining 176 patients underwent adjuvant chemoradiotherapy, resulting in 2- and 5-year survival rates of 38% and 15% respectively, the longest in any reported series. Of the patients with epithelial histologies, negative operative margins, and negative mediastinal nodal involvement, 2- and 5-year survivals of 68% and 46% respectively were recorded. Prognostic indicators for this cohort of patients included histologic subtype, lymph node involvement, extrapleural extension, and integrity of operative margins. No 5-year survival was recorded in patients with sarcomatoid histology, mediastinal node involvement, or positive margins.[317] This experience has yet to be duplicated, but earlier detection of disease combined with further developments of novel therapies, improved chemotherapy, and aggressive surgical approaches may result in improved outcomes in the future.

Some studies have suggested that survival for peritoneal mesotheliomas is worse than that for its pleural counterpart,[306,319] although this observation was not confirmed in a large study of 1475 cases conducted by the Surveillance, Epidemiology, and End Results (SEER) program.[308] The prognosis for this tumor remains poor overall, with median survival of untreated peritoneal mesotheliomas ranging from 4 to 12 months in most series.[320–323] The optimism engendered by some reports of patients with early stage peritoneal mesotheliomas experiencing disease-free intervals following combined modality therapy[321,324] should be tempered by other reports of the not infrequently indolent nature of this disease, especially in women.[279]

References

1. *Stedman's Medical Dictionary*, 22nd ed. Baltimore: Williams & Wilkins, 1972.
2. Roggli VL, Kolbeck J, Sanfilippo F, Shelburne JD: Pathology of human mesothelioma: Etiologic and diagnostic considerations. *Pathol Annu* 22:91–131, 1987.
3. Kuhn C: The cells of the lung and their organelles. In: *The Biochemical Basis of Pulmonary Function* (Crystal RG, ed.), New York: Marcel Dekker, 1976, pp. 3–48.
4. Davis JMG: The histopathology and ultrastructure of pleural mesotheliomas produced in the rat by injections of crocidolite asbestos. *Br J Exp Pathol* 60:642–652, 1979.

5. Roggli VL, Oury TD, Moffatt EJ: Malignant mesothelioma in women. *Anat Pathol* 2:147–163, 1997.

6. Browne K: Asbestos-related disorders. In: *Occupational Lung Disorders*, 3rd ed. (Parkes WR, ed.) London: Butterworths, 1994, pp. 411–504.

7. McDonald JC: Health implications of environmental exposure to asbestos. *Environ Health Perspect* 62:319–328, 1985.

8. Spirtas R, Beebe GW, Connelly RR et al.: Recent trends in mesothelioma incidence in the United States. *Am J Ind Med* 9:397–407, 1986.

9. McDonald AD, McDonald JC: Epidemiology of malignant mesothelioma. In: *Asbestos-Related Malignancy* (Antman K, Aisner J, eds.) Orlando: Harcourt Brace Jovanovich, 1987, pp. 31–55.

10. National Cancer Institute SEER Cancer Statistics review 1973–1993. Bethesda, MD: National Cancer Institute, 1996.

11. Battifora H, McCaughey WTE: Tumors of the serosal membranes. *Atlas of Tumor Pathology*, 3rd Series, Fascicle 15. Washington DC: Armed Forces Institute of Pathology, 1994.

12. Aisner J, Wiernick PH: Malignant mesothelioma: Current status and future prospects. *Chest* 74:438–443, 1978.

13. Chahinian AP: Malignant mesothelioma. In: *Cancer Medicine* (Holland JF, Frei E III, eds.), Philadelphia: Lea & Febiger, 1982, pp. 1744–1751.

14. Wagner E: Das tuberkelahnliche lymphadenom. *Arch d Heilkunde* 11:497–526, 1870.

15. Hammar SP: Pleural diseases. Ch. 34 In: *Pulmonary Pathology*, 2nd ed. (Dail DH, Hammar SP, eds.), New York: Springer-Verlag, 1994, pp. 1463–1580.

16. Craighead JE: Eyes for the epidemiologist: The pathologist's role in shaping our understanding of the asbestos-associated diseases. *Am J Clin Pathol* 89:281–287, 1988.

17. Robertson HE: "Endothelioma" of the pleura. *J Cancer Res* 8:317–375, 1924.

18. Klemperer P, Rabin CB: Primary neoplasms of the pleura: Report of five cases. *Arch Pathol* 11:385–412, 1931.

19. McCaughey WTE, Kannerstein M, Churg J: Tumors and pseudotumors of the serosal membranes. *Atlas of Tumor Pathology*, 2nd Series, Fascicle 20. Washington DC: Armed Forces Institute of Pathology, 1985.

20. Castleman BI: *Asbestos: Medical and Legal Aspects*. New York: Harcourt Brace Jovanovich, 1984.

21. Gloyne SR: The morbid anatomy and histology of asbestosis. *Tubercle* 14:550–558, 1933.

22. Wedler HW: Uber den Lungenkrebs bei Asbestose. *Deutsch Arch Klin Med* 191:189–209, 1943.

23. Mallory TB, Castleman B, Parris EE: Case records of the Massachusetts General Hospital # 33111. *N Engl J Med* 236:407–412, 1947.

24. Lee DHK, Selikoff IJ: Historical background to the asbestos problem. *Environ Res* 18:300–314, 1979.

25. Keal EE: Asbestosis and abdominal neoplasms. *Lancet* 2:1211–1216, 1960.

26. Wagner JC, Sleggs CA, Marchand P: Diffuse pleural mesothelioma and asbestos exposure in Northwestern Cape Province. *Br J Ind Med* 17:260–271, 1960.

27. Edge JR, Choudhoury SL: Malignant mesothelioma of the pleura in Barrow-in-Furness. *Thorax* 33:26–30, 1978.

28. McDonald AD, McDonald JC: Malignant mesothelioma in North America. *Cancer* 46:1650–1656, 1980.

29. Otto H: Das berufsbedingte Mesotheliom in der BRD. *Pathologe* 2:8–18, 1980.

30. Churg A: Malignant mesothelioma in British Columbia in 1982. *Cancer* 5:672–674, 1985.
31. Andersson M, Olsen JH: Trend and distribution of mesothelioma in Denmark. *Br J Cancer* 51:699–705, 1985.
32. Malker HSR, McLaughlin JK, Malker BK: Occupational risks for pleural mesotheliomas in Sweden, 1961–79. *J Natl Cancer Inst* 74:61–66,1985.
33. Connelly RR, Spirtas R, Myers MH, Percy CL, Fraumeni JF: Demographic patterns for mesothelioma in the United States. *J Natl Cancer Inst* 78:1053–1060, 1987.
34. Ferguson DA, Berry G, Jelihovsky T: The Australian Mesothelioma Surveillance Program 1979–1985. *Med J Australia* 147:166–172, 1987.
35. Elmes PC, McCaughey WTE, Wade OL: Diffuse mesothelioma of the pleura and asbestos. *Br Med J* 1:350–353, 1965.
36. Newhouse ML, Thompson H: Mesothelioma of the pleura and peritoneum following exposure to asbestos in London area. *Br J Ind Med* 22:261–269, 1965.
37. McEwen I, Finlayson A, Mair A: Mesothelioma in Scotland. *Br Med J* 4:575–578, 1970.
38. McDonald AD, Harper A, El Attar OA: Epidemiology of primary malignant mesothelial tumors in Canada. *Cancer* 26:914–919, 1970.
39. Rubino GF, Scansetti G, Donna A: Epidemiology of pleural mesothelioma in northwestern Italy (Piedmont). *Br J Ind Med* 29:436, 1972.
40. Ashcroft T: Epidemiologic and quantitative relationships between mesothelioma and asbestos on Tyneside. *J Clin Pathol* 26:832–840, 1973.
41. Hain E, Dalquen P, Bohlig H: Retrospective study of 150 cases of mesothelioma in the Hamburg area. *Arch Arbeitsmed* 33:15–37, 1974.
42. Zielhuis RL, Versteeg JPJ, Planteydt HT: Pleural mesothelioma and exposure to asbestos: A retrospective case control study in the Netherlands. *Arch Occup Environ Health* 36:1–18, 1975.
43. Britton M: The epidemiology of mesothelioma. *Semin Oncol* 29:18–25, 2002.
44. Sheers G, Coles RM: Mesothelioma risks in a naval dockyard. *Arch Environ Health* 35:276–282, 1980.
45. Selikoff IJ, Hammond EC, Seidman H: Mortality experience of insulation workers in the United States and Canada, 1943–1976, In: Health hazards of asbestos exposure (Selikoff IJ, Hammond EC, eds.), *Ann NY Acad Sci* 330:91–116, 1979.
46. Ribak J, Lilis R, Suzuki Y, Penner L, Selikoff IJ: Malignant mesothelioma in a cohort of asbestos insulation workers: Clinical presentation, diagnosis, and causes of death. *Br J Ind Med* 45:182–187, 1988.
47. Churg A: Analysis of asbestos fibers from lung tissue: Research and diagnostic uses. *Sem Respir Med* 7:281–288, 1986.
48. Schenker MB, Garshick E, Munoz A, Woskie SR, Speizer FE: A population-based case-control study of mesothelioma deaths among U.S. railroad workers. *Am Rev Respir Dis* 134:461–465, 1986.
49. Mancuso TF: Relative risk of mesothelioma among railroad machinists exposed to chrysotile. *Am J Ind Med* 13:639–657, 1988.
50. Wolf KM, Piotrowski ZH, Engel JD, et al. Malignant mesotheliomas with occupational and environmental asbestos exposure in an Illinois community hospital. *Arch Intern Med* 147:2145–2149, 1987.
51. Roggli VL, Sharma A, Butnor KJ, Sporn T, Vollmer RT: Malignant mesothelioma and occupational exposure to asbestos: A clinicopathologic correlation of 1445 cases. *Ultrastruct Pathol* 26:1–11, 2002.
52. Antman KH: Malignant mesothelioma. *N Engl J Med* 303:200–202, 1980.

53. Craighead JE, Mossman BT: Pathogenesis of asbestos-associated diseases. *N Engl J Med* 306:1446–1455, 1982.

54. Talcott J, Thurber W, Gaensler E, Antman K, Li FP: Mesothelioma in manufacturers of asbestos-containing cigarette filters. *Lancet* I:392, 1987.

55. Driscoll RJ, Mulligan WJ, Schultz D, Candelaria A: Malignant mesothelioma: A cluster in a Native American pueblo. *N Engl J Med* 318:1437–1438, 1988.

56. Li FP, Dreyfus MG, Antman K: Asbestos-contaminated nappies and familial mesothelioma. *Lancet* I:909–910, 1989

57. National Research Council. *Non-occupational risks of asbestiform fibers.* Washington, DC: National Academy Press, 1984.

58. McDonald AD, McDonald JC: Mesothelioma after crocidolite exposure during gas mask manufacture. *Environ Res* 17:340–347, 1978.

59. Selikoff IJ, Hammond EC, Seidman H: Latency of asbestos disease among insulation workers in the United States and Canada. *Cancer* 46:2736–2740, 1980.

60. Churg A: Neoplastic asbestos-induced disease. Ch. 10 In: *Pathology of Occupational Lung Disease*, 2nd ed. (Churg A, Green FHY, eds.), Baltimore: Williams & Wilkins, 1998, pp. 339–392.

61. Peto J, Seidman H, Selikoff IJ: Mesothelioma mortality in asbestos workers: Implictions for models of carcinogenesis and risk assessment. *Br J Cancer* 45:124–135, 1982.

62. Chronic Hazard Advisory Panel on Asbestos: Report to the U.S. Consumer Product Safety Commission, Directorate for Health Sciences, Washington, DC, 1983.

63. Browne K, Smither WJ: Asbestos-related mesothelioma: Factors discriminating between pleural and peritoneal sites. *Br J Ind Med* 40:145–152, 1983.

64. Jarvholm B, Sanden A: Lung cancer and mesothelioma in the pleura and peritoneum among Swedish insulation workers. *Occup Environ Med* 55:766–770, 1998.

65. Roggli VL: Malignant mesothelioma and duration of asbestos exposure: Correlation with tissue mineral fiber content. *Ann Occup Hyg* 39:363–374, 1995.

66. Roggli VL, Pratt PC, Brody AR: Asbestos fiber types in malignant mesothelioma: An analytical scanning electron microscopic study. *Am J Ind Med* 23:605–614, 1993.

67. Dunnigan J: Linking chrysotile asbestos with mesothelioma. *Am J Ind Med* 14:205–209, 1988.

68. Churg A: On Dr. Dunnigan's commentary linking chrysotile asbestos with mesothelioma. *Am J Ind Med* 14:235–238, 1988.

69. Becklake MR: On Dr Dunnigan's commentary linking chrysotile asbestos with mesothelioma. *Am J Ind Med* 14:239–240, 1988.

70. Craighead JE: Response to Dr Dunnigan's commentary. *Am J Ind Med* 14:241–243, 1988.

71. Roggli VL, Pratt PC: Amphiboles and chrysotile asbestos exposure. *Am J Ind Med* 14:245–246, 1988.

72. McDonald JC: Tremolite, other amphiboles, and mesothelioma. *Am J Ind Med* 14:247–249, 1988.

73. Churg A, Wright JL, Vedal S: Fiber burden and patterns of disease in long term chrysotile miners and millers. *Am Rev Respir Dis* 148:25–31, 1993.

74. Churg A, DiPaoli L, Kempe B, Stevens B: Lung asbestos content in chrysotile workers with mesothelioma. *Am Rev Respir Dis* 130:1042–1045, 1984.

75. Dufresne A, Begin R, Churg A, Masse S. Mineral fibre content of lungs in mesothelioma cases seeking compensation in Quebec. *Am J Respir Crit Care Med* 153:711–718, 1996.
76. Churg A. Chrysotile, tremolite and mesothelioma in man. *Chest* 93:621–628, 1988.
77. Wagner JC, Berry G, Pooley FD: Mesotheliomas and asbestos type in asbestos textile workers: A study of lung contents. *Br Med J* 285:603–606, 1982
78. Green FHY, Harley R, Vallyathan V, et al.: Exposure and mineralogical correlates of pulmonary fibrosis in chrysotile asbestos textile workers. *Occup Environ Med* 54:549–559, 1997.
79. McDonald AD, McDonald JC, Pooley FD: Mineral fiber content of lung in mesothelial tumors in North America. *Ann Occup Hyg* 26:417–422, 1982.
80. Karjalainen A, Meurman LO, Pukkala E: Four cases of mesothelioma among Finnish anthophyllite miners. *Occup Environ Med* 51:212–215, 1994.
81. Carbone M, Kratzke RA, Testa JR: The pathogenesis of mesothelioma. *Semin Oncol* 29:2–17, 2002.
82. Baris YL, Artvinli M, Sahin AA: Environmental mesothelioma in Turkey. *Ann NY Acad Sci* 330:423–432, 1979.
83. Coplu L, Dumortier P, Demir AU, et al.: An epidemiological study in an Anatolian village in Turkey environmentally exposed to tremolite asbestos. *J Environ Pathol* 15:177–182, 1982.
84. Zeren EH, Gumurdulu D, Roggli VL, Zorludemir S, Erkisi M, Tuncer I: Environmental malignant mesothelioma in Southern Anatolia: A study of 50 cases. *Environ Hlth Persp* 108:1047–1050, 2000.
85. Pooley FD: Evaluation of fiber samples taken from the vicinity of two villages in Turkey. In: *Dusts and Disease: Occupational and Environmental Exposures to Selected Fibrous and Particulate Dusts* (Lemen R, Dement JM, eds.), Park Forest South, IL: Pathotox Publishing, 1979, pp. 41–44.
86. Sebastien P, Gaudichet A, Bignon J, Baris YI: Zeolite bodies in human lungs from Turkey. *Lab Invest* 44:420–425, 1981.
87. Rohl AN, Langer AM, Moncure G, Selikoff IJ, Fischbein A: Endemic pleural disease associated with exposure to mixed fibrous dust in Turkey. *Science* 216:518–520, 1982.
88. Maltoni C, Minardi F, Morisi L: Pleural mesotheliomas in Sprague Dawley rats by erionite: First experimental evidence. *Environ Res* 29:238–244, 1982.
89. Suzuki Y, Kohyama N: Malignant mesothelioma induced by asbestos in the mouse peritoneal cavity. *Environ Res* 35:277–292, 1984.
90. Fraire AE, Greenberg SD, Spjut HJ, Dodson RF, Williams G, Lach-Pasko E, Roggli VL: Effect of erionite upon the pleural mesothelium of the Fischer 344 rat. *Chest* 111:1375–1380, 1997.
91. Roushdy-Hammady I, Siegel J, Emri S, et al.: Genetic susceptibility factor and malignant mesothelioma in the Cappadocian region of Turkey. *Lancet* 357:444–445, 2001.
92. Peterson JT, Greenberg SD, Buffler PA: Non-asbestos related mesothelioma: A review. *Cancer* 54:367–369, 1984.
93. Gilks B, Hegedus C, Freeman H, et al.: Malignant mesothelioma after remote abdominal radiation. *Cancer* 61:2019–2021, 1988.
94. Maurer R, Egloff B: Malignant peritoneal mesothelioma after cholangiography with thorotrast. *Cancer* 36:1381–1385, 1975.
95. Antman KH, Ruxer RL, Aisner J, Vawter G: Mesothelioma following Wilms' tumor in childhood. *Cancer* 54:367–369, 1984.
96. Anderson KA, Hurley WC, Hurley BT, Ohrt DW: Malignant pleural mesothelioma following radiotherapy in a 16-year-old boy. *Cancer* 56:273–276, 1985.

97. Austin MB, Fechner RE, Roggli VL: Pleural malignant mesothelioma following Wilms' tumor. *Am J Clin Pathol* 86:227–230, 1986.

98. Neugut AI, Ahsan H, Antman K: Incidence of malignant pleural mesothelioma after thoracic radiation therapy. *Cancer* 80:948–950, 1997.

99. Sanders CI, Jackson TA: Induction of mesotheliomas and sarcomas from hotspots of 239 PuO2 activity. *Health Phys* 22:755–759, 1972.

100. Melato M, Rizzardi C: Malignant pleural mesothelioma after chemotherapy for breast cancer. *Anticancer Res* 21:3093–3096, 2001.

101. Carbone M, Pass HI, Rizzo P: Simian virus 40-like DNA sequences in human pleural mesothelioma. *Oncogene* 9:1781–1790, 1994.

102. Testa JR, Carbone M, Hirvonen A: A multiinstitutional study confirms the presence of and expression of simian virus 40 in human malignant mesotheliomas. *Cancer Res* 58:4505–4509, 1998.

103. Jasani B, Cristaudo A, Emri SA: Association of SV40 with human tumors. *Semin Cancer Biol* 11:43–61, 2001.

104. Cicala C, Pompetti F, Carbone M: SV40 induces mesotheliomas in hamsters. *Am J Pathol* 42:1524–1533, 1993.

105. Carbone M, Fisher S, Powers A, et al.: New molecular and epidemiologic issues in mesothelioma: Role of SV 40. *J Cell Physiol* 180:167–172, 1999.

106. Kops SP: Oral polio vaccine and human cancer: A reassessment of SV40 as a contaminant based upon legal documents. *Anticancer Res* 20:4745–4750, 2000.

107. Rizzo P, Di Resta I, Powers A: Unique strains of SV40 in commercial polio vaccines from 1955 not readily identifiable with current testing for SV40 infection. *Cancer Res* 59:6103–6108, 1999.

108. Mossman BT, Gruenert DC: SV40, growth factors and mesothelioma: Another piece of the puzzle. *Am J Respir Cell Mol Biol* 26:167–170, 2002.

109. Carbone M, Rizzo P, Grimley A: Simian virus 40 large-T antigen binds p53 in human mesotheliomas. *Nat Med* 3:908–912, 1997.

110. DeLuca A, Baldi V, Esposito CM: The retinoblastoma gene family pRb/p105, p107, pRb2/p130 and simian virus 40 large T-antigen in human mesotheliomas. *Nat Med* 3:913–916, 1997.

111. Bocchetta M, Di Resta A, Powers R: Human mesothelial cells are unusually susceptible to simian virus 40-mediated transformation and asbestos cocarcinogenicity. *Proc Natl Acad Sci USA* 97:10214–10219, 2000.

112. Klein G, Powers A, Croce C: Association of SV40 with human tumors. *Oncogene* 21:1141–1149, 2002.

113. Pass H, Donington P, Wu P, Rizzo M: Human mesotheliomas contain the simian virus 40 regulatory region and large tumor antigen DNA sequences. *J Thorac Cardiovasc Surg* 116:854–859, 1998.

114. Caccioti P, Strizzi L, Vianale G: The presence of simian virus 40 sequences in mesothelioma and mesothelial cells is associated with high levels of vascular endothelial growth factor. *Am J Respir Cell Mol Biol* 26:189–193, 2002.

115. Shivapurkar N, Wiethege I, Wistuba E: Presence of simian virus 40 sequences in malignant mesotheliomas and mesothelial cell proliferations. *J Cell Biochem* 76:181–188, 1999.

116. Toyoka S, Pass H, Shivapurkar Y: Aberrant methylation and simian virus 40 tag sequences in malignant mesothelioma. *Cancer Res* 61:5727–5730, 2001.

117. Hirvonen A, Mattson K, Karjalainen A: SV40-like DNA sequences not detectable in Finnish mesothelioma patients not exposed to SV40 contaminated polio vaccines. *Mol Carcinogen* 26:93–99, 1999.

118. Hubner R, Van ME: Reappraisal of the strong association between simian virus 40 and human malignant mesothelioma of the pleura (Belgium). *Cancer Causes Control* 13:121–129, 2002.

119. Pilatte Y, Vivo C, Renier A: Absence of SV40 large T-antigen expression in human mesothelioma cell lines. *Am J Respir Cell Mol Biol* 23:788–793, 2000.

120. Nelson, NJ: Debate on the link between SV40 and human cancer continues. *J Nat Cancer Inst* 93:1284–1286, 2001.

121. Strickler HD, Goedert JJ, Bueno R: A multicenter evaluation of assays for detection of SV40 DNA and results in masked mesothelioma specimens. *Cancer Epidemiol Biomarkers Prev* 10:523–532, 2001.

122. Strickler HD, Rosenberg PS, Devesa SS, Hertel J, Fraumeni JF, Goedert JJ: Contamination of poliovirus vaccines with simian virus 40 (1955–1963) and subsequent cancer rates. *JAMA* 279:292–295, 1998.

123. Hillerdal G, Berg J: Malignant mesothelioma secondary to chronic inflammation and old scars: 2 cases and a review of the literature. *Cancer* 55:1968–1972, 1985.

124. Riddell RH, Goodman MJ, Moosa AR: Peritoneal malignant mesothelioma in a patient with recurrent peritonitis. *Cancer* 48:134–139, 1981.

125. Roggli VL, McGavran MH, Subach JA, Sybers HD, Greenberg SD: Pulmonary asbestos body counts and electron probe analysis of asbestos body cores in patients with mesothelioma: A study of 25 cases. *Cancer* 50:2423–2432, 1982.

126. Gold C: A primary mesothelioma involving the rectovaginal septum and associated with beryllium. *J Path Bact* 93:435–442, 1967.

127. Newman RH: Fine biogenic particulate silica fibres in sugarcane: a possible hazard. *Ann Occup Hyg* 30:365–370, 1986.

128. Risberg B, Nickels J, Wagermark J: Familial clustering of malignant mesothelioma. *Cancer* 45:2422–2427, 1980.

129. Lynch HT, Katz D, Marvicka SE: Familial mesothelioma: Review and family study. *Cancer Genet Cytogenet* 15:25–35, 1985.

130. Hammar SP, Bockus D, Remington F, Freidman S, LaZerte G: Familial mesothelioma: A report of two families. *Hum Pathol* 20:107–112, 1989.

131. Dawson A, Gibbs AR, Browne K, Pooley FD, Griffiths DM: Familial mesotheliomas: Details of 17 cases with histopathologic findings and mineral analysis. *Cancer* 70:1183–1187, 1992.

132. Attanoos RL, Gibbs AR: Pathology of malignant mesothelioma. *Histopathology* 30:403–418, 1997.

133. Otte KE, Sigstaard TI, Kjaerulff J: Malignant mesothelioma: Clustering in the family producing asbestos cement in their home. *Br J Ind Med* 47:10–13, 1990.

134. Fraire AE, Cooper S, Greenberg SD, Buffler P, Langston C: Mesothelioma of childhood. *Cancer* 62:838–847, 1988.

135. Nishioka H, Furusho K, Yasunaga T: Congenital mesothelioma: Case report and electron microscopic study. *Eur J Pediatr* 147:428–430, 1988.

136. Hillerdal G: Malignant mesothelioma 1982: Review of 4710 published cases. *Br J Dis Chest* 77:321–343, 1983.

137. Corson JM: Pathology of diffuse malignant pleural mesothelioma. *Sem Thorac Cardiovasc Surg* 9:347–355, 1997.

138. Boutin C, Rey F, Gouvernet J: Thoracoscopy in pleural mesotheliomas: A prospective study of 188 patients. Part 2. Prognosis and staging. *Cancer* 72:393–404, 1993.

139. McCaughey WTE: Criteria for the diagnosis of diffuse mesothelial tumors. *Ann NY Acad Sci* 132:603–613, 1965.

140. Craighead JE, Abraham JL, Churg A, et al.: Pathology of asbestos-associated diseases of the lungs and pleural cavities: Diagnostic criteria and proposed grading schema (Report of the Pneumoconiosis Committee of the College of American Pathologists and the National Institute for

Occupational Safety and Health). *Arch Pathol Lab Med* 106:544–596, 1982.

141. Sahn SA: State of the Art: The pleura. *Am Rev Respir Dis* 138:184–234, 1988.

142. Adams VI, Unni KK, Muhm JR, Jett JR, Ilstrup DM, Bernatz PE: Diffuse malignant mesothelioma of the pleura: Diagnosis and survival in 92 cases. *Cancer* 58:1540–1551, 1986.

143. Obers VJ, Leiman G, Girdwood RW, Spiro FI: Primary malignant pleural tumors (mesotheliomas) presenting as localized masses: Fine needle aspiration cytologic findings, clinical and radiologic features and a review of the literature. *Acta Cytol* 32:567–575, 1988.

144. Crotty TB, Myers JL, Katzenstein A-LA: Localized malignant mesothelioma: A clinicopathologic and flow cytometric study. *Am J Surg Pathol* 18:357–363, 1994.

145. Solomons K, Polakow R, Marchand P: Diffuse malignant mesothelioma presenting as bilateral malignant lymphangitis. *Thorax* 40:682–683, 1985.

146. Roberts G: Distant visceral metastases in pleural mesothelioma. *Br J Dis Chest* 70:246–250, 1976.

147. Elmes P, Simpson MJC: The clinical aspects of mesothelioma. *Q J Med* 179:427–429, 1976.

148. Marom EH, Erasmus JJ, Pass HI, Patz EF: The role of imaging in malignant pleural mesothelioma. *Sem Oncol* 29:26–35, 2002.

149. Alexander E, Clark RA, Colley DP, Mitchell SE: CT of malignant pleural mesothelioma. *Am J Roentgenol* 137:287–291, 1981.

150. Mirvis S, Dutcher JP, Haney PJ, Whitley NO, Aisner J: CT of malignant pleural mesothelioma. *Am J Roentgenol* 140:665–670, 1983.

151. Lorigan JG, Libshitz HI: MR imaging of malignant pleural mesothelioma. *J Comput Asst Tomogr* 13:617–620, 1989.

152. Harwood TR, Gracey DR, Yokoo H: Pseudomesotheliomatous carcinomas of the lung: A variant of peripheral lung cancer. *Am J Clin Pathol* 65:159–167, 1985.

153. Hammar SP: The pathology of benign and malignant pleural diseases. *Chest Surg Clin N Am* 4:405–430, 1994.

154. Koss M, Travis W, Moran C, Hochholzer L: Pseudomesotheliomatous adenocarcinoma: A reappraisal. *Sem Diagn Pathol* 9:117–123, 1992.

155. Sporn TA, Butnor KJ, Roggli VL: Epithelioid hemangioendothelioma of the pleura: An aggressive vascular malignancy and clinical mimic of malignant mesothelioma. *Histopathology* 41 [Suppl 2]:173–177, 2002.

156. Zhang PJ, LiVolsi VA, Brooks JJ: Malignant epithelioid vascular tumors of the pleura: Report of a series and literature review. *Hum Pathol* 31:29–34, 2000.

157. Lin B, Colby T, Gown AM, et al.: Vascular tumors of the serosal membranes: A report of 14 cases. *Am J Surg Pathol* 20:1431–1439, 1999.

158. Attanoos RL, Suvarna SK, Rhead: Malignant vascular tumors of the pleura in "asbestos workers" and endothelial differentiation in mesothelioma. *Thorax* 55:860–863, 2000.

159. Renshaw AA, Dean BR, Antman KH, Sugarbaker DJ, Cibas ES: The role of cytologic evaluation of pleural fluid in the diagnosis of malignant mesothelioma. *Chest* 111:106–109, 1997.

160. Travis WD, Colby TV, Corrin B, Shimosato Y, Brambilla E: *World Health Organization International Histological Classification of Tumours: Histological Typing of Lung and Pleural Tumors.* Berlin Heidelberg: Springer Verlag, pp. 51–54, 1999.

161. Kannerstein M, Churg J: Peritoneal mesothelioma. *Hum Pathol* 8:83–93, 1977.

162. Churg J, Rosen SH, Moolten S: Histological characteristics of mesothelioma associated with asbestos. *Ann NY Acad Sci* 132:614–622, 1965.

163. Mayall FG, Gibbs AR: The histology and immunohistochemistry of small cell mesotheliomas. *Histopathology* 20:47–51, 1992.

164. Nascimento GA, Keeney GL, Fletcher CDM: Deciduoid peritoneal mesothelioma: An unusual phenotype affecting young females. *Am J Surg Pathol* 18:439–445, 1994.

165. Puttagunta L, Vriend RA, Nguyen GK: Deciduoid epithelial mesothelioma of the pleura with focal rhabdoid change. *Am J Surg Pathol* 24:1440–1443, 2000.

166. Ordonez NG: Epithelial mesothelioma with deciduoid features: Report of four cases. *Am J Surg Pathol* 24:816–823, 2000.

167. Shanks JH, Harris M, Banerjee SS, et al.: Mesotheliomas with deciduoid morphology: A morphologic spectrum and a variant not confined to young females. *Am J Surg Pathol* 24:285–294, 2000.

168. Serio G, Scattone A, Pennella A, Giardina C, Musti M, Valente T, Pollice L: Malignant deciduoid mesothelioma of the pleura: Report of two cases with long survival. *Histopathology* 40:348–352, 2002.

169. Monaghan H, Al-Nafussi A: Deciduoid pleural mesothelioma. *Histopathology* 39:104–105, 2001.

170. Reis-Filho JS, Pope LZB, Milanezi F, Balderrama CMSR, Serapiao MJ, Schmitt FC: Primary epithelial malignant mesothelioma of the pleura with deciduoid features: Cytohistologic and immunohistochemical study. *Diagn Cytopathol* 26:117–122, 2002.

171. Henderson DW: Pleomorphic malignant mesothelioma. *Histopathology* 41 [Suppl 2]:149–154, 2002.

172. Daya D, McCaughey WT: Well differentiated papillary mesothelioma of the peritoneum: A clinicopathologic study of 22 cases. *Cancer* 65:292–296, 1990.

173. Goldblum J, Hart WR: Localized and diffuse mesotheliomas of the genital tract and peritoneum in women: A clinicopathologic study of nineteen true mesothelial neoplasms, other than adenomatoid tumors, multicystic mesotheliomas and localized fibrous tumors. *Am J Surg Pathol* 19:1124–1137, 1995.

174. Butnor KJ, Sporn TA, Hammar SP, Roggli VL: Well-differentiated papillary mesothelioma. *Am J Surg Pathol* 25:1304–1309, 2001.

175. Gallateau-Salle F: Well differentiated papillary mesothelioma. *Histopathology* 41 [Suppl 2]:154–156, 2002.

176. Yousem SA, Hochholzer L: Malignant mesotheliomas with osseous and cartilaginous differentiation. *Arch Pathol Lab Med* 111:62–66, 1987.

177. Andrion A, Mazzucco G, Bernardi P, Mollo F: Sarcomatous tumor of the chest wall with osteochondroid differentiation: Evidence of mesothelial origin. *Am J Surg Pathol* 13:707–712, 1989.

178. Henderson DW, Attwood HD, Constance TJ, Shilkin KB, Steele RH: Lymphohistiocytoid mesothelioma: A rare lymphomatoid variant of predominantly sarcomatoid mesothelioma. *Ultrastruct Pathol* 12:367–384, 1988.

179. Kannerstein M, Churg J: Desmoplastic diffuse mesothelioma. In: *Progress in Surgical Pathology* (Fenoglio CM, Wolff M, eds.), New York: Masson Pub., 1980, pp. 19–29.

180. Cantin R, Al-Jabi M, McCaughey WTE: Desmoplastic diffuse mesothelioma. *Am J Surg Pathol* 6:215–222, 1982.

181. Mangano WE, Cagle PT, Churg A, Vollmer RT, Roggli VL: The diagnosis of desmoplastic malignant mesothelioma and its distinction from fibrous pleurisy: A histologic and immunohistochemical analysis of 31 cases including p53 immunostaining. *Am J Clin Pathol* 110:191–199, 1998.

182. Stout A: Biological effects of asbestos. *Ann NY Acad Sci* 130:680–682, 1965.

183. Adams VI, Unni KK: Diffuse malignant mesothelioma of the pleura: Diagnostic criteria based on an autopsy study. *Am J Clin Pathol* 82:15–23, 1984.

184. Churg A, Colby TV, Cagle PT, Corson JM, Gibbs AR, Gilks B, Grimes MM, Hammar SP, Roggli VL, Travis WD: The separation of benign and malignant mesothelial proliferations. *Am J Surg Pathol* 24:1183–1200, 2000.

185. Cagle P, Brown R, Lebovitz R: p53 immunostaining in the differentiation of reactive processes from malignancy in pleural biopsy specimens. *Hum Pathol* 5:443–448, 1994.

186. Harrison RN: Sarcomatous pleural mesotheliomas and cerebral metastases: Case report and review of eight cases. *Eur J Respir Dis* 65:185–188, 1984.

187. Huncharek M, Muscat J: Metastases in diffuse pleural mesotheliomas: Influence of histologic type. *Thorax* 42:897–898, 1987.

188. Huncharek M, Smith K: Extrathoracic lymph node metastases in malignant pleural mesothelioma. *Chest* 93:443–444, 1988.

189. Machin T, Mashiyama ET, Henderson JAM, McCaughey WTE: Bony metastases in desmoplastic pleural mesothelioma. *Thorax* 43:155–156, 1988.

190. Waxler B, Eisenstein R, Battifora H: Electrophoresis of tissue glycosaminoglycans as an aid in the diagnosis of mesotheliomas. *Cancer* 44:221–227, 1979.

191. MacDougall DB, Wang SE, Zidar BL: Mucin-positive epithelial mesothelioma. *Arch Pathol Lab Med* 116:874–880, 1992.

192. Cooke DS, Attanoos RL, Jalloh SS, Gibbs AR: "Mucin-positive" epithelial mesotheliomas of the peritoneum: An unusual diagnostic pitfall. *Histopathology* 37:33–36, 1999.

193. Hammar SP, Bockus DE, Remington FL, Rohrbach KA: Mucin-positive epithelial mesotheliomas: A histochemical, immunohistochemical and ultrastructural comparison with mucin-producing pulmonary adenocarcinoma. *Ultrastruct Pathol* 20:293–325, 1996.

194. Wang NS, Huang SN, Gold P: Absence of carcinoembryonic antigen material in mesothelioma. *Cancer* 44:937–943, 1979.

195. Blobel GA, Moll R, Franke WW, Kayser KW, Gould VE: The intermediate filament cytoskeleton of malignant mesotheliomas and its diagnostic significance. *Am J Pathol* 121:235–247, 1985.

196. Battifora H, Kopinski MI: Distinction of mesothelioma from adenocarcinoma: An immunohistochemical approach. *Cancer* 55:1679–1685, 1985.

197. Gibbs AR, Harach R, Wagner JC, Jasani B: Comparison of tumour markers in malignant mesothelioma and pulmonary adenocarcinoma. *Thorax* 40:91–95, 1985.

198. Holden J, Churg A: Immunohistochemical staining for keratin and carcinoembryonic antigen in the diagnosis of malignant mesothelioma. *Am J Surg Pathol* 8:277–279, 1984.

199. Loosli H, Hurlimann J: Immunohistological study of malignant diffuse mesotheliomas of the pleura. *Histopathology* 8:793–803, 1984.

200. van Muijen GNP, Ruiter DJ, Ponec M, Huiskens van der Mey C, Warnaar SO: Monoclonal antibodies with different specificities against cytokeratins: An immunohistochemical study of normal tissues and tumors. *Am J Pathol* 114:9–17, 1984.

201. Bolen JW, Hammar SP, McNutt MA: Reactive and neoplastic serosal tissue: A light-microscopic, ultrastructural, and immunocytochemical study. *Am J Surg Pathol* 10:34–47, 1986.

202. Montag AG, Pinkus GS, Corson JM: Keratin protein immunoreactivity of sarcomatoid and mixed types of diffuse malignant mesotheliomas: An immunoperoxidase study of 30 cases. *Hum Pathol* 19:336–342, 1988.

203. Epstein JI, Budin RE: Keratin and epithelial membrane antigen immunoreactivity in nonneoplastic fibrous pleural lesions: Implications for the diagnosis of desmoplastic mesothelioma. *Hum Pathol* 17:514–519, 1986.

204. Cagle PT, Truong L, Roggli VL, Greenberg SD: Immunohistochemical differentiation of sarcomatoid mesotheliomas from other spindle cell neoplasms. *Am J Clin Pathol* 92:66–71, 1989.

205. Wick MR, Loy T, Mills SE: Malignant epithelioid pleural mesothelioma versus peripheral pulmonary adenocarcinoma: a histochemical, ultrastructural, and immunohistologic study of 103 cases. *Hum Pathol* 21:759–766, 1990.

206. Ordonez NG: Value of cytokeratin 5/6 immunostaining in distinguishing epithelial mesothelioma of the pleura from lung adenocarcinoma. *Am J Surg Pathol* 22:1215–1221, 1998.

207. Cury PM, Butcher DN, Fisher C: Value of the mesothelium-associated antibodies thrombomodulin, cytokeratin 5/6, calretinin, and CD44H in distinguishing epithelioid pleural mesothelioma from adenocarcinoma metastatic to the pleura. *Mod Pathol* 13:107–112, 2000.

208. Chu P, Wu E, Weiss LM: Cytokeratin 7 and cytokeratin 20 expression in epithelial neoplasms: A survey of 435 cases. *Mod Pathol* 13:962–972, 2000.

209. Moran CA, Wick MR, Suster S: The role of immunohistochemistry in the diagnosis of malignant mesothelioma. *Sem Diagn Pathol* 17:178–183, 2000.

210. Corson JM, Pinkus GS: Mesothelioma: profile of keratin and carcinoembryonic antigen: An immunoperoxidase study of 20 cases and comparison with pulmonary adenocarcinoma. *Am J Pathol* 108:80–87, 1982.

211. Sheibani K, Battifora H, Burke JS: Antigenic phenotype of malignant mesotheliomas and pulmonary adenocarcinomas: An immunohistologic analysis demonstrating the value of Leu M1 antigen. *Am J Pathol* 123:212–219, 1986.

212. Metzger J, Lamerz R, Permanetter W: Diagnostic significance of carcinoembryonic antigen in the differential diagnosis of malignant mesothelioma. *J Cardiovasc Surg* 100:860–866, 1990.

213. Ordonez NG: The immunohistochemical diagnosis of epithelial mesothelioma. *Hum Pathol* 30:313–323, 1999.

214. Ordonez NG: Role of immunohistochemistry in differentiating epithelial mesothelioma from adenocarcinoma: Review and update. *Am J Clin Pathol* 112:75–89, 1989.

215. Latza U, Niedobitek G, Schwarting R: Ber-Ep4: new monoclonal antibody which distinguishes epithelia from mesothelia. *J Clin Pathol* 43:213–219, 1990.

216. Ordonez NG: Value of the BerEP4 antibody in differentiating epithelial pleural mesothelioma from adenocarcinoma. *Am J Clin Pathol* 109:85–89, 1998.

217. Arber DA, Weiss LM: CD15: A review. *Appl Immunohistochem* 1:17–30, 1993.

218. Sheibani K, Battifora H, Burke JS: LeuM1 antigen in human neoplasms: An immunohistochemical study of 400 cases. *Am J Surg Pathol* 10:227–236, 1986.

219. Lefebvre MP, Rodriguez F, Schlom J: The application of a monoclonal antibody to the differentiation of benign and malignant mesothelial proliferations from adenocarcinoma. (abstr) *Lab Invest* 52:38A, 1985.

220. Szpak CA, Johnston WW, Roggli V: The diagnostic distinction between malignant mesothelioma of the pleura and adenocarcinoma of the lung as defined by a monoclonal antibody, B72.3. *Am J Pathol* 122:252–260, 1986.

221. Ordonez NG: The immunohistochemical diagnosis of mesothelioma and lung adenocarcinoma. *Am J Surg Pathol* 13:276–291, 1985.
222. Riera JR, Astengo-Osuna C, Longmate JA, et al.: The immunohistochemical diagnostic panel for epithelial mesothelioma: A reevaluation after heat induced epitope retrieval. *Am J Surg Pathol* 21:1409–1419, 1997.
223. Leong ASY, Vernon-Roberts E: The immunohistochemistry of malignant mesothelioma. *Pathol Annu* 29:157–179, 1994.
224. Marshall RJ, Herbert A, Braye SG: Use of antibodies to carcinoembryonic antigen and human milk fat globule to distinguish carcinoma, mesothelioma and reactive mesothelium. *J Clin Pathol* 37:1215–1221, 1984.
225. Doglioni C, Dei Tos AP, Laurino L: Calretinin: A novel immunocytochemical marker for mesothelioma. *Am J Surg Pathol* 20:1037–1046, 1996.
226. Leers MPG, Aarts MMJ, Theunissen PHMH: E-cadherin and calretinin: A useful combination of immunohistochemical markers for differentiation between mesothelioma and metastatic adenocarcinoma. *Histopathology* 32:209–216, 1998.
227. Barberis MCP, Faleri M, Veronese S: Calretinin: A selective marker of normal and neoplastic mesothelial cells in serous effusions. *Acta Cytol* 41:1757–1761, 1997.
228. Ordonez NG: Value of calretinin immunostaining in differentiating epithelial mesothelioma from lung adenocarcinoma. *Mod Pathol* 11:929–933, 1998.
229. Collins CL, Ordonez NG, Schaefer R: Thrombomodulin expression in malignant pleural mesothelioma and pulmonary adenocarcinoma. *Am J Pathol* 141:827–833, 1992.
230. Ordonez NG: The value of antibodies 44-3A6, SM3, HBME-1, and thrombomodulin in differentiating epithelial pleural mesothelioma from lung adenocarcinoma: A comparative study with other commonly used antibodies. *Am J Surg Pathol* 21:1399–1408, 1997.
231. Sheibani K, Esteban JM, Bailey A, Battifora H, Weiss LM: Immunopathologic and molecular studies as an aid to the diagnosis of malignant mesothelioma. *Hum Pathol* 23:107–116, 1992.
232. Miettinen M, Kobatich AJ: HBME-1: a monoclonal antibody useful in the differential diagnosis of mesothelioma, adenocarcinoma, and soft-tissue and bone tumors. *Appel Immunohistochem* 3:115–122, 1995.
233. Takeichi M: Cadherin cell adhesion receptors as morphogenetic regulators. *Science* 251:1451–1455, 1991.
234. Soler AP, Knudsen KA, Jaurand M-C: The differential expression of N-Cadherin and E-Cadherin distinguishes pleural mesotheliomas from lung adenocarcinomas. *Hum Pathol* 26:1363–1369, 1995.
235. Ordonez NG: Value of thyroid transcription factor-1, E-cadherin, BG8, WT1, and CD44S immunostaining in distinguishing epithelial pleural mesotheliomas from pulmonary and nonpulmonary adenocarcinomas. *Am J Surg Pathol* 24:598–606, 2000.
236. Soler AP, Knudsen KA, Teeson-Miguel A: Expression of E-cadherin and N-cadherin in surface epithelial-stromal tumors of the ovary distinguishes mucinous from serous and endometrioid tumors. *Hum Pathol* 28:734–739, 1997.
237. Bejarano PA, Baughman RP, Biddinger PW, et al.: Surfactant proteins and thyroid transcription factor-1 in pulmonary and breast carcinomas. *Mod Pathol* 9:445–452, 1996.
238. Di Loreto C, Puglisi F, Di Luro V, Damante G, Beltrami CA: TTF-1 protein expression in pleural malignant mesotheliomas and adenocarcinomas of the lung. *Cancer Letts* 124:73–78, 1998.

239. Wang NS: Electron microscopy in the diagnosis of pleural mesotheliomas. *Cancer* 31:1046–1054, 1973.
240. Davis JMG: Ultrastructure of human mesotheliomas. *J Natl Cancer Inst* 52:1715–1725, 1974.
241. Dardick I, El-Jabbi M, McCaughey WT, et al: Ultrastructure of poorly differentiated diffuse epithelial mesotheliomas. *Ultrastruct Pathol* 7:151–160, 1984.
242. Warhol MJ, Hickey WF, Corson JM: Malignant mesothelioma: Ultrastructural distinction from adenocarcinoma. *Am J Surg Pathol* 6:307–314, 1982.
243. Warhol MJ, Corson JM: An ultrastructural comparison of mesotheliomas with adenocarcinomas of the lung and breast. *Hum Pathol* 16:50–55, 1985.
244. Burns TR, Greenberg SD, Mace ML, Johnson EH: Ultrastructural diagnosis of epithelial malignant mesothelioma. *Cancer* 56:2036–2040, 1985.
245. Dardick I, El-Jabbi M, McCaughey WT: Diffuse epithelial mesothelioma: A review of the ultrastructural spectrum. *Ultrastruct Pathol* 11:503–533, 1987.
246. Oury TD, Hammar SP, Roggli VL: Ultrastructural features of diffuse malignant mesotheliomas. *Hum Pathol* 29:1382–1392, 1998.
247. Dewar A, Valente M, Ring NP, et al.: Pleural mesothelioma of epithelial type and pulmonary adenocarcinoma: An ultrastructural and cytochemical comparison. *J Pathol* 152:309–316, 1987.
248. Jandik WR, Landas SK, Bray CK, Lager DJ: Scanning electron microscopic distinction of pleural mesotheliomas from adenocarcinomas. *Mod Pathol* 6:761–764, 1993.
249. Burns TR, Johnson EH, Cartwright J, Greenberg SD: Desmosomes of epithelial malignant mesothelioma. *Ultrastruct Pathol* 12:385–388, 1988.
250. Ghadially FN, Rippstein PU: Giant desmosomes in tumors. *Ultrastruct Pathol* 19:469–474, 1995.
251. Mukherjee TM, Swift JG, Henderson DW: Freeze-fracture study of intercellular junctions in benign and malignant mesothelial cells in effusions and a comparison with those seen in pleural mesotheliomas (solid tumor). *J Submicrosc Cytol Pathol* 20:195–208, 1988.
252. Roggli VL, Sanfilippo F, Shelburne JD: Mesothelioma. Ch. 5 In: *Pathology of Asbestos-Associated Diseases* (Roggli VL, Greenberg SD, Pratt PC, eds.), Boston: Little, Brown & Co., 1992, pp. 109–164.
253. Klima M, Bossart MI: Sarcomatous type of malignant mesothelioma. *Ultrastruct Pathol* 4:349–358, 1983.
254. Ordonez NG, Ro JY, Ayala AG: Lesions described as nodular mesothelial hyperplasia are primarily composed of histiocytes. *Am J Surg Pathol* 22:285–292, 1998.
255. Taylor DR, Page W, Hughes D, Varghese G: Metastatic renal cell carcinoma mimicking pleural mesothelioma. *Thorax* 42:901–902, 1987.
256. Weiss SW, Enzinger FM: Epithelioid hemangioendothelioma: A vascular tumor often mistaken for an adenocarcinoma. *Cancer* 50:970–981, 1982.
257. Dail DH, Liebow AA, Gmelich JT: Intravascular, bronchiolar, and alveolar tumor of the lung (IVBAT): An analysis of twenty cases of a peculiar sclerosing endothelial tumor. *Cancer* 51:452–464, 1983.
258. Corrin B, Manners B, Millard M, Weaver L: Histogenesis of the so-called "intravascular bronchioloalveolar tumor." *J Pathol* 128:163–167, 1979.
259. Miettinen M, Limon J, Niezabitowski A, Lasota J: Calretinin and other mesothelioma markers in synovial sarcoma: Analysis of antigenic similarities and differences with malignant mesothelioma. *Am J Surg Pathol* 25:610–617, 2001.

260. Gaertner E, Zeren EH, Fleming MV, Colby TV, Travis WD: Biphasic synovial sarcomas arising in the pleural cavity: A clinicopathologic study of five cases. *Am J Surg Pathol* 20:36–45, 1996.

261. Aubry M-C, Bridge JA, Wickert R, Tazelaar HD: Primary monophasic synovial sarcoma of the pleura: Five cases confirmed by the presence of SYT-SSX fusion transcript. *Am J Surg Pathol* 25:776–781, 2001.

262. Praet M, Forsyth R, Dhaene K, Hermans G, Remmelinck M, Goethem JV, Verbeken E, Weynand B: Synovial sarcoma of the pleura: Report of four cases. *Histopathology* 41 [Suppl 2]:147–149, 2002.

263. De Leeuw B, Balemans M, Olde Weghuis D, Geurts van Kessel A: Identification of two alternative fusion genes, SYT-SSX1 and SYT-SSX2 in t(8: 18) (p1 1.2:q1 1.2) positive synovial sarcoma. *Hum Mol Genet* 4:1097–1099, 1995.

264. Winslow TJ, Taylor HB: Malignant peritoneal mesotheliomas: A clinicopathological analysis of 12 fatal cases. *Cancer* 13:127–136, 1960.

265. Whitley NO, Brenner DE, Antman KH, et al.: Computed tomographic evaluation of peritoneal mesothelioma: An analysis of eight cases. *Am J Roentgenol* 138:531–535, 1982.

266. Fukuda T, Hayashi K, Mori M, et al.: Radiologic manifestations of peritoneal mesothelioma. *Nippon Igaku Hoshasen Gakkai Zasshi* 51:643–647, 1991.

267. Piccigallo E, Jeffers LJ, Reddy KR, Caldironi MW, Parenti A, Schiff ER: Malignant peritoneal mesothelioma: A clinical and laparoscopic study of ten cases. *Dig Dis Sci* 33:633–639, 1988.

268. Mennemeyer R, Smith M: Multicystic peritoneal mesothelioma: A report with electron microscopy of a case mimicking intra-abdominal cystic hygroma (lymphangioma). *Cancer* 44:692–698, 1979.

269. Moore JH, Crum CP, Chandler JG, Feldman PS: Benign cystic mesothelioma. *Cancer* 45:2395–2399, 1980.

270. Weiss SW, Tavassoli FA: Multicystic mesothelioma: An analysis of pathologic findings and biologic behavior in 37 cases. *Am J Surg Pathol* 12:737–746, 1988.

271. Ross MJ, Welsh WR, Scully RE: Multilocular peritoneal inclusion cysts (so-called cystic mesothelioma). *Cancer* 64:1326–1346, 1989.

272. Greengard O, Head JF, Chahinian AP, Goldberg SL: Enzyme pathology of human mesotheliomas. *J Natl Cancer Inst* 78:617–622, 1987.

273. Talerman A, Montero JR, Chilcote RR, Okagaki T: Diffuse malignant peritoneal mesothelioma in a 13-year-old girl: Report of a case and review of the literature. *Am J Surg Pathol* 9:73–80, 1985.

274. Santucci M, Biancalani M, Dini S: Multicystic peritoneal mesothelioma: A fine structure study with special reference to the spectrum of phenotypic differentiation exhibited by mesothelial cells. *J Submicrosc Cytol Pathol* 21:749–764, 1989.

275. Rosai J: Peritoneum, Retroperitoneum, and Related Structures, Ch. 26, In: *Ackerman's Surgical Pathology*, 8th ed. (Rosai J, ed.), St. Louis: Mosby, 1996, pp. 2135–2172.

276. Gilks CB, Bell DA, Scully RE: Serous psammocarcinoma of the ovary and peritoneum. *Int J Gyn Pathol* 9:110–121, 1990.

277. Chu PG, Weiss LM: Expression of cytokeratin 5/6 in epithelial neoplasms: An immunohistochemical study of 509 cases. *Mod Pathol* 15:6–10, 2002.

278. Armstrong GR, Raafat F, Ingram L, Mann JR: Malignant peritoneal mesothelioma in childhood. *Arch Pathol Lab Med* 112:1159–1162, 1988.

279. Kerrigan SAJ, Turnnir RT, Clement PB, et al.: Diffuse malignant epithelial mesotheliomas of the peritoneum in women: A clinicopathologic study of 25 patients. *Cancer* 94:378–385, 2002.

280. Hodgson JT, Darnton A: The quantitative risks of mesothelioma and lung cancer in relation to asbestos exposure. *Ann Occup Hyg* 44:565–601, 2000.

281. Barbera V, Rubino M: Papillary mesothelioma of the tunica vaginalis. *Cancer* 10:182–189, 1957.

282. Jones MA, Young RH, Scully RE: Malignant mesothelioma of the tunica vaginalis: A clinicopathologic analysis of 11 cases with review of the literature. *Am J Surg Pathol* 19:815–825, 1995.

283. Plas E, Riedl CR, Pflueger H: Malignant mesothelioma of the tunica vaginalis testis: Review of the literature and assessment of prognostic parameters. *Cancer* 83:2437–2446, 1998.

284. Japko L, Horta AA, Schreiber K, Mitsudo S, Karwa GL, Singh G, Koss LG: Malignant mesothelioma of the tunica vaginalis testis: Report of first case with preoperative diagnosis. *Cancer* 49:119–127, 1982.

285. Khan MA, Puri P, Devaney D: Mesothelioma of the tunica vaginalis testis in a child. *J Urol* 158:198–199, 1997.

286. Nochomowitz LE, Orenstein JM: Adenocarcinoma of the rete testis: Case report, ultrastructural observations and clinicopathologic correlates. *Am J Surg Pathol* 8:625–634, 1984.

287. Taxy JB, Battifora H, Ovasu R: Adenomatoid tumors: A light microscopic, histochemical and ultrastructural study. *Cancer* 34:306–316, 1974.

288. Thompson R, Schlegel W, Lucca M: Primary malignant mesothelioma of the pericardium: Case report and literature review. *Texas Heart Inst J* 21:170–174, 1994.

289. Vigneswaran WT, Stefanacci PR: Pericardial mesothelioma. *Curr Treat Options Oncol* 1:299–302, 2000.

290. Nomori H, Shimosato Y, Tsuchiya R: Diffuse malignant pericardial mesothelioma. *Acta Pathol Jpn* 35:1475–1481, 1985.

291. Llewellyn MJ, Atkinson MW, Fabri B: Pericardial constriction caused by pericardial mesothelioma. *Br Heart J* 57:54–57, 1987.

292. Nishikimi T, Ochi H, Hirota K, Ikuno Y, Oku H, Takeuchi K, Takeda T: Primary pericardial mesothelioma detected by gallium-67 scintigraphy. *J Nucl Med* 28:1210–1212, 1987.

293. Gossinger HD, Siostrzonek P, Zangeneh M, Neuhold A, Herold C, Schmoliner R, Laczkovics A, Tscholakoff D, Mosslacher H: Magnetic resonance imaging findings in a patient with pericardial mesothelioma. *Am Heart J* 115:1321–1322, 1988.

294. Naramoto A, Itoh N, Nakano M, Shigematsu H: An autopsy case of tuberous sclerosis associated with primary pericardial mesothelioma. *Acta Pathol Jpn* 39:400–406, 1989.

295. Burke A, Virmani R: Tumors of the heart and great vessels. In: *Atlas of Tumor Pathology*. Series 3, Fasc 16. Washington, DC: Armed Forces Institute of Pathology, 1996.

296. Smith C: Tumors of the heart. *Arch Pathol Lab Med* 110:371–374, 1986.

297. Linder J, Shelburne JD, Sorge JP, Whalen RE, Hackel DB: Congenital endodermal heterotopia of the atrioventricular node: Evidence for the endodermal origin of so-called mesotheliomas of the atrioventricular node. *Hum Pathol* 15:1093–1098, 1984.

298. Sopher IM, Spitz WU: Endodermal inclusions of the heart: So-called mesotheliomas of the atrioventricular node. *Arch Pathol* 92:180–186, 1971.

299. Fine G, Raju U: Congenital polycystic tumor of the atrioventricular node (endodermal heterotopia, mesothelioma): A histogenetic appraisal with evidence for its endodermal origin. *Hum Pathol* 18:791–795, 1987.

300. Beck B, Konetzke G, Ludwig V, et al.: Malignant pericardial mesotheliomas and asbestos exposure: A case report. *Am J Ind Med* 3:149–159, 1982.

301. Kahn EI, Rohl A, Barnett EW, Suzuki Y: Primary pericardial mesothelioma following exposure to asbestos. *Environ Res* 23:270–281, 1980.

302. Churg A, Warnock ML, Bersch KG: Malignant mesothelioma arising after direct application of asbestos and fiberglass to the pericardium. *Am Rev Respir Dis* 118:419–424, 1978.

303. Roggli VL: Pericardial mesothelioma after exposure to asbestos. *N Engl J Med* 304:1045, 1981.

304. Steele JPC: Prognostic factors in mesothelioma. *Semin Oncol* 29:36–40, 2002.

305. Steele JPC, Rudd RM: Malignant mesothelioma: Predictors of prognosis and clinical trials. *Thorax* 55:725–726, 2000.

306. Chahinian AP, Pajak TF, Holland JF, Norton L, Ambinder RM, Mandel EM: Diffuse malignant mesothelioma: Prospective evaluation of 69 patients. *Ann Int Med* 96:746–755, 1982.

307. Ruffie P, Feld R, Minkin S: Diffuse malignant mesothelioma of the pleura in Ontario and Quebec: A retrospective study of 188 consecutive patients. *Cancer* 72:410–417, 1993.

308. Spirtas R, Connelly RR, Tucker MA: Survival patterns for malignant mesothelioma: The SEER experience. *Int J Cancer* 41:525–530, 1988.

309. Herndon JE, Green MR, Chahinian AP: Factors predictive of survival among 337 patients with mesothelioma treated between 1984 and 1994 by the Cancer and Leukemia Group B. *Chest* 113:723–731, 1998.

310. Curran D, Sahmoud T, Therasse P: Prognostic factors in patients with pleural mesotheliomas: The European Organization for Research and Treatment of Cancer experience. *J Clin Oncol* 16:145–152, 1998.

311. Edwards JG, Abrams KR, Leverment JN: Prognostic factors for malignant mesothelioma in 142 patients: Validation of CALGB and EORTC prognostic scoring systems. *Thorax* 55:723–731, 2000.

312. Antman K, Blum R, Greenberger J, et al.: Multimodality therapy for mesothelioma based on a study of natural history. *Am J Med* 68:356–362, 1980.

313. Antman KH: Current concepts: Malignant mesothelioma. *N Engl J Med* 303:200–202, 1980.

314. Ceresoli GL, Locati LdeB, Ferreri AJ: Therapeutic outcome according to histologic subtype in 121 patients with malignant pleural mesothelioma. *Lung Cancer* 34:279–287, 2001.

315. Antman KH, Shemin R, Ryan L: Malignant mesothelioma: Prognostic variables in a registry of 180 patients, the Dana-Farber Cancer Institute and Brigham and Women's Hospital experience over two decades 1965–1985. *J Clin Oncol* 6:147–153, 1988.

316. Butchart EG, Ashcroft T, Barnsley WC, Holden MP: Pleuropneumonectomy in the management of diffuse malignant mesothelioma of the pleura: Experience with 29 patients. *Thorax* 31:15–24, 1976.

317. Sugarbaker DJ, Flores R, Jacklitsch M: Resection margins, extrapleural nodal status and cell type determine post-operative long term survival in trimodality therapy of malignant pleural mesothelioma: Results in 183 patients. *J Thorac Cardiovasc Surg* 117:54–65, 1999.

318. Rusch VW: A proposed new international TNM staging system for malignant pleural mesothelioma from the International Mesothelioma Interest Group. *Chest* 108:1122–1128, 1995.

319. Lerner HJ, Schoenfeld DA, Martin AM, Falson G, Borden E: Malignant mesothelioma: The Eastern Cooperative Oncology Group (ECOG) experience. *Cancer* 52:1981–1985, 1983.

320. Moertel C: Peritoneal mesothelioma. *Gastroenterology* 63:346–350, 1972.

321. Antman K, Klegar K, Pomfret EA, et al.: Early peritoneal mesothelioma: a treatable malignancy. *Lancet* 2:977–981, 1985.
322. Weissman L, Osteen R, Corson J: Combined modality therapy for intraperitoneal mesothelioma (abstr). *Proc Am Soc Clin Oncol* 7:274, 1988.
323. Antman K, Pomfret E, Aisner J: Peritoneal mesothelioma: Natural history and response to chemotherapy. *J Clin Oncol* 1:386–391, 1983.
324. Sugarbaker PH, Acherman YIZ, Gonzalez-Moreno S, Ortega-Perez G: Diagnosis and treatment of peritoneal mesothelioma: The Washington Cancer Institute Experience. *Semin Oncol* 29:51–61, 2002.

6

Benign Asbestos-Related Pleural Disease

Tim D. Oury

Introduction

Benign asbestos-related pleural diseases are the most common pathologic and clinical abnormalities related to asbestos exposure. Solomon
et al.[1] emphasized that the pleural manifestations of asbestos exposure
include four specific entities: parietal pleural plaques, diffuse pleural
fibrosis, rounded atelectasis, and benign asbestos effusion. Notably,
there is considerable overlap among these four disease processes
(Figure 6-1), with various combinations manifesting simultaneously or
sequentially in a single individual. For example, a patient with benign
asbestos effusion may subsequently be found to have diffuse pleural
fibrosis, or a patient with parietal pleural plaques may develop
rounded atelectasis. Benign asbestos-related pleural diseases may
occur after low-level, indirect, or even environmental exposures to
asbestos. However, the prevalence of these abnormalities is clearly
greatest in those who are exposed to asbestos in an occupational
setting.

The pathogenesis of these disorders is poorly understood,[2] but it
undoubtedly involves transport of asbestos fibers to the pleura, either
directly through the lung parenchyma or through lymphatic pathways.[3] In the former, asbestos fibers inhaled into the lung pass into the
alveoli, where they eventually work their way to the visceral pleural
surface. The mechanical theory suggests that this transport occurs
when the needlelike fibers work their way through the lung tissue as
a result of the lung's motion during inhalation and exhalation.[4] Alternatively, fibers reach the pulmonary interstitium through a process of
translocation across the alveolar epithelium.[5] Within the interstitium,
the fibers would have access to pulmonary lymphatics, which in the
outer third of the lung drain centripetally to the pleura. Fibers reaching the visceral pleura can then penetrate this structure and hence reach
the parietal pleura, which normally is directly apposed to the visceral
pleura, separated only by a potential space. The presence of fibers
within the pleura elicits an inflammatory response, which may
undergo organization or healing with subsequent fibrosis. In this

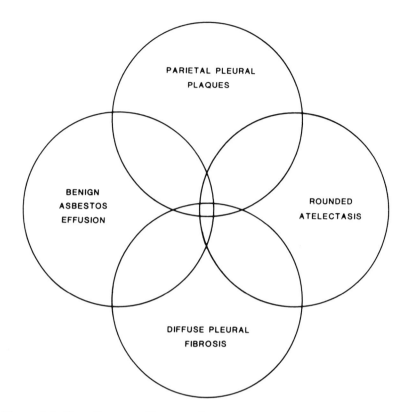

Figure 6-1. Venn diagram of benign asbestos-related pleural diseases, showing the overlap among these four specific disorders.

regard, it is of interest that one study has shown that pleural mesothelial cells in culture release a chemotactic factor for neutrophils when stimulated with asbestos fibers.[6] A recent study also indicates that asbestos fibers also induce mesothelial release of chemoattractants for monocytes.[7] Clinical manifestations will then depend on the intensity of the initial inflammatory reaction and the degree and extent of any consequent pleural fibrosis.

Parietal Pleural Plaques

Historical Background

Pleural plaques consist of circumscribed areas of dense, firm, gray-white fibrous tissue usually free of any inflammatory reaction. While most pleural plaques occur on the parietal pleura, they may occur on the visceral pleura as well.[1] They are most commonly located on the parietal pleural surface opposite the dependant portions of the lungs.

Cartilage-like plaques on the costal pleura have long been recognized by pathologists. They were considered to be remnants of inflammation, similar to "sugar icing" (*Zuckerguss*). The first description of pleural plaques in connection with asbestos workers was made by Sparks in 1931, who described irregular, small, calcified plaques in the lower lung zones.[8] In 1938, Gloyne reported visceral pleural plaques that were hornlike and stiff.[8] The first description of pleural plaques in talc workers was made by Porro et al. in 1942.[9] Siegal et al. reported the initial observation of pleural plaques in tremolite talc workers.[10] In the 1950s, several reports of pleural plaques in asbestos- and talc-exposed workers appeared.[11,12]

Talcosis is very similar clinically and roentgenologically to asbestosis, and it is probably the asbestos found in almost all types of talc that causes the pulmonary and pleural changes.[13–15] Indeed, some of the first studies of pleural plaques were made among talc workers.[10,11] Animal experiments with "pure" talc (i.e., free of asbestos) have resulted in both pulmonary fibrosis and pleural reactions.[16] Also, talc particles have been found in pleural plaques. Talc also induces mesothelial cells to release several chemokines, which induce inflammation.[17,18] Therefore, it is possible that talc itself may have some effect in the formation of pleural plaques.

Radiographic Features

Parietal pleural plaques appear on chest x-ray as discrete areas of pleural thickening, usually in the lower lung zones or on the diaphragms. They are best observed when viewed tangentially (Figure 6-2), but may appear as a hazy density when viewed *en face*. The plaques often calcify, which usually does not occur until two to three decades after the initial exposure to asbestos.[19,20] Calcification greatly

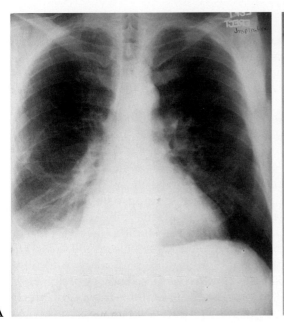
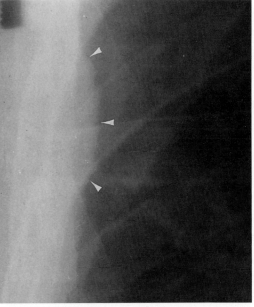

A   B

Figure 6-2. (A) Chest radiograph shows mild bilateral increase in interstitial markings most prominent in the lung bases, right pleural effusion, and pleural thickening with focal plaque formation. **(B)** The outline of this plaque viewed tangentially is seen to better advantage in this magnified view of the periphery of the right mid-lung field (*arrowheads*). (Reprinted from Ref. 40, with permission.)

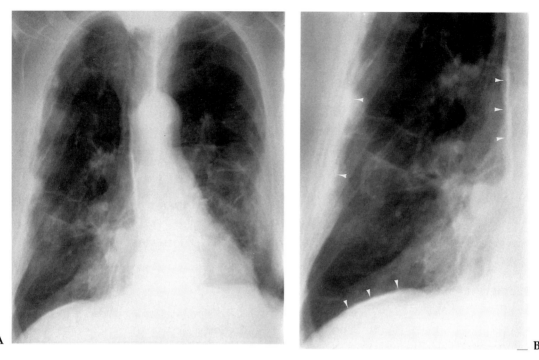

Figure 6-3. (A) Chest radiograph showing parietal pleural plaque formation with extensive bilateral pleural calcification. **(B)** The pleural calcification is seen to better advantage in this magnified view of the right hemithorax (*arrowheads*) (Courtesy Dr. William F. Foster, Department of Radiology, Durham VA Medical Center, Durham, NC.)

enhances plaque detectability with routine chest films (Figure 6-3). In addition, oblique views are useful for detecting plaques, especially noncalcified ones.[21] Plaques generally spare the costophrenic angles. When blunting is observed, one should suspect the presence of pleural effusions or adhesions. Pleural plaques are most often bilateral. Left-sided predominance of unilateral plaques on chest x-rays has been reported by some authors,[22,23] but has not been confirmed by thoracic computerized tomography (CT) studies.[24]

Radiographic surveys of populations have shown that 1% to 2% of men and less than 1% of women have pleural plaques. There is, however, a high rate of false negative results, because autopsy surveys have indicated that the postmortem prevalence of plaques ranges from 4% to as high as 39% (Table 6-1).[25] In these autopsy studies, the percentage of plaques that were detected on premortem chest films ranged from 8% to 40%. Noncalcified diaphragmatic plaques are particularly difficult to visualize on routine chest films, and were observed in none of eight cases in the series of Wain et al.[25] One must also use caution to avoid overinterpretation of films as showing pleural plaques (i.e., false positives), which can occur secondary to shadows produced by the serratus anterior in particularly muscular individuals, or due to subpleural adipose tissue in the obese. Notably, a study by Miller and Zurlo suggests that even when plaques are radiographically evident, they are frequently overlooked or

Table 6-1. Summary of previously reported pathologic x-ray correlation studies of patients with pleural plaques

Author	Country	Population composition	No. of autopsies	% Pleural plaques*	% Detected on chest films*
Rubino et al.[19]	Italy	General population in asbestos industrial region	862	7.8%	40.3%
Hourihane et al.[42]	England	General urban population	381	4.1	13.7
Hillerdal and Lindgren[13]	Sweden	General population screen	437	6.8	12.5
Meurman[26]	Finland	General population in coastal, urban, and asbestos mining region	438	39.3	8.3
Wain et al.[25]	U.S.A.	Male veterans	434	5.8	28

Source: Reprinted from Ref. 25, with permission
*These values are calculated from published data.

misdiagnosed and the patients are not followed as carefully as they should be with proper recognition of this process.[27]

Computed tomography has been shown to improve both the specificity and sensitivity of routine chest films with respect to identification of asbestos-related pleural disease (Figure 6-4).[28-30] A study comparing CT scanning to chest radiography found that CT was able to detect approximately 60% more plaques than chest x-ray[30] and high resolution CT may even be better.[31] However, another study comparing conventional CT to high resolution CT found that conventional CT was more sensitive for detecting plaques.[32] As the cost of CT becomes increasingly affordable compared to chest x-rays, this will become a much more useful tool in identification of patients with asbestos-related pleural disease.[33]

Pathologic Findings

Grossly, parietal pleural plaques are yellow-white, elevated, firm, and glistening and have sharply circumscribed borders.[34,35] They are frequently bilateral and are usually seen within the costal pleura, where they lie parallel to the ribs. They are also seen on the domes of the diaphragm (Figures 6-5 and 6-6). Pleural plaques vary in size from those that are just visible to the naked eye to structures that are 12 or more centimeters across.[36] They are frequently calcified. These ivory-colored structures may have either a smooth surface or a knobby appearance, consisting of multiple 5 mm nodules that create a "candle-wax dripping" appearance.[36] The thickness of the plaques varies from a few millimeters to a centimeter or more. Visceral pleural plaques have been described as well, but are considerably less frequent.[1] Plaques have also been described within the peritoneum on the surface of the spleen or liver, and some of these are related to prior asbestos exposure.[37,38] In rare instances, calcified plaques or asbestos-induced diffuse pericardial fibrosis may involve the pericardium.[37,39] Adhesions between the surface of parietal pleural plaques and the adjacent visceral pleura are uncommon.

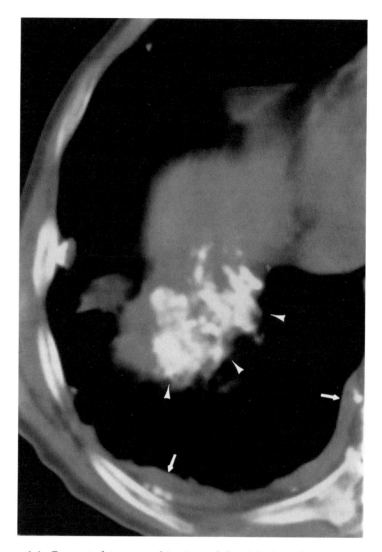

Figure 6-4. Computed tomographic view of the right hemithorax shows partially calcified parietal pleural plaques viewed tangentially (*arrows*) as well as an extensively calcified diaphragmatic plaque viewed *en face* (*arrowheads*). (Courtesy Dr. William F. Foster, Department of Radiology, Durham VA Medical Center, Durham, NC.)

Microscopically, plaques are predominantly collagenous with scant cellularity (Figures 6-7 to 6-10). This dense fibrous tissue often shows a "basket-weave" pattern (Figures 6-8 and 6-9).[34,35] However, plaques with a solid appearance lacking the "basket-weave" pattern may also be observed (Figure 6-10). These solid appearing plaques accounted for almost one-third of the plaques studied histologically by Wain et al.[25] Rarely, a row of cuboidal mesothelial cells may be seen on the surface of the plaque. Although inflammatory cells are not observed within the

plaque, small clusters of lymphocytes are invariably found at the edge
of the plaque or at the interface between the plaque and the subjacent
chest wall (Figure 6-9).[40] Foci of dystrophic calcification are also commonly observed within the plaque. With light microscopy, neither

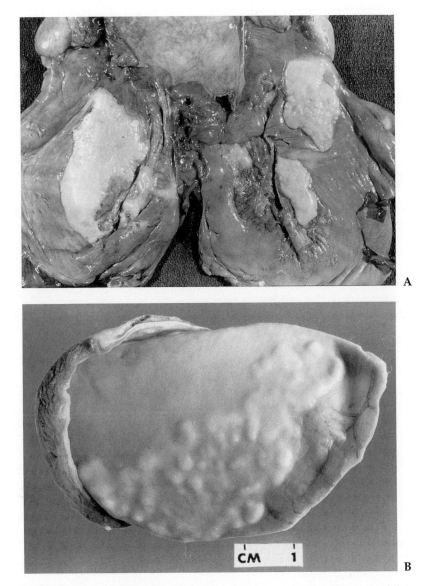

Figure 6-5. (A) Gross photograph from autopsy examination illustrates bilateral elevated white plaques on the diaphragmatic pleura. **(B)** Close view of a
parietal diaphragmatic plaque showing smooth areas as well as knobby areas
resembling "candle-wax drippings."

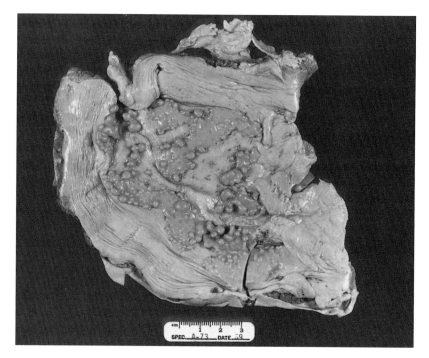

Figure 6-6. Gross appearance of diaphragm with parietal pleural plaque shows irregular, 10 cm plaque with smooth and nodular areas. (Reprinted from Ref. 25, with permission.)

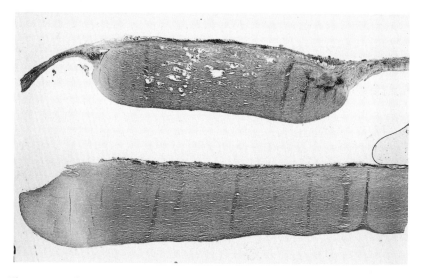

Figure 6-7. Low power H&E photomicrograph showing fibrous parietal pleural plaques as they appeared at autopsy.

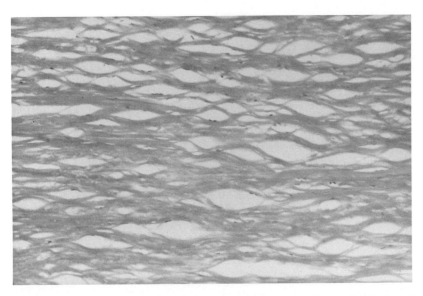

Figure 6-8. High magnification H&E photomicrograph of a parietal pleural plaque. Note the lack of cellularity and the "basket-weave" pattern of the collagen fibers.

asbestos bodies nor fibers are seen. With electron microscopy, asbestos fibers may be found.[20]

Examination of histologic sections of lung parenchyma from patients with pleural plaques may show normal lung or a variety of pathologic

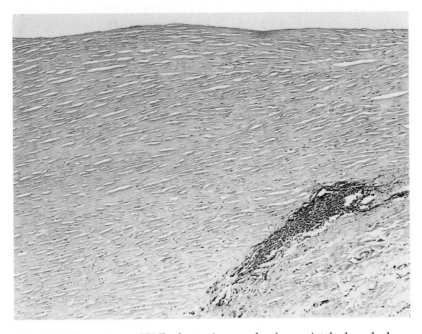

Figure 6-9. Low power H&E photomicrograph of a parietal pleural plaque showing the "basket-weave" pattern of the collagen and a focal collection of lymphocytes at the interface between the plaque and the underlying connective tissue of the chest wall. (Reprinted from Ref. 97, with permission.)

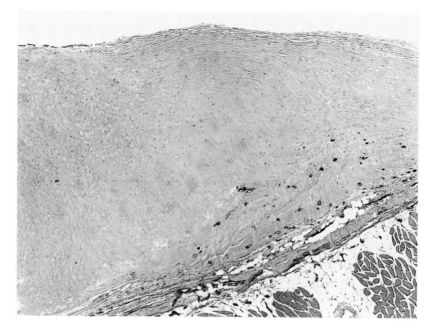

Figure 6-10. H&E photomicrograph of a parietal pleural plaque showing dense collagenous tissue without a "basket-weave" pattern (i.e., solid variant).

features, including peribronchiolar fibrosis, visceral pleural thickening, organizing pneumonia, focal parenchymal scarring, paracicatricial emphysema, or asbestos bodies.[41] The presence of peribronchiolar fibrosis *and* asbestos bodies in histologic sections is diagnostic of asbestosis (see Chapter 4). However, the term asbestosis, which refers to pulmonary interstitial fibrosis, should not be applied to parietal pleural plaques or any of the other benign asbestos-related pleural diseases.

Epidemiologic Considerations

Various epidemiological studies have clearly established the role of inhaled asbestos fibers in the formation of parietal pleural plaques.[20,25,42–51] By means of tissue digests, it has been shown that it is primarily amphibole asbestos fibers that are found in abnormal amounts in the lungs of patients with plaques.[25,45,49–51] The quantity of asbestos present in the lungs of patients with plaques who lack the histologic criteria for the diagnosis of asbestosis (see Chapter 4) is intermediate between that of the general population and that of individuals with asbestosis (see Chapter 11). These data agree well with the epidemiological observations that pleural plaques often occur in individuals with brief, intermittent, or low-level asbestos exposure.[20,25,36] They also occur in individuals exposed to asbestos indirectly, such as family members exposed to dust brought home on an asbestos worker's clothes[46] or individuals living near an asbestos mine or production plant. Outbreaks of pleural plaques and calcification have also been observed in populations exposed to asbestos fibers from an environmental source. For example, a high prevalence of pleural plaques has been noted among Finnish immigrants, believed to be exposed to anthophyllite asbestos in rocks used to heat sauna baths or in insulation materials for the baths.[52] Similarly, a high prevalence of plaques has been described among inhabitants of the island of Cyprus[53] and in the Metsovo region of Greece,[54] where tremolite occurs naturally. In the Metsovo region of Greece, long, thin tremolite fibers are found in the whitewash materials used inside and outside the homes of the inhabitants.[54] More recent environmental exposures leading to plaque formation have been documented,[55,56] and additional epidemics of pleural disease because of environmental asbestos exposure undoubtedly await discovery.

Fibrous zeolites found in the soil and rocks in rural areas of Turkey are also causally associated with bilateral pleural plaques. Although nonasbestiform, these zeolite fibers have length/width ratios that simulate those of asbestos fibers.[57] A detailed epidemiological study of the fibrous zeolite (erionite) in Turkey was reported by Artvinli and Baris in 1982. In Tuzkoy, one of the villages with environmental zeolite exposure, the fibrous mineral was found in soil samples from roads and fields, as well as in building stones. Tissues of lung and pleura from the inhabitants of Tuzkoy also revealed the effects of zeolites, with 17% showing calcified pleural plaques, 10% showing fibrous pleural thickening, and 12% revealing interstitial pulmonary fibrosis.[57] These Anatolian villages also have one of the highest rates of pleural mesothelioma yet identified anywhere in the world (see Chapter 5).

In addition to the observations of pleural plaques caused by asbestos and erionite, Hillerdal lists talc as another environmental mineral that may produce bilateral pleural plaques. However, talc is often contaminated with noncommercial amphiboles (anthophyllite and tremolite), so its exact role is unclear. It is of interest that cigarette smoking interacts with asbestos to greatly increase the risk for development of pleural plaques.[50,58,59] The mechanism is unknown, since smoking has no apparent effect on mesothelioma rates (see Chapter 5). Finally, whereas the vast majority of cases with bilateral parietal pleural plaques are the result of asbestos exposure, unilateral plaques with or without calcification may be the result of other causes, including trauma with organized hemothorax, old empyema, or tuberculous pleuritis.[25,45]

Clinical Implications

The clinical implications of parietal pleural plaques are twofold: (1) the implications of plaques with regard to functional disability, and (2) the prognostic implications with regard to other asbestos-related diseases. The great majority of individuals with pleural plaques alone have no symptoms or physiologic changes.[60–64] In cases where either symptoms or clinical impairment is present, one must carefully consider contributions from diffuse pleural fibrosis (see below), cigarette smoking, or from radiographically inapparent parenchymal fibrosis. Impairment from cigarette smoking is most often due to emphysema, which can be recognized radiographically.[65] Pulmonary interstitial fibrosis (i.e., asbestosis) in the presence of a negative chest x-ray occurs in 10% to 18% of cases.[66,67] Although Schwartz et al.[68] in a study of more than 1200 sheet metal workers found a significant correlation between radiographically detected parietal pleural plaques and restrictive ventilatory defects, these authors concede that the most probable explanation is subclinical alveolitis or interstitial fibrosis not detected by routine chest radiographs.[69] The lack of symptoms or signs in the majority of patients with pleural plaques alone leads one to ask whether pleural plaques should be considered a disease. *Stedman's Medical Dictionary*[70] defines a disease entity as characterized by at least two of the following criteria: (1) a recognized etiologic agent (or agents); (2) an identifiable group of signs or symptoms; and (3) consistent anatomical alterations. Because pleural plaques clearly satisfy the first and third criteria, plaques, by this definition, constitute a disease entity. However, the asymptomatic nature of plaques is not necessarily applicable to other benign asbestos-related pleural disease (see later discussion).

The second issue regards the prognostic implications of plaques with respect to other potentially fatal asbestos-related diseases. Hourihane et al.[42] state that pleural mesotheliomas are more common in patients with pleural plaques, an observation confirmed by others.[71,72] Hillerdal found an 11-fold increased risk of mesothelioma among individuals with bilateral pleural plaques.[71] However, there is no evidence that pleural plaques are a precursor lesion of mesothelioma. Mollo et al.[48] reported that patients with bilateral plaques are more likely to develop asbestosis than those without plaques. Three different studies have independently shown a strong association between pleural plaques and laryngeal carcinoma.[25,48,73] Thus, plaques seem to be a predictor of increased risk for some asbestos-related disorders.

More controversial is the relationship between plaques and carcinoma of the lung. Studies from the United Kingdom have suggested that shipyard workers with pleural plaques are at increased risk for development of carcinoma of the lung.[74,75] Others have found no increased risk of lung cancer associated with plaques alone,[25,48,76] and Kiviluoto et al.,[77] in a study of 700 workers with pleural plaques, found an increased risk for bronchogenic carcinoma only when there was concomitant parenchymal fibrosis (i.e., asbestosis). Hillerdal reported a relative risk for lung cancer of 1.43 for patients with bilateral pleural plaques, and this finding was statistically significant when controlled for asbestosis and cigarette smoking.[75] More recently, Roggli and Sanders showed that only 10% of patients with pleural plaques in the absence of asbestosis had a fiber burden that has been associated with an increased lung cancer risk.[78] A consensus of experts from a meeting in Helsinki, Finland, in 1997 concluded that plaques alone are insufficient to relate lung cancer to prior asbestos exposure.[79]

Diffuse Pleural Fibrosis

Radiographic Features

Diffuse thickening of the visceral pleura can be detected on routine chest films but is better identified by computed tomography.[80] It may occur as a consequence of a connective tissue disorder, such as rheumatoid arthritis or systemic lupus erythematosus.[81] However, in the absence of clinical evidence of a connective tissue disorder, the chest x-ray showing bilateral pleural fibrosis usually indicates prior asbestos exposure.[43,44] Diffuse pleural fibrosis must be distinguished on the one hand from the more localized and often calcified parietal pleural plaque, and on the other hand from malignant pleural mesothelioma. The latter usually shows asymmetrical involvement of the hemithoraces, irregular thickening of the pleura, and invasion or destruction of portions of the chest wall. These features can often be seen to better advantage with computed tomography of the thorax.[82,83] Diffuse pleural thickening may follow benign asbestos effusion,[84] and is often unilateral (Figure 6-11).

Pathologic Findings

Diffuse pleural fibrosis is typically of varying and uneven thickness and can surround the entire lung.[85] The inferior and dorsal portions of

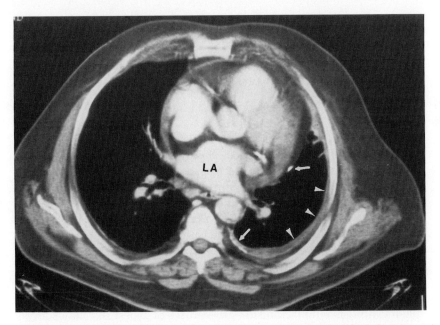

Figure 6-11. Computed tomography of the thorax at the level of the left atrium (LA) showing unilateral diffuse pleural thickening (*arrowheads*) in a 74-year-old manufacturer of asbestos cloth. Calcification is present posteriorly on the parietal pleural surface and also adjacent to the left heart border (*arrows*). No tumor was found at open thoracotomy and pleural biopsy. (Courtesy of Dr. Caroline Chiles, Department of Radiology, Duke University Medical Center, Durham, NC.)

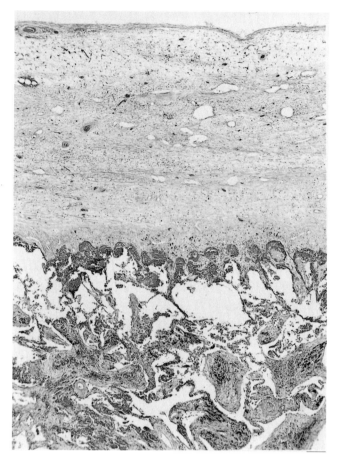

Figure 6-12. H&E photomicrograph showing diffuse fibrosis of the visceral pleura in an insulator with asbestosis. Asbestos bodies in adjacent lung parenchyma are just beyond resolution at this magnification.

the lung are the areas most frequently affected, and the process may extend into the major fissures (see Figure 4-5). A constrictive pleuritis may occur and contribute to decreased vital capacity.[84,86] With time, diffuse pleural fibrosis may progress.[20] Differential diagnosis of such lesions should include infectious pleuritis, rheumatoid arthritis, and systemic lupus erythematosus. The fibrous thickening of the visceral pleura is bland and nonspecific, consisting of dense collagenous tissue and varying numbers of chronic inflammatory cells (lymphocytes, macrophages, and plasma cells) (Figure 6-12). Fibrin deposits may be observed on the surface of the collagenous tissue. Analysis of tissue asbestos content in the lung parenchyma of patients with diffuse pleural fibrosis who lack histologic features of asbestosis shows levels intermediate between those of the general population and those of individuals with asbestosis (see Chapter 11).[85] A dose-response relationship has been demonstrated between the degree of asbestos exposure and the extent of pleural thickening.[47] With light microscopy, neither asbestos bodies nor fibers are seen within the fibrotic visceral pleura. With electron microscopy, asbestos fibers may be found.[20]

Clinical Implications

Diffuse pleural fibrosis may be asymptomatic, but in some cases may be of sufficient extent and severity as to result in functional impairment.[67,84,86,87] This usually manifests as restrictive changes on pulmonary function tests, with a diminished vital capacity.[88] Picado et al.[89] described six patients with extensive asbestos-related pleural disease that manifested diminished exercise tolerance. These investigators felt that parenchymal fibrosis was unlikely, although lung parenchyma was not available for histologic examination in any of the cases. Although some of the patients were characterized as having parietal pleural plaques, it is likely that most or all had some degree of diffuse visceral pleural fibrosis. A study by Schwartz et al.[90] found a correlation between the degree of pleural fibrosis detected by computed tomography and the restrictive lung function in the patients. Surgical decortication is rarely indicated in these patients, because postoperative improvement is usually only marginal.[20]

Rounded Atelectasis

Radiologic Features

Blesovsky originally described rounded atelectasis, also known as the folded lung syndrome, in 1966.[91] It is characterized radiographically as a peripheral rounded mass, 2 to 7 cm in diameter, that is pleural based.[92] Pleural thickening that is greatest near the mass and interposition of lung parenchyma between the mass and the diaphragm are invariably present (Figure 6-13). One of the most useful diagnostic features is the presence of curvilinear shadows extending from the mass toward the hilum.[92,93] The intrapulmonary location of the mass is indicated by the acute angle formed between the pleura and mass. The intralobar fissure is frequently thickened. When sequential films are available for review, the static nature of the lesion can be demonstrated. In cases where bronchography has been performed, bronchi have been demonstrated to curve toward the lower pole of the mass.[92] Computed tomography and high resolution CT are much better at detecting this lesion[93] and may also detect other asbestos-related pleural changes, such as calcification (Figure 6-14).[32,94] Rounded atelectasis may be bilateral in some instances,[95] and cases with spontaneous resolution have also been reported.[96]

Pathologic Findings

Pathologists must be aware of the gross and microscopic features of rounded atelectasis, because they may be called upon to make the diagnosis at frozen section. The lesion is characterized by dense pleural fibrosis that is of greatest thickness overlying the mass (see Figure 6-14). The pleura may be buckled or puckered and thus drawn into the underlying lung parenchyma. The lung itself may contain some fibrosis but is largely atelectatic. Because of the frequent association with asbestos exposure,[92] asbestos bodies should be searched for within the

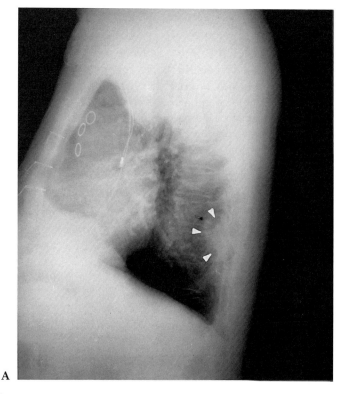

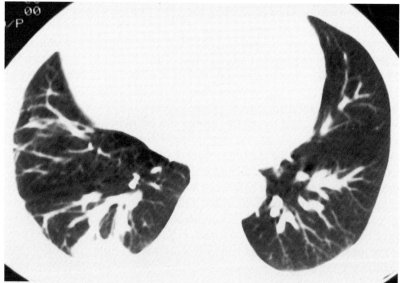

Figure 6-13. **(A)** Lateral chest radiograph showing a posterior, pleural-based mass (*arrowheads*). **(B)** Computed tomogram of the thorax shows the typical features of rounded atelectasis, with a pleural-based mass and curvilinear bronchovascular structures entering the mass. (Reprinted from Ref. 97, with permission.)

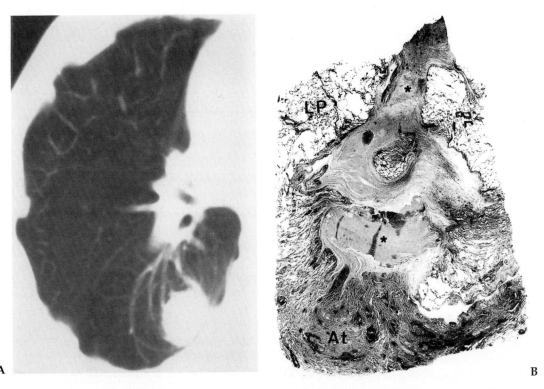

A   B

Figure 6-14. (A) Computed tomography of the left hemithorax in a patient with a left lower lobe mass on chest x-ray. Note the curvilinear bronchovascular structures entering the pleural-based mass, which is characteristic of rounded atelectasis. (B) Low power H&E photomicrograph of the resected lesion shown in A, with pleural surface toward the top. There is localized thickening and fibrosis of the visceral pleura, which has buckled inward (*). Adjacent lung parenchyma is atelectatic (At). Elsewhere, the lung parenchyma (LP) is normally expanded.

lung parenchyma.[97] However, care must be taken not to diagnose asbestosis based on changes secondary to the pleural lesion. Blesovsky believed that the mechanism of formation of rounded atelectasis involved localized visceral pleural thickening and fibrosis in which adhesion between visceral and parietal pleura was prevented from forming because of an associated pleural effusion. Contraction and buckling of the fibrotic visceral pleura then led to atelectasis and folding of the immediately adjacent lung parenchyma. In support of this pathogenetic concept, it was observed at thoracotomy that the collapsed lung reexpanded when the thickened pleura was dissected away.[91]

Clinical Implications

The strong association between rounded atelectasis and prior asbestos exposure has been emphasized.[92] Indeed, all three of the original cases described by Blesovsky had been occupationally exposed to asbestos.[92] Because of this association and the increased risk of lung cancer in asbestos workers (see Chapter 7), rounded atelectasis may be confused with lung cancer clinically and radiographially.[98] Recognition of the clinical and radiographic features of rounded atelectasis is important, because the rendering of the correct diagnosis can spare the patient a thoracotomy.[99]

Benign Asbestos Pleural Effusion

Clinical Criteria

Eisenstadt reported the first case of benign asbestos-related pleural effusion in 1964.[100] This was a unilateral effusion in an asbestos worker. Dr. Eisenstadt stated that a diagnosis of benign asbestos pleural effusion should only be made after biopsies of the lung and pleura were performed to rule out other disease processes. More than 250 additional cases have subsequently been reported, and it is now recognized that asbestos pleural effusion (pleurisy) is the most common asbestos-related lesion during the first decade after exposure. However, it can occur at a later date.[101] It is usually a moderate-sized effusion of up to 2000 ml that may be clear to hemorrhagic and of variable cellularity. Hillerdal lists three diagnostic criteria of an asbestos effusion: (1) tuberculosis, infection, or malignancy must be ruled out; (2) the individual must be followed for two years to verify the effusion is benign; and (3) there must be an occupational exposure to asbestos (Table 6-2). The asbestos effusion tends to recur and can last for months. Recurrence on the same or opposite side is common, and clinical symptoms are only mild to absent.[20,84] In addition to this tendency to recur, another feature characteristic of benign asbestos effusion is the presence of either rounded atelectasis or converging pleural linear structures (so-called "crow's feet") on the chest radiograph at the initial presentation.[101]

Epler et al., in 1982, reviewed chest x-rays of 1135 employees in the asbestos industry. The prevalence of asbestos effusions was 7.0%, 3.7%, and 0.2%, depending on whether the asbestos work exposure was, respectively, severe, indirect, or peripheral.[102] The latency for asbestos effusions was shorter than for asbestos plaques and was the only manifestation seen within 10 years of exposure. The incidence ranged from less than one to as many as nine cases of asbestos effusion per 1000 person-years of observation, depending on the degree of exposure. The recurrence rate was 29%. In 66% of the effusions, the workers were asymptomatic. In a related article, Gaensler et al.[99] reported on 68 patients with benign asbestos pleural effusions, the majority of whom had no symptoms. These investigators stated that benign asbestos pleural effusions were the most common asbestos-related disorder

Table 6-2. Clinical criteria for benign asbestos pleural effusion

1. Clinically documented pleural effusion
2. History of exposure to asbestos
3. Elimination of other causes of effusion (infection, collagen vascular disease, malignancy, etc.)
4. Follow-up of two or three years to verify benign nature of process

Source: Modified from Refs. 20 and 99

during the first 20 years after initial exposure and were seen in approximately 5% of all heavily exposed persons.[99] Robinson and Musk reported on still another cohort of 22 asbestos workers with asbestos pleural effusion.[103] Their mean work exposure was five years, their time between work exposure and occurrence of pleurisy was 16 years, and the mean duration of the effusion was four months. The pleural fluid was blood tinged and rarely greater than 500 ml.

Hillerdal emphasized the benign course of these effusions even though they may be bloody and of large volume.[104] An exception was a very small group of more heavily exposed individuals who sometimes developed progressive pleural fibrosis after an initial effusion. This observation was confirmed by McLoud et al.,[105] and in some cases may result in respiratory failure.[106] Lilis et al.[107] described 20 patients in a series of 2815 insulation workers (0.7%) who had a history of symptomatic pleural effusion. Sixteen of these 20 (80%) had diffuse pleural fibrosis radiographically, whereas 5.0% of the total group had diffuse pleural fibrosis. These observations suggest that diffuse pleural fibrosis in the patients without a history of benign asbestos effusion may be the residua of asymptomatic pleural effusion in at least some of these individuals.[107] In another article, Hillerdal made the observation that asbestos workers in Finland are exposed to anthophyllite asbestos, and there is a low incidence among them of both asbestos effusion and pleural mesothelioma.[108]

Pathologic Findings

The pathologic features of benign asbestos effusion have not been well defined. Core needle biopsy of the pleura in a few of the cases in the series of Robinson and Musk[103] showed pleural fibrosis with or without an inflammatory infiltrate. Decortication in four of the cases of Mattson[109] showed chronic nonspecific fibrotic pleurisy. In one of these four cases, asbestos bodies and pulmonary fibrosis were observed in the adjacent lung parenchyma. The effusion itself is characteristically an exudate, with glucose and protein levels similar to that of plasma.[110] In more than half the cases, the fluid is grossly hemorrhagic. The cell count usually is less than 6000/mm^3, with either a mononuclear or neutrophil predominance.[111] In about one-fourth of the cases, esoinophils are a prominent feature. In this regard, it should be noted that injection of asbestos fibers into the pleural cavities of experimental animals results in an exudative effusion.[2] Bilaterality of benign asbestos effusion is common, occurring in eleven of 60 patients studied by Hillerdal and Ozesmi.[110] In three cases the effusions were synchronous, whereas in the remaining eight cases they were metachronous, separated by an interval ranging from one to 15 years.

References

1. Solomon A, Sluis-Cremer GK, Goldstein B: Visceral pleural plaque formation in asbestosis. *Environ Res* 19:258–264, 1979.
2. Sahn SA, Antony VB: Pathogenesis of pleural plaques. Relationship of early cellular response and pathology. *Am Rev Respir Dis* 130:884–887, 1984.

3. Craighead JE: Current pathogenetic concepts of diffuse malignant mesothelioma. *Hum Pathol* 18:544–557, 1987.
4. Greenberg S: Asbestos lung disease. *Sem Respir Med* 4:130–137, 1982.
5. Brody AR, Hill LH, Adkins B Jr, O'Connor RW: Chrysotile asbestos inhalation in rats: deposition pattern and reaction of alveolar epithelium and pulmonary macrophages. *Am Rev Respir Dis* 123:670–679, 1981.
6. Antony VB, Owen CL, Hadley KJ: Pleural mesothelial cells stimulated by asbestos release chemotactic activity for neutrophils in vitro. *Am Rev Respir Dis* 139:199–206, 1989.
7. Tanaka S, Choe N, Iwagaki A, Hemenway DR, Kagan E: Asbestos exposure induces MCP-1 secretion by pleural mesothelial cells. *Exp Lung Res* 26:241–255, 2000.
8. Gloyne S: Pathology. In: *Silicosis and Asbestosis* (Lanza A, ed.), New York: Oxford University Press, 1938, pp. 120–135.
9. Porro F, Patten J, Hobbs A: Pneumoconiosis in the talc industry. *Am J Roentgenol* 47:507–524, 1942.
10. Siegal W, Smith A, Greenberg L: Dust hazard in tremolite talc mining, including roentgenologic findings in talc workers. *Am J Roentgenol* 49:11–29, 1943.
11. Smith A: Pleural calcification resulting from exposure to certain dusts. *Am J Roentgenol* 69:375–382, 1952.
12. Frost J, George J, Moller P: Asbestosis with pleural calcification among insulation workers. *Danish Med Bull* 3:202–204, 1956.
13. Hillerdal G, Lindgren A: Pleural plaques: correlation of autopsy findings to radiographic findings and occupational history. *Eur J Respir Dis* 61:315–319, 1980.
14. Rohl AN: Asbestos in talc. *Environ Health Perspect* 9:129–132, 1974.
15. Gamble JF, Fellner W, Dimeo MJ: An epidemiologic study of a group of talc workers. *Am Rev Respir Dis* 119:741–753, 1979.
16. Wagner J, Berry G, Cooke T, Hill R, Pooley F, Skidmore J: Animal experiments with talc, In: *Inhaled particles IV. Proceedings of the International Symposium* (Walton, W, ed.), Edinburgh: Pergamon Press, 1977, pp. 647–654.
17. van den Heuvel MM, Smit HJ, Barbierato SB, Havenith CE, Beelen RH, Postmus PE: Talc-induced inflammation in the pleural cavity. *Eur Respir J* 12:1419–1423, 1998.
18. Nasreen N, Hartman DL, Mohammed KA, Antony VB: Talc-induced expression of C-C and C-X-C chemokines and intercellular adhesion molecule-1 in mesothelial cells. *Am J Respir Crit Care Med* 158:971–978, 1998.
19. Rubino G, Scansetti G, Piro E, Piolatto G, Mollo F, Andrion A, Colombo A, Bentasso L: Pleural plaques and lung asbestos bodies in the general population: An autoptical and clinical-radiologic survey, In: *Biological Effects of Mineral Fibers* (Wagner J, ed.), *Ann Sci Pub* I:545–551, 1980.
20. Hillerdal G: Nonmalignant pleural disease related to asbestos exposure. *Clin Chest Med* 6:141–152, 1985.
21. Svenes KB, Borgersen A, Haaversen O, Holten K: Parietal pleural plaques: A comparison between autopsy and X-ray findings. *Eur J Respir Dis* 69:10–15, 1986.
22. Withers BF, Ducatman AM, Yang WN: Roentgenographic evidence for predominant left-sided location of unilateral pleural plaques. *Chest* 95:1262–1264, 1989.
23. Hu H, Beckett L, Kelsey K, Christiani D: The left-sided predominance of asbestos-related pleural disease. *Am Rev Respir Dis* 148:981–984, 1993.
24. Gallego JC: Absence of left-sided predominance in asbestos-related pleural plaques: A CT study. *Chest* 113:1034–1036, 1998.

25. Wain SL, Roggli VL, Foster WL: Parietal pleural plaques, asbestos bodies, and neoplasia. A clinical, pathologic, and roentgenographic correlation of 25 consecutive cases. *Chest* 86:707–713, 1984.

26. Meurman L: Asbestos bodies and pleural plaques in a Finnish series of autopsy cases. *Acta Path Microbiol Scand* 181 [Suppl]:1–107, 1966.

27. Miller JA, Zurlo JV: Asbestos plaques in a typical Veteran's hospital population. *Am J Ind Med* 30:726–729, 1996.

28. Aberle DR, Gamsu G, Ray CS: High-resolution CT of benign asbestos-related diseases: clinical and radiographic correlation. *Am J Roentgenol* 151:883–891, 1988.

29. Friedman AC, Fiel SB, Fisher MS, Radecki PD, Lev-Toaff AS, Caroline DF: Asbestos-related pleural disease and asbestosis: a comparison of CT and chest radiography. *Am J Roentgenol* 150:269–275, 1988.

30. al Jarad N, Poulakis N, Pearson MC, Rubens MB, Rudd RM: Assessment of asbestos-induced pleural disease by computed tomography—correlation with chest radiograph and lung function. *Respir Med* 85:203–208, 1991.

31. Jarad NA, Wilkinson P, Pearson MC, Rudd RM: A new high resolution computed tomography scoring system for pulmonary fibrosis, pleural disease, and emphysema in patients with asbestos related disease. *Br J Ind Med* 49:73–84, 1992.

32. Gevenois PA, De Vuyst P, Dedeire S, Cosaert J, Vande Weyer R, Struyven J: Conventional and high-resolution CT in asymptomatic asbestos-exposed workers. *Acta Radiol* 35:226–229, 1994.

33. Aberle DR: High-resolution computed tomography of asbestos-related diseases. *Semin Roentgenol* 26:118–131, 1991.

34. Hammar SP: Pleural diseases, In: *Pulmonary Pathology*, 2nd ed. (Dail DH, Hammar SP, eds.), New York: Springer-Verlag, 1994, pp. 1463–1579.

35. Hammar SP: The pathology of benign and malignant pleural disease. *Chest Surg Clin N Am* 4:405–430, 1994.

36. Craighead JE, Abraham JL, Churg A, Green FH, Kleinerman J, Pratt PC, Seemayer TA, Vallyathan V, Weill H: The pathology of asbestos-associated diseases of the lungs and pleural cavities: diagnostic criteria and proposed grading schema. *Arch Pathol Lab Med* 106:544–596, 1982.

37. Fischbein L, Namade M, Sachs RN, Robineau M, Lanfranchi J: Chronic constrictive pericarditis associated with asbestosis. *Chest* 94:646–647, 1988.

38. Mollo F, Bellis D, Magnani C, Delsedime L, Andrion A: Hyaline splenic and hepatic plaques. Correlation with cirrhosis, pulmonary tuberculosis, and asbestos exposure. *Arch Pathol Lab Med* 117:1017–1021, 1993.

39. Davies D, Andrews MI, Jones JS: Asbestos induced pericardial effusion and constrictive pericarditis. *Thorax* 46:429–432, 1991.

40. Roggli VL, Shelburne JD: New concepts in the diagnosis of mineral pneumoconioses. *Sem Respir Med* 4:138–148, 1982.

41. Sison RF, Hruban RH, Moore GW, Kuhlman JE, Wheeler PS, Hutchins GM: Pulmonary disease associated with pleural "asbestos" plaques. *Chest* 95:831–835, 1989.

42. Hourihane D, Lessof L, Richardson P: Hyaline and calcified pleural plaques as an index of exposure to asbestos: A study of radiological and pathological features of 100 cases with consideration of epidemiology. *Brit Med J* 1:1069–1074, 1966.

43. Albelda SM, Epstein DM, Gefter WB, Miller WT: Pleural thickening: Its significance and relationship to asbestos dust exposure. *Am Rev Respir Dis* 126:621–624, 1982.

44. Andrion A, Colombo A, Dacorsi M, Mollo F: Pleural plaques at autopsy in Turin: A study on 1,019 adult subjects. *Eur J Respir Dis* 63:107–12, 1982.

45. Churg A: Asbestos fibers and pleural plaques in a general autopsy population. *Am J Pathol* 109:88–96, 1982.
46. Kilburn KH, Lilis R, Anderson HA, Boylen CT, Einstein HE, Johnson SJ, Warshaw R: Asbestos disease in family contacts of shipyard workers. *Am J Public Health* 75:615–617, 1985.
47. Lundorf E, Aagaard MT, Andresen J, Silberschmid M, Sabro S, Coutte A, Bolvig L: Radiological evaluation of early pleural and pulmonary changes in light asbestos exposure. *Eur J Respir Dis* 70:145–149, 1987.
48. Mollo F, Andrion A, Colombo A, Segnan N, Pira E: Pleural plaques and risk of cancer in Turin, northwestern Italy. An autopsy study. *Cancer* 54:1418–1422, 1984.
49. Warnock ML, Prescott BT, Kuwahara TJ: Numbers and types of asbestos fibers in subjects with pleural plaques. *Am J Pathol* 109:37–46, 1982.
50. Karjalainen A, Karhunen PJ, Lalu K, Penttila A, Vanhala E, Kyyronen P, Tossavainen A: Pleural plaques and exposure to mineral fibres in a male urban necropsy population. *Occup Environ Med* 51:456–460, 1994.
51. Murai Y, Kitagawa M, Hiraoka T: Fiber analysis in lungs of residents of a Japanese town with endemic pleural plaques. *Arch Environ Health* 52:263–269, 1997.
52. Hillerdal G: Pleural plaques in Sweden among immigrants from Finland—with an editorial note. *Eur J Respir Dis* 64:386–390, 1983.
53. McConnochie K, Simonato L, Mavrides P, Christofides P, Pooley FD, Wagner JC: Mesothelioma in Cyprus: The role of tremolite. *Thorax* 42:342–347, 1987.
54. Langer AM, Nolan RP, Constantopoulos SH, Moutsopoulos HM: Association of Metsovo lung and pleural mesothelioma with exposure to tremolite-containing whitewash. *Lancet* 1:965–967, 1987.
55. Rey F, Boutin C, Steinbauer J, Viallat JR, Alessandroni P, Jutisz P, Di Giambattista D, Billon-Galland MA, Hereng P, Dumortier P: Environmental pleural plaques in an asbestos exposed population of northeast Corsica. *Eur J Respir Dis* 6:978–982, 1993.
56. Hiraoka T, Ohkura M, Morinaga K, Kohyama N, Shimazu K, Ando M: Anthophyllite exposure and endemic pleural plaques in Kumamoto, Japan. *Scand J Work Environ Health* 24:392–397, 1998.
57. Artvinli M, Baris YI: Environmental fiber-induced pleuro-pulmonary diseases in an Anatolian village: An epidemiologic study. *Arch Environ Health* 37:177–181, 1982.
58. Andrion A, Pira E, Mollo F: Pleural plaques at autopsy, smoking habits, and asbestos exposure. *Eur J Respir Dis* 65:125–130, 1984.
59. McMillan GH, Pethybridge RJ, Sheers G: Effect of smoking on attack rates of pulmonary and pleural lesions related to exposure to asbestos dust. *Br J Ind Med* 37:268–272, 1980.
60. Lumley K: Physiological changes in asbestos pleural diseases, In: *Inhaled Particles* (Walton W, ed.), Pergamon Press: Oxford, 1977, pp. 781–788.
61. Jarvholm B, Arvidsson H, Bake B, Hillerdal G, Westrin CG: Pleural plaques–asbestos–ill-health. *Eur J Respir Dis Suppl* 145:1–59, 1986.
62. Jarvholm B, Sanden A: Pleural plaques and respiratory function. *Am J Ind Med* 10:419–426, 1986.
63. Copley SJ, Wells AU, Rubens MB, Chabat F, Sheehan RE, Musk AW, Hansell DM: Functional consequences of pleural disease evaluated with chest radiography and CT. *Radiology* 220:237–243, 2001.
64. Van Cleemput J, De Raeve H, Verschakelen JA, Rombouts J, Lacquet LM, Nemery B: Surface of localized pleural plaques quantitated by computed tomography scanning: No relation with cumulative asbestos exposure and no effect on lung function. *Am J Respir Crit Care Med* 163:705–710, 2001.
65. Pratt PC: Role of conventional chest radiography in diagnosis and exclusion of emphysema. *Am J Med* 82:998–1006, 1987.

66. Epler, GR, McLoud TC, Gaensler EA, Mikus JP, Carrington CB: Normal chest roentgenograms in chronic diffuse infiltrative lung disease. *N Engl J Med* 298:934–939, 1978.
67. Kipen HM, Lilis R, Suzuki Y, Valciukas JA, Selikoff IJ: Pulmonary fibrosis in asbestos insulation workers with lung cancer: a radiological and histopathological evaluation. *Br J Ind Med* 44:96–100, 1987.
68. Schwartz DA, Fuortes LJ, Galvin JR, Burmeister LF, Schmidt LE, Leistikow BN, LaMarte FP, Merchant JA: Asbestos-induced pleural fibrosis and impaired lung function. *Am Rev Respir Dis* 141:321–326, 1990.
69. Shih JF, Wilson JS, Broderick A, Watt JL, Galvin JR, Merchant JA, Schwartz DA: Asbestos-induced pleural fibrosis and impaired exercise physiology. *Chest* 105:1370–1376, 1994.
70. Steadman's Medical *Dictionary*: Baltimore: Williams & Wilkins, 1972, pp. 358.
71. Hillerdal G: Pleural plaques and risk for bronchial carcinoma and mesothelioma. A prospective study. *Chest* 105:144–150, 1994.
72. Bianchi C, Brollo A, Ramani L, Zuch C: Pleural plaques as risk indicators for malignant pleural mesothelioma: a necropsy-based study. *Am J Ind Med* 32:445–449, 1997.
73. Hillerdal G: Pleural plaques and risks for cancer in the county of Uppsala. *Eur J Respir Dis* 61 (Suppl 107):111–117, 1980.
74. Fletcher DE: A mortality study of shipyard workers with pleural plaques. *Br J Ind Med* 29:142–145, 1972.
75. Edge JR: Incidence of bronchial carcinoma in shipyard workers with pleural plaques. *Ann N Y Acad Sci* 330:289–294, 1979.
76. Weiss W: Asbestos-related pleural plaques and lung cancer. *Chest* 103:1854–1859, 1993.
77. Kiviluoto R, Meurman LO, Hakama M: Pleural plaques and neoplasia in Finland. *Ann N Y Acad Sci* 330:31–33, 1979.
78. Roggli VL, Sanders LL: Asbestos content of lung tissue and carcinoma of the lung: a clinicopathologic correlation and mineral fiber analysis of 234 cases. *Ann Occup Hyg* 44:109–117, 2000.
79. Henderson D, Rantanen J, Barnhart S, Dement J, DeVuyst P, Hillerdal G, Huuskonen M, Kivisaari L, Kusaha Y, Lahdensuo A, Langard S, Mowe G, Okubo T, Parker J, Roggli V, Rodelsperger K, Rosler J, Tossavainen A, Woitowitz H: Asbestos, asbestosis, and cancer: The Helsinki criteria for diagnosis and attribution: A consensus report of an international expert group. *Scand J Work Environ Health* 23:311–316, 1997.
80. Ameille J, Brochard P, Brechot JM, Pascano T, Cherin A, Raix A, Fredy M, Bignon J: Pleural thickening: a comparison of oblique chest radiographs and high-resolution computed tomography in subjects exposed to low levels of asbestos pollution. *Int Arch Occup Environ Health* 64:545–548, 1993.
81. Lie J: Rheumatic connective tissue disease. In: *Pulmonary Pathology*, 2nd ed. (Dail D, Hammar S, eds.), New York: Springer-Verlag, 1994, pp. 679–705.
82. Alexander E, Clark RA, Colley DP, Mitchell SE: CT of malignant pleural mesothelioma. *Am J Roentgenol* 137:287–291, 1981.
83. Mirvis S, Dutcher JP, Haney PJ, Whitley NO, Aisner J: CT of malignant pleural mesothelioma. *Am J Roentgenol* 140:665–670, 1983.
84. Anonymous: Benign asbestos pleural effusions. *Lancet* 1:1145–1146, 1988.
85. Stephens M, Gibbs AR, Pooley FD, Wagner JC: Asbestos induced diffuse pleural fibrosis: Pathology and mineralogy. *Thorax* 42:583–588, 1987.
86. Britton MG: Asbestos pleural disease. *Br J Dis Chest* 76:1–10, 1982.
87. Lilis R, Miller A, Godbold J, Benkert S, Wu X, Selikoff IJ: Comparative quantitative evaluation of pleural fibrosis and its effects on pulmonary function in two large asbestos-exposed occupational groups—insulators and sheet metal workers. *Environ Res* 59:49–66, 1992.

88. Kee ST, Gamsu G, Blanc P: Causes of pulmonary impairment in asbestos-exposed individuals with diffuse pleural thickening. *Am J Respir Crit Care Med* 154:789–793, 1996.

89. Picado C, Laporta D, Grassino A, Cosio M, Thibodeau M, Becklake MR: Mechanisms affecting exercise performance in subjects with asbestos-related pleural fibrosis. *Lung* 165:45–57, 1987.

90. Schwartz DA, Galvin JR, Yagla SJ, Speakman SB, Merchant JA, Hunninghake GW: Restrictive lung function and asbestos-induced pleural fibrosis. A quantitative approach. *J Clin Invest* 91:2685–2692, 1993.

91. Blesovsky A: The folded lung. *Br J Dis Chest* 60:19–22, 1966.

92. Mintzer RA, Cugell DW: The association of asbestos-induced pleural disease and rounded atelectasis. *Chest* 81:457–460, 1982.

93. Batra P, Brown K, Hayashi K, Mori M: Rounded atelectasis. *J Thorac Imaging* 11:187–197, 1996.

94. Lynch DA, Gamsu G, Ray CS, Aberle DR: Asbestos-related focal lung masses: manifestations on conventional and high-resolution CT scans. *Radiology* 169:603–607, 1988.

95. Gevenois PA, de Maertelaer V, Madani A, Winant C, Sergent G, De Vuyst P: Asbestosis, pleural plaques and diffuse pleural thickening: Three distinct benign responses to asbestos exposure. *Eur Respir J* 11:1021–1027, 1998.

96. Hillerdal G: Rounded atelectasis. Clinical experience with 74 patients. *Chest* 95:836–841, 1989.

97. Roggli V: Pathology of human asbestosis: A critical review. In: *Advances in Pathology* (Fenoglio-Preiser C, ed.), Chicago: Yearbook Pub., 1989, pp. 28–47.

98. Payne CR, Jaques P, Kerr IH: Lung folding simulating peripheral pulmonary neoplasm (Blesovsky's syndrome). *Thorax* 35:936–940, 1980.

99. Gaensler EA, McLoud TC, Carrington CB: Thoracic surgical problems in asbestos-related disorders. *Ann Thorac Surg* 40:82–96, 1985.

100. Eisenstadt H: Asbestos pleurisy. *Dis Chest* 46:78–81, 1964.

101. Martensson G, Hagberg S, Pettersson K, Thiringer G: Asbestos pleural effusion: A clinical entity. *Thorax* 42:646–651, 1987.

102. Epler GR, McLoud TC, Gaensler EA: Prevalence and incidence of benign asbestos pleural effusion in a working population. *JAMA* 247:617–622, 1982.

103. Robinson BW, Musk AW: Benign asbestos pleural effusion: Diagnosis and course. *Thorax* 36:896–900, 1981.

104. Hillerdal G: Non-malignant asbestos pleural disease. *Thorax* 36:669–75, 1981.

105. McLoud TC, Woods BO, Carrington CB, Epler GR, Gaensler EA: Diffuse pleural thickening in an asbestos-exposed population: Prevalence and causes. *Am J Roentgenol* 144:9–18, 1985.

106. Miller A, Teirstein AS, Selikoff IJ: Ventilatory failure due to asbestos pleurisy. *Am J Med* 75:911–919, 1983.

107. Lilis R, Lerman Y, Selikoff IJ: Symptomatic benign pleural effusions among asbestos insulation workers: residual radiographic abnormalities. *Br J Ind Med* 45:443–449, 1988.

108. Hillerdal G, Zitting A, van Assendelft AH, Kuusela T: Rarity of mineral fibre pleurisy among persons exposed to Finnish anthophyllite and with low risk of mesothelioma. *Thorax* 39:608–611, 1984.

109. Mattson SB: Monosymptomatic exudative pleurisy in persons exposed to asbestos dust. *Scand J Respir Dis* 56:263–272, 1975.

110. Hillerdal G, Ozesmi M: Benign asbestos pleural effusion: 73 exudates in 60 patients. *Eur J Respir Dis* 71:113–121, 1987.

111. Sahn SA: State of the art. The pleura. *Am Rev Respir Dis* 138:184–234, 1988.

7

Carcinoma of the Lung

Victor L. Roggli

Introduction

During the past fifty years, the United States and other industrialized nations have witnessed a remarkable increase in mortality from carcinoma of the lung. Today, this disease is the number one cause of cancer mortality in the United States, accounting for 170,000 deaths annually.[1] Unraveling the various causes of this increased risk has required painstaking epidemiologic studies, but it has become apparent that cigarette smoking is the single largest preventable cause of lung cancer in the world today.[2] It has been estimated that between 85% and 95% of deaths from lung cancer are directly attributable to smoking.[1,2] Cigarettes are the leading offenders, but pipe and cigar smokers are also at risk, though only if they inhale the smoke.[1-3] Asbestos workers are also at increased risk for lung cancer, particularly those who smoke tobacco products.[4,5] This chapter will review the characteristics of asbestos-associated lung cancers and discuss the role of the pathologist in recognizing asbestos as a causative factor. The historical context in which asbestos was recognized to be a carcinogen for the lower respiratory tract will be reviewed first, followed by a discussion of the epidemiologic features of asbestos-related lung cancer, including the role of asbestosis, synergism with cigarette smoking, and asbestos fiber type. The role of cytopathology in the diagnosis of lung cancer in asbestos workers is discussed in Chapter 9, experimental models of pulmonary carcinogenesis in Chapter 10, and lung fiber burdens in asbestos workers with lung cancer in Chapter 11.

Historical Background

The first report of carcinoma of the lung in an asbestos worker was that of Lynch and Smith in 1935, a squamous carcinoma in a patient with asbestosis.[6] In 1943, Homburger reported three additional cases of bronchogenic carcinoma associated with asbestosis, bringing the world total reported to that date to 19 cases.[7] In his annual report for 1947 as chief inspector of factories in England and Wales, Merewether noted that among 235 deaths attributed at autopsy to asbestosis, 13% had a lung or pleural cancer.[8] During the 20-year period following Lynch and Smith's initial case report, some 26 reports were published covering approximately 90 cases of carcinoma of the lung found at autopsy in asbestos workers.[9] Then in 1955, Sir Richard Doll published his classic study, which was the first systematic combined epidemiologic and pathologic study of lung cancer among asbestos workers.[10] Doll concluded that carcinoma of the lung was a specific industrial hazard of asbestos workers. Also in 1955, Breslow published a case control study of asbestosis and lung cancer from California hospitals.[11] In 1968, Selikoff published data from a cohort of asbestos insulation workers that showed that insulators who smoked had a 92-fold increased risk of carcinoma of the lung over nonasbestos-exposed, nonsmoking individuals.[12] This was also the first study to suggest that there is a multiplicative, or synergistic, effect between cigarette smoking and asbestos exposure in the production of pulmonary carcinomas. Buchanan noted that more than half of all patients with asbestosis would eventually die of respiratory tract cancer.[13] Since these pioneering studies, numerous reports have confirmed the association between asbestos exposure and carcinoma of the lung.[14–23]

Epidemiology

Asbestos or Asbestosis?

Epidemiologic studies have demonstrated a dose-response relationship between asbestos exposure and lung cancer risk, and there is a long latency period between initial exposure and manifestation of disease, usually beginning more than 15 years after initial exposure.[4,5,9,19] Three primary hypotheses have been put forward to describe the relationship between asbestos exposure and lung cancer risk.[24] The first hypothesis [H1] is that there is only an increased risk of lung cancer in asbestos workers who also have asbestosis. The second hypothesis [H2] is that it is the dose of asbestos rather than the occurrence of fibrosis that is the determinant of lung cancer risk. The third hypothesis [H3] is that there is a no threshold, linear dose response relationship between asbestos exposure and subsequent lung cancer risk, with any level of exposure potentially increasing one's risk of disease. Whether there is a threshold for asbestos-induced carcinoma of the lung and whether asbestosis is a prerequisite precursor lesion are issues of more than academic importance,[25] because the number of individuals exposed to low levels of asbestos greatly exceeds the numbers of individuals with asbestosis.

All investigators are in agreement that a dose-response relationship exists between asbestos exposure and lung cancer risk,[26] and that the highest risk occurs among those workers who also have asbestosis. Proponents of [H1] believe that only those with asbestosis have an increased lung cancer risk.[27–31] In the original study by Doll,[10] all 11 of the asbestos workers dying of carcinoma of the lung had pathologically confirmed asbestosis. Furthermore, in the review by An and Koprowska of asbestos associated carcinoma of the lung reported from 1935 to 1962, all 41 cases occurred in individuals with asbestosis.[32] Published mortality data reveal a close correlation between relative risks of death from lung cancer and from asbestosis.[14,16,33–38] In addition, a longitudinal study of Quebec chrysotile miners indicated that most of the observed cancers have occurred in subgroups of workers with prior radiographic evidence of asbestosis.[39]

Further support for this hypothesis includes studies of Louisiana asbestos cement workers, South African asbestos miners, insulators, and individuals with nonasbestos-related interstitial lung disease. The Hughes–Weill study of 839 asbestos cement workers found a statistically significant increased risk of lung cancer among workers with radiographic evidence of asbestosis (International Labor Organization score ≥1/0), but not among those with pleural disease only or with no radiographic abnormality.[19] Sluis-Cremer and Bezuidenout reported on an autopsy study of 399 amphibole miners, in which increased lung cancer rates were observed in cases with pathological asbestosis, but not in those lacking asbestosis.[40] Kipen et al. studied 138 insulators with lung cancer and tissue samples available for histologic review and found evidence for asbestosis in all 138 cases.[41] In addition, the risk of lung cancer increases among patients with interstitial lung disease other than asbestosis.[42,43]

The hypothesis that asbestosis is a prerequisite for asbestos-induced lung cancer has a number of weaknesses. First, the Hughes–Weill[19] study lacks the statistical power to detect an increased risk of lung cancer among patients without radiographic evidence of asbestosis.[44] Second, the studies by Sluis-Cremer[40] and Kipen[41] have unconventional definitions for the histologic diagnosis of asbestosis.[45,46] For example, the Kipen study diagnosed asbestosis in eight cases lacking asbestos bodies in histologic sections.[41] Third, the rates of lung cancer among individuals with asbestosis (from 40% to more than 50%) are much higher than the rates in cases with idiopathic pulmonary fibrosis (approximately 10% to 15%).[13,42,43,47] Fourth, the vast majority of lung cancers among asbestos workers are bronchogenic carcinomas not distinguishable on the basis of their morphology or histological features from those occurring in nonexposed smokers and not the peripheral adenocarcinomas typically associated with diffuse interstitial fibrosis. It is difficult to reconcile the requirement for the peripheral fibrosis of asbestosis with the proximal bronchogenic carcinomas seen in the majority of asbestos workers (including those with asbestosis). Finally, it is difficult to explain the synergistic effect between asbestos exposure and cigarette smoking in lung cancer induction on the basis of [H1].[25]

Proponents of [H2] believe that lung cancer and asbestosis are independent manifestations of asbestos exposure, each following a dose-response relationship with exposure. Hence, both diseases are likely to occur among individuals with the heaviest exposures. Accordingly, it is the dose of asbestos rather than the development of fibrosis per se that is the determining factor. Asbestosis is not invariably present in cohorts of asbestos workers with a demonstrable excess risk of lung cancer.[25,39,48,49] In addition, studies with greater statistical power than that of the Hughes-Weill study[19] have shown an increased risk of lung cancer among asbestos workers without radiographic evidence of asbestosis.[50,51] Furthermore, studies have shown an increased risk of lung cancer based on the fiber burden within the lung, independent of asbestosis and cigarette smoking.[52,53] For example, Karjalainen studied 113 surgically treated male lung cancer patients versus 297 autopsy cases on males as referents.[53] For subjects with amphibole fiber counts exceeding one million per gram of dry lung, the adjusted odds ratio was 4.0 for adenocarcinoma and 1.6 for squamous cell carcinoma. The odds ratio for a lower lobe carcinoma was 2.8 for patients with a fiber count between one and five million and 8.0 for those with fiber concentrations greater than or equal to five million per gram of dry lung.

There are also several weaknesses to the hypothesis that fiber burden rather than asbestosis is the primary determinant of lung cancer risk among asbestos workers. First, the studies by Hillerdal[50] and Wilkinson[51] do not exclude the possibility that the patients with an increased lung cancer risk but no radiographic evidence of asbestosis actually had subclinical asbestosis that would have been detected histologically. Second, it is difficult to reconcile the preferential association between fiber burden and a specific histologic type (i.e., adenocarcinoma) and location (i.e., lower lobe tumors), when studies have not consistently shown an association between any histologic pattern or tumor location and asbestos exposure (see below). Third, there are few epidemiologic studies that have examined the relationship between fiber burden and lung cancer risk. Finally, the fiber burden levels in patients without asbestosis did not have a statistically significant odds ratio for lung cancer in the Karjalainen study.[53] However, the study did show a trend from a low to a higher odds ratio, with transition from an intermediate to a higher level fiber count. Furthermore, the odds ratio for adenocarcinoma did show a statistically significant elevation with fiber burden greater than one million, even when all cases with any fibrosis were excluded.[44]

Proponents of [H3] believe that asbestos exposure rather than asbestosis is the key element in lung cancer induction by asbestos and that any level of exposure increases one's risk for cancer. Hence there is no threshold for asbestos exposure and increased lung cancer risk according to this hypothesis. In published cohorts with the steepest dose-response relationship, excess lung cancers were detected even in the groups with the very lowest level of exposure.[33,48] Although some investigators have suggested that there is a threshold level of exposure to asbestos below which no excess deaths from carcinoma of the lung will occur,[17,54] investigation of the consequences of low level exposures is the Achilles' heel of epidemiological studies because it requires large cohorts followed for extended periods of time to detect statistically significant associations.[55,56] Nonetheless, the consensus based on a number of cohort mortality studies, as well as studies of populations with environmental asbestos exposure, is that there is some level of exposure below which no statistical excess of lung cancers can be demonstrated.[25,57-65]

Experimental animal studies also bear on the issue of the mechanism of asbestos-induced carcinogenesis,[25] and this subject is reviewed in detail in Chapter 10. The author's view is that the literature in this regard indicates that fibrogenesis and carcinogenesis are separate and distinct effects of asbestos pathobiology, which have as a common denominator a dose-response relationship with respect to asbestos exposure and a dependence upon fiber length.

In summary, the weight of the evidence at this time seems to favor [H2]: asbestos-induced lung cancer is a function of fiber dose (and hence fiber burden), with a threshold for increased lung cancer risk.[44] Therefore, to attribute a substantial contributing role for asbestos in the causation of lung cancer, asbestosis must be present clinically or histologically or there should be a tissue asbestos burden within the range of values observed in patients with asbestosis[66] (see Chapter 11). The mere presence of parietal pleural plaques is not sufficient to establish causation (see Chapter 6). Furthermore, recent studies have shown a very close correlation between fiber burden levels associated with an increased lung cancer risk and the presence of histologically confirmed asbestosis. A fiber burden in the range determined by Karjalainen[52] to be associated with an increased lung cancer risk was found in 82% of 70 cases with histologic asbestosis, but in only 6% of 164 cases without asbestosis.[67] Hence it is unlikely that the distinction between [H1] and [H2] can be resolved by epidemiologic studies.

Cigarette Smoking and Synergism

Epidemiologic studies have indicated that there is a synergistic effect between cigarette smoking and asbestos exposure in the production of lung cancer.[5,12,68,69] This concept is well illustrated in the study by Hammond et al.,[5] in which cancer mortality in 17,800 asbestos insulators was compared with cancer death rates in the general population. This study noted that cigarette smoking increases one's risk of lung cancer approximately 11-fold, whereas asbestos exposure increases the risk about fivefold, when compared to a nonsmoking, nonexposed reference population. If these two effects were merely additive, one would expect an approximately 16-fold increase in lung cancer risk among cigarette-smoking asbestos insulators. Instead, what is actually observed is a 55-fold increased risk, indicating that the two effects are multiplicative rather than additive.[5] Other investigators have also indicated that the interaction between asbestos and cigarette smoke in increasing the lung cancer risk is a synergistic or multiplicative effect.[14,70–82] Some studies have reported an additive effect,[83,84] or an effect that was intermediate between additive and multiplicative.[84–86] Possible mechanisms for synergism are discussed in Chapter 10.

The U.S. Surgeon General's report on the effects of smoking cessation on the risk of developing carcinoma of the lung indicates that former smokers have a risk that is intermediate between that of current smokers and nonsmokers.[87] The magnitude of the decrease in risk is related to a number of factors, including the age when the patient started smoking, total duration and intensity of smoking, the age at cessation of smoking, and the time elapsed since the individual quit smoking. In this regard, studies have indicated that the risk of developing lung cancer in an ex-smoker is still greater than that of a lifelong nonsmoker even 20 or more years after cessation of smoking.[87] These factors must be considered in the evaluation of the role of asbestos exposure in the development of carcinoma of the lung in an ex-smoker. Because most lung cancers among asbestos-exposed individuals occur in workers who also smoke, it is difficult to obtain information regarding the lung cancer risk among nonsmoking asbestos workers. Hammond et al.[5] reported four such cases among their asbestos insulators, with an expected value of 0.8; hence their calculation of a fivefold increase in risk among nonsmoking asbestos workers. Berry et al.[84] reported four additional cases of lung cancer among nonsmoking asbestos factory workers. They concluded that after allowance had been made for the effect of smoking on lung cancer, the relative risk as a result of asbestos was highest for those who had never smoked, lowest for current smokers, and intermediate for former smokers (p < 0.05). Lemen[88] reported four more cases of lung cancer among nonsmoking women in a predominantly chrysotile asbestos textile plant.

The author has also observed 17 additional cases of lung cancer in nonsmokers with some history of asbestos exposure in which fiber burden analyses had been performed. Of these cases, 11 have been reported previously.[67] Fifteen of the 17 were adenocarcinomas, including two bronchioloalveolar cell carcinomas, one pseudomesotheliomatous carcinoma, and one adenosquamous carcinoma. The other two were large cell carcinoma and pleomorphic carcinoma. Two cases occurred in the setting of idiopathic pulmonary fibrosis (usual interstitial pneumonia), including one bronchioloalveolar cell carcinoma. Two of the patients had pleural plaques, including the one pseudomesotheliomatous carcinoma. One patient with adenocarcinoma had asbestosis. Only the latter case of the 17 had a fiber burden within the range described by Karjalainen et al., as being associated with an increased odds ratio for lung cancer.[53] Carcinoma of the lung is quite rare among nonsmokers.[89] In such cases, one must consider other possible factors such as the effects of passive smoking[90] and of household radon gas exposure.[91]

Role of Fiber Type

Epidemiologic data indicate that carcinoma of the lung may develop in response to exposure to any of the types of asbestos.[4,9,14,33,74,92] However, there is considerable controversy regarding the relative potency of the various fiber types for the production of pulmonary neoplasms.[25] Individuals who believe that chrysotile is less potent as a lung carcinogen than the amphiboles amosite and crocidolite, cite as evidence the relatively low rate of carcinoma of the lung among chrysotile miners and millers,[57,93] asbestos cement workers,[17,94] and friction-product manufacturers.[58,59] On the other hand, some chrysotile asbestos textile plants have reported extremely high lung cancer rates, with exceptionally steep dose-response curves.[33,35,95] Although it has been suggested that contamination of the asbestos fibers with mineral oil might explain the high rate of carcinoma of the lung among asbestos textile workers,[9] the steep dose-response relationship among these workers also holds for asbestosis, which is difficult to explain on the basis of contaminating oil. One major difficulty for studies trying to assess the relative potency of asbestos fiber types is the inaccuracy of historic estimates of asbestos exposure.[25,96] In this regard, Newhouse[97] noted that chrysotile textile plants were particularly dusty when compared with other types of occupational exposure to chrysotile. Furthermore, in comparing the cancer mortality for two different asbestos textile plants, Finkelstein concluded that the risk of death from asbestos-associated cancer in factories manufacturing similar products is unrelated to the type of asbestos fiber used.[35,95,96]

The author suspects that much of the variation in lung cancer rates among chrysotile workers can be explained on the basis of dose and relative fiber size, with longer fibers being more potent. For example, the low rate of lung cancer among automotive maintenance and brake repair workers[98] can be explained on the basis of relatively low dust levels, the low proportion of asbestos in the dust generated, and the preponderance of very short chrysotile fibers in brake dust.[99,100] The relative ability of fibers to penetrate the bronchial mucosa may also be an important factor. Churg and Stevens in a study of smokers and nonsmokers with similar exposure histories and similar fiber burdens in the lung parenchyma examined this question.[101] These investigators found that the amosite content was six times greater in the bronchial mucosa of smokers as compared to nonsmokers, and the chrysotile content was 50 times greater. Thus, evidence exists that cigarette smoking increases the penetration of fibers into the bronchial mucosa, and this effect appears to be greater for chrysotile than for the amphiboles.

Pathology of Asbestos-Related Carcinoma of the Lung

Gross Morphology

Lung carcinomas have been classically divided into the proximal bronchogenic carcinomas, which arise from a mainstem, segmental, or subsegmental bronchus and typically present as a hilar mass, and peripheral carcinomas, arising from small airways (i.e., bronchioles or peripheral bronchi) and presenting as a "coin" lesion on chest roentgenogram.[102] Asbestos-related lung cancers can assume either of these gross appearances. In fact, there are no discernible differences between the macroscopic appearance of carcinomas of the lung among asbestos workers and those in individuals not exposed to asbestos.[28,45,102,103] One possible exception to this observation is the lobar distribution, with carcinomas among cigarette smokers from the general population occurring about twice as often in the upper as compared to the lower lobes, whereas the reverse is true for carcinomas among asbestos workers.[52,53,104] However, more recent studies have failed to confirm this observation and have found instead that lung cancers in asbestos workers occur more commonly in the upper lobe.[67,105] At any rate, the overlap is great enough that the lobar distribution is hardly sufficient to assign attribution to asbestos exposure in the individual case.[67,103]

Typical examples of carcinoma of the lung in asbestosis patients are illustrated in Figures 7-1 through 7-3. One shows a proximal bronchogenic carcinoma (Figure 7-1) from a Tyler, Texas, asbestos plant worker who was a guard at the Tyler plant for seven years and developed the neoplasm 21 years after initial exposure. This plant made pipe insulation material from amosite asbestos.[106,107] The second example is a lower lobe cavitating cancer (Figure 7-2) from a shipyard insulator and boiler scaler for 30 years. The third example shows a massively enlarged hilar lymph node secondary to metastatic bronchogenic carcinoma (primary tumor not visible in the section). Very fine interstitial fibrosis was just visible to the unaided eye in the lower lobes

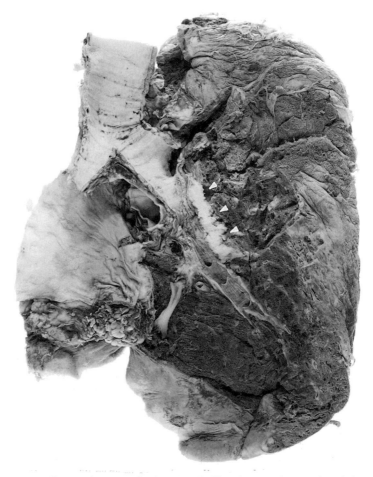

Figure 7-1. Gross photograph showing infiltrating carcinoma involving the bronchus intermedius of the right lung (*arrowheads*). The patient was a guard in a plant that manufactured amosite pipe insulation for seven years. (Reprinted from Ref. 106, with permission.)

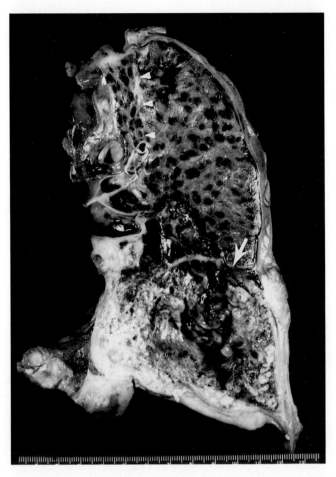

Figure 7-2. Gross photograph showing a cavitating carcinoma of the right lower lobe (*arrow*). The patient was an asbestos insulator in a shipyard for 30 years (same case as Figure 4-4). Radiation fibrosis is present in the medial aspect of the right upper lobe (*arrowheads*), and a few scattered silicotic nodules were also palpable in the right upper lobe.

(Figure 7-3). This patient was admitted comatose and died shortly thereafter, without providing any occupational history; asbestosis was confirmed upon histologic examination. All three examples are squamous cell carcinomas (Figure 7-4), and two of the individuals also smoked cigarettes (180 and 50 pack-years, respectively). The smoking history of the third is unknown.

Histopathology

Carcinomas of the lung have conventionally been categorized into four histologic patterns: squamous cell carcinoma, small cell carcinoma, adenocarcinoma, and large cell carcinoma.[102,108,109] These patterns are illustrated in Figure 7-5. The most recently revised WHO classification for the more common lung cancer types is summarized in Table 7-1.[110] Squamous cell carcinomas are characterized by keratinization or

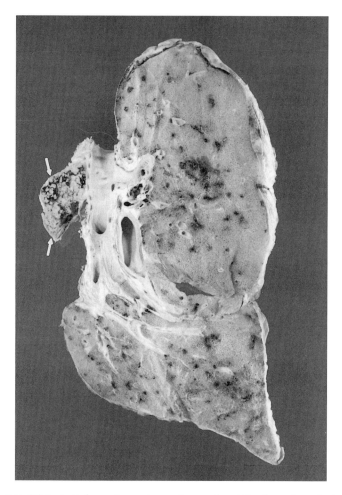

Figure 7-3. Metastatic bronchogenic carcinoma in a hilar lymph node (*arrows*). Asbestosis was present in histologic sections.

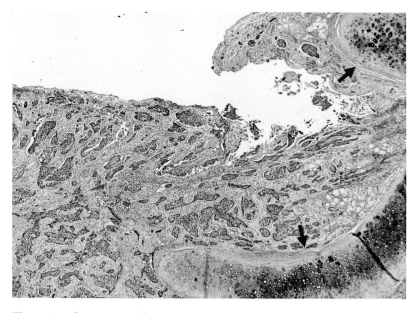

Figure 7-4. Squamous cell carcinoma of the right lung invading the wall of the bronchus intermedius in close proximity to the bronchial cartilages (*arrows*). Same case as Figure 7-1. Hematoxylin and eosin, ×39. (Reprinted from Ref. 107, with permission.)

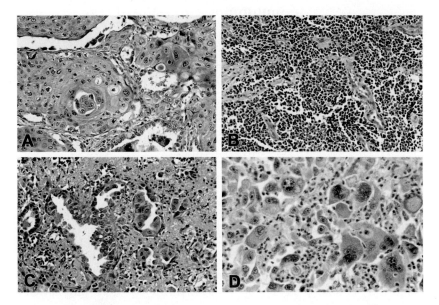

Figure 7-5. High magnification photomicrographs illustrating the four major cell types of carcinoma of the lung. **(A)** squamous carcinoma, **(B)** small cell carcinoma, **(C)** adenocarcinoma, and **(D)** large cell carcinoma. Hematoxylin and eosin, ×600.

intercellular bridges. In well-differentiated tumors, keratinization manifests in the form of keratin pearls, and, in more poorly differentiated tumors, as individual cell keratinization (Figure 7-5A). Squamous cell carcinomas account for approximately 30% of primary lung carcinomas

Table 7-1. Histologic typing of lung cancer[a]

I.   Squamous cell carcinoma
A. Papillary
B. Clear cell
C. Small cell
D. Basaloid
II. Small cell carcinoma
A. Combined small cell carcinoma
III. Adenocarcinoma
A. Acinar type
B. Papillary type
C. Bronchioloalveolar cell carcinoma
D. Solid adenocarcinoma with mucin
E. Adenocarcinoma with mixed subtypes
IV. Large cell carcinoma
A. Large cell neuroendocrine carcinoma
B. Basaloid carcinoma
C. Lymphoepithelioma-like carcinoma
D. Clear cell carcinoma
E. Large cell carcinoma with rhabdoid phenotype
V.   Adenosquamous carcinoma
VI. Carcinomas with pleomorphic, sarcomatoid or sarcomatous elements

[a] Modified after WHO classification of lung tumors[110]

and usually present as proximal hilar masses. Small cell carcinomas have scant amounts of cytoplasm with high nuclear-to-cytoplasmic ratios. The nuclei are often hyperchromatic or else have finely stippled chromatin with inconspicuous nucleoli (Figure 7-5B). Small cell carcinomas account for about 15% to 20% of primary lung carcinomas and also present as proximal tumors. Adenocarcinomas are recognized by their tendency to form glandular, acinar, or papillary structures (Figure 7-5C). In some cases, the tumor cells form solid sheets and can only be distinguished from large cell carcinoma by means of special stains for mucosubstances. Adenocarcinomas account for approximately 40% of primary lung carcinomas and usually present as peripheral nodules or masses. An uncommon variant of adenocarcinoma, known as bronchioloalveolar cell carcinoma, consists of tall columnar tumor cells that tend to grow along intact alveolar septa without invasion (Figure 7-6). This variant accounts for approximately 1% to 2% of lung cancers. Large cell carcinomas consist of sheets or nests of tumor cells with moderately abundant cytoplasm, anaplastic nuclei, and prominent nucleoli (Figure 7-5D). They do not keratinize, form glandular or papillary

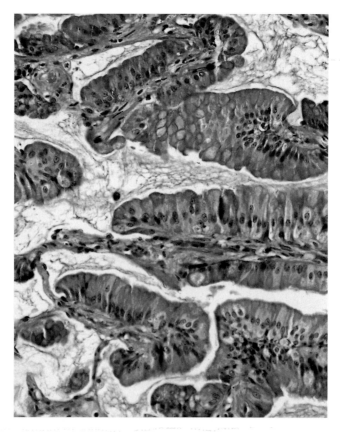

Figure 7-6. Bronchioloalveolar cell carcinoma of the left upper lobe in a 73-year-old housewife of an asbestos worker. Tissue asbestos analysis of nontumorous lung parenchyma indicated an elevated content of amosite and chrysotile asbestos. Hematoxylin and eosin, ×130.

structures, or produce mucosubstances. Large cell carcinomas account for approxmately 10% to 15% of primary lung carcinomas and more often present as a peripheral mass. All of the major lung cancer histologic types are associated with cigarette smoking, although adenocarcinoma is the type most likely to occur in a nonsmoker.[89]

Some pulmonary carcinomas may have a pleomorphic or sarcomatoid appearance.[110,111] We have seen examples of such carcinomas in asbestos workers presenting as superior sulcus (Pancoast) tumors (Figure 7-7) or as proximal hilar masses (Figure 7-8). These tumors may invade the pleura or chest wall and thus must be distinguished from sarcomatoid or biphasic malignant mesotheliomas (see below). Mixtures of the major histologic cell types may also occur, resulting in a heterogeneous histologic appearance of many primary carcinomas of the lung. With thorough sampling, various combinations of the four major histologic patterns can be found in almost half of the cases.[112] In addition, the authors have encountered examples of asbestos workers with synchronous primary lung neoplasms of differing histologic type (e.g., a patient with asbestosis and adenosquamous carcinoma and small cell carcinoma in the same lung).[67]

All of the histologic patterns of lung cancer described above may occur in asbestos workers.[45,47,102,103,113,114] However, there is some confusion in the literature regarding the distribution of histologic types in asbestos workers as compared to nonexposed individuals. A number of studies described an excess of adenocarcinomas among asbestos workers with carcinoma of the lung.[13,53,115-118] Other investigators have reported that the distribution of histologic types of lung cancer was similar for asbestos workers and members of the general population.[47,67,105,119-123] Possible reasons for these discrepancies include selection bias for surgical resection (with patients with peripheral adenocarcinomas more likely to be surgical candidates) or to referral bias. In the author's opinion, the histologic features of a lung tumor are of no particular value in deciding whether or not it is an asbestos-related malignancy.[45,103]

The distribution of histologic types of lung cancer in 895 patients from the author's series is shown in Table 7-2. The first column includes patients with carcinoma of the lung in which asbestosis was confirmed histologically, whereas the second column includes patients with parietal pleural plaques but without asbestosis. The third column includes cases with no histologic evidence of asbestosis or cases for which only a biopsy of the tumor was available (no lung tissue sampled). The fourth column includes 100 consecutive lung cancer resections or autopsies collected at Baylor Affiliated Hospitals, Houston, from 1979 to 1980.[112] The percentage of adenocarcinoma cases is similar across all four groups (38%–41%). The data in Table 7-2 are consistent with the proposition that most carcinomas of the lung occurring in asbestos workers are histologically similar to those occurring in nonexposed cigarette smokers. Adenocarcinomas derived from the scarring process account for only a small proportion of cases, resulting in a statistically insignificant increase in the percentage of adenocarcinomas.

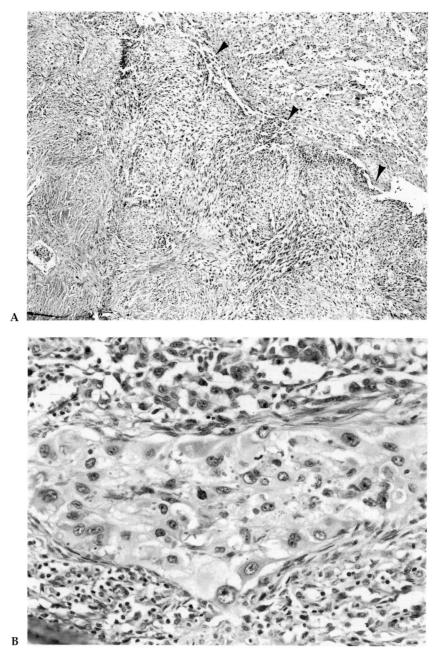

Figure 7-7. **(A)** Predominantly spindle cell carcinoma of right upper lobe of an asbestos worker, presenting as a superior sulcus tumor. The margin of tumor invading the underlying lung parenchyma can be discerned (*arrowheads*). **(B)** Higher magnification elsewhere in the tumor shows epithelial component composed of large anaplastic cells with abundant cytoplasm. Hematoxylin and eosin, (A) ×40, (B) ×250.

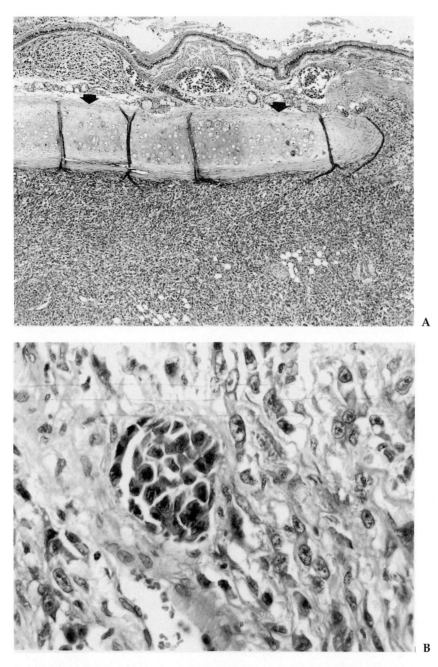

Figure 7-8. **(A)** Predominantly spindle cell carcinoma invading the right main-stem bronchus in close proximity to the bronchial cartilages (*arrows*). Asbestosis was confirmed histologically in the pneumonectomy specimen. **(B)** Higher magnification elsewhere in the tumor shows epithelial component composed of a nest of loosely cohesive polygonal shaped tumor cells which were strongly positive for cytokeratins. Hematoxylin and eosin, (A) ×40, (B) ×400.

Table 7-2. Distribution of histological types in 895 lung cancer cases with and without asbestosis*

	Asbestos	PPP[a]	Other[b]	Ref. Pop[c]
Squamous cell carcinoma	56 (29%)	10 (24%)	182 (33%)	31 (31%)
Small cell carcinoma	30 (15)	9 (21)	69 (12)	11 (11)
Adenocarcinoma	79 (41)	16 (38)	226 (41)	39 (39)
Large cell carcinoma	22 (11)	7 (17)	70 (13)	19 (19)
Adenosquamous carcinoma	8 (4)	0 (0)	11 (2)	—
Total	195	42	558	100

[a] PPP = parietal pleural plaques, no evidence of asbestosis
[b] No histologic evidence of asbestosis or biopsy of tumor only (no lung tissue sampled)
[c] 100 consecutive lung cancer cases collected at Baylor Affiliated Hospitals, 1979–1980.[112]

Differential Diagnosis

Primary lung carcinomas must be distinguished from pulmonary metastases and from other primary intrathoracic malignancies. Knowledge of the clinical information and radiographic findings is often useful in this regard. Primary lung carcinomas usually present as a solitary pulmonary mass or nodule, whereas metastatic disease most often manifests as multiple and bilateral nodules of similar size, most numerous in the lower lobes. A history of a primary malignancy in an extrapulmonary location is of obvious significance in this regard. The histologic appearance of the tumor is of limited use in determining whether a lung neoplasm is primary or metastatic. For example, most small cell carcinomas are primary to the lung, whereas adenocarcinomas are common histologic patterns in a number of primary sites, and histologic features alone (especially on a small biopsy) usually are not indicative of a primary site of origin. Similarly, for tumors with a prominent clear cell component, a renal primary source needs to be excluded.

Primary lung carcinomas must also be distinguished from other pulmonary neoplasms, most of which are distinctly uncommon.[124] Peripheral carcinomas that invade the pleura must be distinguished from malignant mesothelioma (see Chapter 5). The gross features of the tumor may be of limited utility in this regard,[125,126] and the pathologist must rely on histological, histochemical, immunohistochemical, or ultrastructural features of the tumor to make this distinction. Uncommonly, a pulmonary carcinoma with a prominent spindle cell component may occur in the lung periphery and invade the pleura, mimicking a biphasic pleural mesothelioma (Figures 7-7 and 7-8). The localized nature of the tumor with a prominent pulmonary parenchymal component, or the presence of a hilar mass with prominent involvement of a proximal bronchus, are useful differentiating features in this regard.

The Pathologist's Role in Identification of Asbestos-Associated Carcinoma of the Lung

It has been estimated that in the 25-year period from 1985 to 2009, there will have been 76,700 deaths from asbestos-related carcinomas of the lung in the United States alone.[127] In contrast, there are 170,000 lung cancer deaths annually (or 4.25 million over the same time period), the great majority of which are related to cigarette smoking.[1,2] Thus it is clear that a major challenge for the medical profession and society in general will be to determine which lung cancers are related to asbestos exposure so that appropriate compensation may be provided where indicated. This will require careful consideration of clinical, radiographic, and pathological data in the individual case, as well as epidemiologic and relevant experimental animal studies. As noted in the previous discussion, there are no pathologic features of carcinoma of the lung in asbestos workers that permit their distinction in the individual case from the much more common tobacco-related cancers in nonasbestos exposed individuals. Therefore, the primary role of the pathologist is to render an accurate and precise diagnosis of carcinoma of the lung based on available pathological materials and to help exclude other differential diagnostic considerations.

Another important aspect of the pathologists' role has been referred to as the "second diagnosis";[128] that is, the identification of other abnormalities that are related to inhalation of asbestos fibers. These include the identification of benign asbestos-related pleural diseases, such as parietal pleural plaques or diffuse pleural fibrosis (Chapter 6), asbestosis (Chapter 4), and asbestos bodies in histologic sections.[129] Similarly, the pathologist should search for evidence of tissue injury related to inhalation of tobacco smoke, including centrilobular emphysema, chronic bronchitis, and small airways disease.[130] This requires adequate sampling of lung parenchyma at a distance well removed from the primary tumor and its effects on immediately adjacent tissues.[103,131] These changes are best observed with lungs that have been fixed by intrabronchial instillation of formalin,[45,130] which procedure should be employed when feasible on lobectomy or pneumonectomy specimens. In addition, lung cancer cases for which a role for asbestos is suspected should have portions of formalin-fixed lung tissue uninvolved by tumor preserved for possible tissue asbestos analysis at some subsequent time if indicated (Chapter 11). Such analyses should preferably be performed at specialized centers with experience with these procedures, since proper interpretation of results requires determination of a normal range of expected values.

It has been suggested that in the future, molecular genetic markers may be found that specifically link a lung cancer to asbestos exposure.[132] Because asbestos acts primarily as a promoter for cigarette smoke carcinogens, it is the opinion of this author that it is unlikely that a molecular marker for asbestos-related lung cancer distinct from tobacco-associated markers will ever be identified.

References

1. Rom WN, Hay JG, Lee TC, Jiang Y, Tchou-Wong K-M: Molecular and genetic aspects of lung cancer. *Am J Respir Crit Care Med* 161:1355–1367, 2000.
2. World Health Organization: Tobacco or health: A global status report. Geneva: World Health Organization, 1997.
3. Rodenstein DO, Stănescu DC: Pattern of inhalation of tobacco smoke in pipe, cigarette, and never smokers. *Am Rev Respir Dis* 132:628–632, 1985.
4. Selikoff IJ, Lee DHK: *Asbestos and Disease*. New York: Academic Press, 1978.
5. Hammond EC, Selikoff IJ, Seidman H: Asbestos exposure, cigarette smoking, and death rates. In: *Health Hazards of Asbestos Exposure* (Selikoff IJ, Hammond EC, eds.), *Ann NY Acad Sci* 330:473–490, 1979.
6. Lynch KM, Smith WA: Pulmonary asbestosis. Carcinoma of the lung in asbestos silicosis. *Am J Cancer* 24:56–64, 1985.
7. Homburger F: The coincidence of primary carcinoma of the lungs and pulmonary asbestosis. Analysis of literature and report of three cases. *Am J Pathol* 19:797–807, 1943.
8. Merewether ERA: Annual report to the chief inspector of factories for the year 1947. London: Her Majesty's Stationery Office, 1949, pp. 79–87.
9. McDonald JC, McDonald AD: Epidemiology of asbestos-related lung cancer. In: *Asbestos Related Malignancy* (Antman K, Aisner J, eds.), Orlando, FL: Grune & Stratton, 1987, pp. 57–79.
10. Doll R: Mortality from lung cancer in asbestos workers. *Br J Ind Med* 12:81–86, 1955.
11. Breslow L: Industrial aspects of bronchogenic neoplasms. *Dis Chest* 28:421–430, 1955.
12. Selikoff IJ, Churg J, Hammond EC: Asbestos exposure, smoking and neoplasia. *JAMA* 204:104–110, 1968.
13. Buchanan WD: Asbestosis and primary intrathoracic neoplasms. *Ann NY Acad Sci* 132:507–518, 1965.
14. Acheson ED, Gardner MJ, Winter PD, Bennett C: Cancer in a factory using amosite asbestos. *Int J Epidemiol* 13:3–10, 1984.
15. Finkelstein MM: Mortality among employees of an Ontario asbestos-cement factory. *Am Rev Respir Dis* 129:754–761, 1984.
16. Newhouse ML, Berry G, Wagner JC: Mortality of factory workers in east London 1933–80. *Br J Ind Med* 42: 4–11, 1985.
17. Ohlson CG, Hogstedt C: Lung cancer among asbestos cement workers: A Swedish cohort study and a review. *Br J Ind Med* 42:397–402, 1985.
18. Botha JL, Irwig LM, Strebel PM: Excess mortality from stomach cancer, lung cancer, and asbestosis and/or mesothelioma in crocidolite mining districts in South Africa. *Am J Epidemiol* 123:30–40, 1986.
19. Hughes JM, Weill H, Hammad YY: Mortality of workers employed in two asbestos cement manufacturing plants. *Br J Ind Med* 44:161–174, 1987.
20. Enterline PE, Hartley J, Henderson V: Asbestos and cancer: A cohort followed up to death. *Br J Ind Med* 44:396–401, 1987.
21. Raffn E, Lynge E, Juel K, Korsgaard B: Incidence of cancer and mortality among employees in the asbestos cement industry in Denmark. *Br J Ind Med* 46:90–96, 1989.
22. Karjalainen A: Occupational asbestos exposure, pulmonary fiber burden and lung cancer in the Finnish population. PhD Thesis: University of Helsinki, 1994.

23. Rösler JA, Woitowitz H-J, Lange H-J: Forschungsbericht Asbest IV: Asbesteinwirkung am Arbetzplatz und Sterblichkeit an bösartigen Tumoren in der Bundersrepublik Deutschland. Eingrenzung von Hochrisikogruppen anhand Standardisierter proportionale Mortalitäts-raten der "Berufskrebsstudie Asbest". HVBG, Abteilung Offentlichkeits-arbeit, 1993.

24. Henderson DW, Roggli VL, Shilkin KB, et al.: Is asbestosis an obligate pre-cursor for asbestos-induced lung cancer? Fiber burden and the changing balance of evidence: a preliminary discussion document. In: *Sourcebook on Asbestos Diseases, Vol. 11* (Peters GA, Peters BJ, eds.), Charlottesville: Michie Pub. Co., 1995, pp. 97–168.

25. Cullen MR: Controversies in asbestos-related lung cancer. *Occup Med State Art Revs* 2:259–272, 1987.

26. Peto J: Dose-response relationships for asbestos-related disease: Implica-tions for hygiene standards. Part II. Mortality. *Ann NY Acad Sci* 330: 195–203, 1979.

27. Churg A: Asbestos, asbestosis, and lung cancer. *Mod Pathol* 6: 509–510, 1983.

28. Churg A: Neoplastic Asbestos-Induced Disease. Ch. 10 In: *Pathology of Occupational Lung Disease*, 2nd ed. (Churg A, Green FHY, eds.), Baltimore: Williams & Wilkins, 1998, pp. 339–391.

29. Weill H, Hughes JM, Jones RN: Asbestos: a risk too far? (letter) *Lancet* 346:304, 1995.

30. Weiss W: Asbestos-related pleural plaques and lung cancer. *Chest* 103:1854–1859, 1993.

31. Browne K: Is asbestos or asbestosis the cause of the increased risk of lung cancer in asbestos workers? *Br J Ind Med* 43:145–149, 1986.

32. An SH, Koprowska I: Primary cytologic diagnosis of asbestosis associated with bronchogenic carcinoma: Case report and review of literature. *Acta Cytolo* 6:391–398, 1962.

33. Dement JM, Harns RL, Symons MJ, Shy CM: Exposures and mortality among chrysotile asbestos workers. Part II: Mortality. *Am J Ind Med* 4:421–434, 1983.

34. Hodgson JT, Jones RD: Mortality of asbestos workers in England and Wales 1971–81. *Br J Ind Med* 43:158–164, 1986.

35. McDonald AD, Fry JS, Woolley AJ, McDonald JC: Dust exposure and mor-tality in an American factory using chrysotile, amosite and crocidolite in mainly textile manufacture. *Br J Ind Med* 40:368–374, 1983.

36. Puntoni R, Vercelli M, Merlo F, Valerio F, Santi L: Mortality among ship-yard workers in Genoa, Italy. *Ann NY Acad Sci* 330:353–377, 1979.

37. Rubino GF, Piolatto G, Newhouse ML, Scansetti G, Aresini GA, Murray R: Mortality of chrysotile asbestos miners at the Balangero Mine, North-ern Italy. *Br J Ind Med* 36:187–194, 1979.

38. Selikoff IJ, Hammond EC, Seidman H: Mortality experience of insulation workers in the United States and Canada 1943–1976. *Ann NY Acad Sci* 330:91–116, 1979.

39. Liddell FDK, McDonald JC: Radiologic findings as predictors of mortal-ity in Quebec asbestos workers. *Br J Ind Med* 37:257–267, 1980.

40. Sluis-Cremer GK, Bezuidenhout BN: Relation between asbestosis and bronchial cancer in amphibole asbestos miners. *Br J Ind Med* 46:537–540, 1989.

41. Kipen HM, Lilis R, Suzuki Y, Valciukas JA, Selikoff IJ: Pulmonary fibrosis in asbestos insulation workers with lung cancer: A radiological and histopathological evaluation. *Br J Ind Med* 44:96–100, 1987.

42. Fraire AE, Greenberg SD: Carcinoma and diffuse interstitial fibrosis of lung. *Cancer* 31:1078–1086, 1973.

43. Hubbard R, Venn A, Lewis S, Britton J: Lung cancer and cryptogenic fibrosing alveolitis: A population-based cohort study. *Am J Respir Crit Care Med* 161:5–8, 2000.

44. Henderson DW, de Klerk NH, Hammar SP, Hillerdal G, Huuskonen MS, Karjalainen A, Leigh J, Pott F, Roggli VL, Shilkin KB, Tossavainen A: Asbestos and lung cancer: Is it attributable to asbestosis or to asbestos fibre burden? Ch. 6 In: *Pathology of Lung Tumors* (Corrin B, ed.), London: Churchill Livingstone, 1997, pp. 83–118.

45. Craighead JE, Abraham JL, Churg A, Green FHY, Kleinerman J, Pratt PC, Seemayer TA, Vallyathan V, Weill H: The pathology of asbestos-associated diseases of the lungs and pleural cavities: Diagnostic criteria and proposed grading schema. *Arch Pathol Lab Med* 106:544–596, 1982.

46. Roggli VL: Pathology of human asbestosis: A critical review. In: *Advances in Pathology*, (Vol. 2) (Fenoglio CM, ed.), Chicago: Yearbook Pub. Co, 1989, pp. 31–60.

47. Roggli VL, Pratt PC, Brody AR: Asbestos content of lung tissue in asbestos-associated diseases: A study of 110 cases. *Br J Ind Med* 43:18–28, 1986.

48. Seidman H, Selikoff IJ, Hammond EC: Short-term asbestos work exposure and long-term observations. *Ann NY Acad Sci* 330:61–89, 1979.

49. Becklake MR: Asbestos-related diseases of the lung and other organs: Their epidemiology and implications for clinical practice. *Am Rev Respir Dis* 114:187–227, 1976.

50. Hillerdal G: Pleural plaques and risk for bronchial carcinoma and mesothelioma: A prospective study. *Chest* 105:144–150, 1994.

51. Wilkinson P, Hansell DM, Janssens J, Rubens M, Rudd RM, Taylor AN, McDonald C: Is lung cancer associated with asbestos exposure without small opacities on the chest radiograph? *Lancet* 345:1074–1078, 1995.

52. Anttila S, Karjalainen A, Taikina-aho O, Kyyronen P, Vainio H: Lung cancer in the lower lobe is associated with pulmonary asbestos fiber count and fiber size. *Environ Health Persp* 101:166–170, 1993.

53. Karjalainen A, Anttila S, Vanhala E, Vainio H: Asbestos exposure and the risk of lung cancer in a general urban population. *Scand J Work Environ Health* 20:243–250, 1994.

54. Browne K: A threshold for asbestos related lung cancer. *Br J Ind Med* 43:556–558, 1986.

55. McDonald JC: Health implications of environmental exposure to asbestos. *Environ Health Persp* 62:319–328, 1985.

56. Mossman BT, Gee JBL: Asbestos-related diseases. *N Engl J Med* 320: 1721–1730, 1989.

57. McDonald JC, Liddell FDK, Gibbs GW, Eyssen GE, McDonald AD: Dust exposure and mortality in chrysotile mining, 1910–1975. *Br J Ind Med* 37:11–24, 1980.

58. McDonald AD, Fry JS, Woolley AJ, McDonald JC: Dust exposure and mortality in an American chrysotile asbestos friction products plant. *Br J Ind Med* 41:151–157, 1984.

59. Berry G, Newhouse ML: Mortality of workers manufacturing friction materials using asbestos. *Br J Ind Med* 40:1–7, 1983.

60. Enterline P, DeCoufle P, Henderson V: Respiratory cancer in relation to occupational exposures among retired asbestos workers. *Br J Ind Med* 30:162–166, 1973.

61. Hughes J, Weill H: Lung cancer risk associated with manufacture of asbestos cement products. In: *Biological Effects of Mineral Fibers* (Wagner JC, ed.), IARC Scientific Publications No. 30, Lyon, 1980, pp. 627–635.

62. Peto J, Doll R, Herman G, Binns R, Goffe T, Clayton R: Relationship of mortality to measures of environmental pollution in an asbestos textile factory. *Ann Occup Hyg* 29:305–355, 1985.

63. Pampalon R, Siemiatycki J, Blanchet M: Environmental asbestos pollution and public health in Quebec. *Union Med Can* 111:475–489, 1982.

64. Camus M, Siematycki J, Meek B: Nonoccupational exposure to chrysotile asbestos and the risk of lung cancer. *N Engl J Med* 338:1565–1571, 1998.

65. Weiss W: Asbestosis: A marker for the increased risk of lung cancer among workers exposed to asbestos. *Chest* 115:536–549, 1999.

66. Henderson DW, Rantanen J, Barnhart S, Dement JM, De Vuyst P, Hillerdal G, Huuskonen MS, Kivisaari L, Kusaka Y, Lahdensuo A, Langard S, Mowe G, Okubo T, Parker JE, Roggli VL, Rodelsperger K, Rösler J, Tossavainen A, Woitowitz HJ: Asbestos, asbestosis, and cancer: The Helsinki criteria for diagnosis and attribution. A consensus report of an international expert group. *Scand J Work Environ Health* 23:311–316, 1997.

67. Roggli VL, Sanders LL: Asbestos content of lung tissue and carcinoma of the lung: A clinicopathologic correlation and mineral fiber analysis of 234 cases. *Ann Occup Hyg* 44:109–117, 2000.

68. Selikoff IJ, Hammond EC: Asbestos and smoking. *JAMA* 242:458, 1979.

69. Selikoff IJ, Seidman H, Hammond EC: Mortality effects of cigarette smoking among amosite asbestos factory workers. *J Natl Cancer Inst* 65:507–513, 1980.

70. Berry G, Newhouse ML, Turok M: Combined effect of asbestos exposure and smoking on mortality from lung cancer in factory workers. *Lancet* 2:476–479, 1972.

71. Saracci R: Asbestos and lung cancer: An analysis of the epidemiological evidence on the asbestos-smoking interaction. *Int J Cancer* 20:323–331, 1977.

72. Martischnig KM, Newell DJ, Barnsley WC, Cowan WK, Feinmann EL, Oliver E: Unsuspected exposure to asbestos and bronchogenic carcinoma. *Br Med J* 1: 746–749, 1977.

73. Blot WJ, Harrington M, Toledo A, Hoover R, Heath CW Jr., Fraumeni JF Jr.: Lung cancer after employment in shipyards during World War II. *N Engl J Med* 299:620–624, 1978.

74. Meurman LO, Kiviluoto R, Hakama M: Combined effect of asbestos exposure and tobacco smoking on Finnish anthophyllite miners and millers. *Ann NY Acad Sci* 330:491–495, 1979.

75. Blot WJ, Morris LE, Stroube R, et al: Lung and laryngeal cancer in relation to shipyard employment in coastal Virginia. *J Natl Cancer Inst* 65:571–575, 1980.

76. Newhouse M: Epidemiology of asbestos-related tumors. *Sem Oncol* 8:250–257, 1981.

77. Huuskonen MS: Asbestos and cancer. *Eur J Respir Dis* 63 [Suppl 123]:145–152, 1982.

78. Baker JE: Lung cancer incidence amongst previous employees of an asbestos mine in relationship to crocidolite exposure and tobacco smoking. PhD Thesis: Department of Medicine, University of Western Australia, 1985.

79. Hilt B, Langärd S, Anderson A, Rosenberg J: Asbestos exposure, smoking habits, and cancer incidence among production and maintenance workers in an electrochemical plant. *Am J Ind Med* 8:565–577, 1985.

80. Kjuus H, Skjaerven R, Langård S, et al.: A case-referent study of lung cancer, occupational exposures and smoking. II. Role of asbestos exposure. *Scand J Work Environ Health* 12:203–209, 1986.

81. de Klerk NH, Musk AW, Armstrong BK, Hobbs MST. Smoking, exposure to crocidolite, and the incidence of lung cancer and asbestosis. *Br J Ind Med* 48:412–417, 1991.

82. Cheng WN, Kong J: A retrospective mortality cohort study of chrysotile asbestos products workers in Tianjin 1972–1987. *Environ Res* 59:271–278, 1992.

83. Liddell FDK, Thomas DC, Gibbs JW, McDonald JC: Fibre exposure and mortality from pneumoconiosis, respiratory and abdominal malignancies in chrysotile production in Quebec, 1926–1975. *Ann Acad Med Singapore* 13 [suppl 2]:340–344, 1984.

84. Berry G, Newhouse ML, Antonis P: Combined effect of asbestos and smoking on mortality from lung cancer and mesothelioma in factory workers. *Br J Ind Med* 42:12–18, 1985.

85. Selikoff IJ, Seidman H, Hammond EC: Mortality effects of cigarette smoking among amosite asbestos factory workers. *J Natl Cancer Inst* 65:507–513, 1980.

86. Pastorino U, Berrino F, Gervasio A, et al.: Proportion of lung cancers due to occupational exposures. *Int J Cancer* 33:231–237, 1984.

87. Surgeon General. Smoking Cessation and Respiratory Cancers. Ch. 4 In: *The Health Benefits of Smoking Cessation.* Rockville, MD: U.S. Dept. of Health and Human Services, Publication No. 90–8416, 1990, pp. 107–141.

88. Lemen RA: Occupationally induced lung cancer epidemiology. In: *Occupational Respiratory Diseases* (Merchant JA, ed.), U.S. Dept. of Health and Human Services, Publication No. 86–102, 1986, pp. 629–656.

89. Kabat GC, Wynder EL: Lung cancer in nonsmokers. *Cancer* 53:1214–1221, 1984.

90. Zhong L, Goldberg MS, Parent M-E, Hanley JA: Exposure to environmental tobacco smoke and the risk of lung cancer: a meta-analysis. *Lung Cancer* 27:3–18, 2000.

91. Samet JM: Radon and lung cancer. *J Natl Cancer Inst* 81:745–757, 1989.

92. Roggli VL, Greenberg SD, Seitzman LH, McGavran MH, Hurst GA, Spivey CG, Nelson KG, Hieger LR: Pulmonary fibrosis, carcinoma, and ferruginous body counts in amosite asbestos workers: A study of six cases. *Am J Clin Pathol* 73:496–503, 1980.

93. McDonald JC, Becklake MR, Gibbs GW, McDonald A, Rossiter CE: The health of chrysotile asbestos mine and mill workers of Quebec. *Arch Environ Health* 26:61–68, 1974.

94. Weiss W: Mortality of a cohort exposed to chrysotile asbestos. *J Occup Med* 19:737–740, 1977.

95. McDonald AD, Fry JS, Woolley AJ, McDonald J: Dust exposure and mortality in an American chrysotile textile plant. *Br J Ind Med* 40:361–367, 1983.

96. Finkelstein M: On the relative toxicity of asbestos fibres. *Br J Ind Med* 42:69–72, 1985.

97. Newhouse ML: Cancer among workers in the asbestos textile industry. In: *Biological Effects of Asbestos* (Bogovski P, Gilson JC, Timbrell V, Wagner JC, eds.), Lyon: IARC Scientific Publications. No. 8, Lyon, 1973, pp. 203–208.

98. Rushton L, Alderson MR, Nagarajah CR: Epidemiological survey of maintenance workers in London Transport Executive bus garages and Chiswick Works. *Br J Ind Med* 40:340–345, 1983.

99. Cheng VKI, O'Kelly FJ: Asbestos exposure in the motor vehicle repair and servicing industry in Hong Kong. *J Soc Occup Med* 36:104–106, 1986.

100. Williams RL, Muhlbaier JL: Asbestos brake emissions. *Environ Res* 29: 70–82, 1982.

101. Churg A, Stevens B: Enhanced retention of asbestos fibers in the airways of human smokers. *Am J Respir Crit Care Med* 151:1409–1413, 1995.

102. Green FHY, Vallyathan V: Pathology of occupational lung cancer, In: *Occupational Respiratory Diseases* (Merchant JA, ed.), U.S. Dept. of Health and Human Services (NIOSH) Pub. No. 86–102, 1986, pp. 657–668.

103. Churg A, Golden J: Current problems in the pathology of asbestos-related disease. *Pathol Annu* 17(2):33–66, 1982.

104. Weiss W: Lobe of origin in the attribution of lung cancer to asbestos. *Br J Ind Med* 45:544–547, 1988.

105. Lee BW, Waih JC, Lesley KT, Wieneke JK, Christiani DC: Association of cigarette smoking and asbestos exposure with location and histology of lung cancer. *Am J Respir Crit Care Med* 157:748–755, 1998.

106. Greenberg SD, Hurst GA, Matlage WT, Christianson CS, Hurst IJ, Mabry LC: Sputum cytopathological findings in former asbestos workers. *Tex Med* 72:1–5, 1976.

107. Greenberg SD, Hurst GA, Matlage WT, Miller JM, Hurst IJ, Mabry LC: Tyler asbestos workers program. *Ann NY Acad Sci* 271:353–364, 1976.

108. Colby TV, Koss MN, Travis WD: Tumors of the Lower Respiratory Tract. Atlas of Tumor Pathology, Series. 3, Fasc 13. Washington, DC: Armed Forces Institute of Pathology, 1995.

109. Hammar SP: Common Neoplasms. Ch. 32 In: *Pulmonary Pathology*, 2nd ed. (Dail DH, Hammar SP, eds.), New York: Springer-Verlag, 1994, pp. 1123–1278.

110. Travis WD, Colby TV, Corrin B, Shimosato Y, Brambilla E: *The World Health Organization Histological Typing of Lung and Pleural Tumours*, 3rd ed., Berlin: Springer-Verlag, 1999.

111. Humphrey PA, Scroggs MS, Roggli VL, Shelburne JD: Pulmonary carcinomas with a sarcomatoid element: An immunocytochemical and ultrastructural analysis. *Hum Pathol* 19:155–165, 1988.

112. Roggli VL, Vollmer RT, Greenberg SD, McGavran MH, Spjut HJ, Yesner R: Lung cancer heterogeneity: A blinded and randomized study of 100 consecutive cases. *Hum Pathol* 16:569–579, 1985.

113. Greenberg SD: Asbestos lung disease. *Sem Respir Med* 4:130–137, 1982.

114. Greenberg SD: Asbestos. Ch. 22 In: *Pulmonary Pathology* (Dail DH, Hammar SP, eds.), New York: Springer-Verlag, 1988, pp. 619–636.

115. Whitwell F, Newhouse ML, Bennett DR: A study of the histologic cell types of lung cancer in workers suffering from asbestosis in the United Kingdom. *Br J Ind Med* 31:298–303, 1974.

116. Hourihane DO'B, McCaughey WTE: Pathological aspects of asbestosis. *Postgrad Med J* 42:613–622, 1966.

117. Hasan FM, Nash G, Kazemi H: Asbestos exposure and related neoplasia: The 28 year experience of a major urban hospital. *Am J Med* 65:649–654, 1978.

118. Johansson L, Albin M, Jakobsson K, Mikoczy Z: Histological type of lung carcinoma in asbestos cement workers and matched controls. *Br J Ind Med* 49:626–630, 1992.

119. Kannerstein M, Churg J: Pathology of carcinoma of the lung associated with asbestos exposure. *Cancer* 30:14–21, 1972.

120. Ives JC, Buffler PA, Greenberg SD: Environmental associations and histopathologic patterns of carcinoma of the lung: The challenge and dilemma in epidemiologic studies. *Am Rev Respir Dis* 128:195–209, 1983.

121. Auerbach O, Garfinkel L, Parks VR, Conston AS, Galdi VA, Joubert L: Histologic type of lung cancer and asbestos exposure. *Cancer* 54:3017–3021, 1984.

122. Vena JE, Byers TE, Cookfair D, Swanson M: Occupation and lung cancer risk: An analysis of histologic subtypes. *Cancer* 56:910–917, 1985.

123. Churg A: Lung cancer cell type and asbestos exposure. *JAMA* 253: 2984–2985, 1985.

124. Dail DH: Uncommon Tumors. Ch. 33 In: *Pulmonary Pathology*, 2nd ed. (Dail DH, Hammar SP, eds.), New York: Springer-Verlag, 1994, pp. 1279–1461.

125. Harwood TR, Gracey DR, Yokoo H: Pseudomesotheliomatous carcinoma of the lung—A variant of peripheral lung cancer. *Am J Clin Pathol* 65:159–167, 1976.

126. Koss M, Travis W, Moran C, Hochholzer L. Pseudomesotheliomatous adenocarcinoma: A reappraisal. *Sem Diag Pathol* 9:117–123, 1992.

127. Lilienfeld DE, Mandel JS, Coin P, Schuman LM: Projection of asbestos related diseases in the United States, 1985–2009. 1. Cancer. *Br J Ind Med* 45:283–291, 1988.

128. Mark EJ: The second diagnosis: The role of the pathologist in identifying pneumoconioses in lungs excised for tumor. *Hum Pathol* 12:585–587, 1981.

129. Mollo F, Magnani C, Bo P, Burlo P, Cravello M: The attribution of lung cancers to asbestos exposure: A pathologic study of 924 unselected cases. *Am J Clin Pathol* 117: 90–95, 2002.

130. Pratt PC: Emphysema and chronic airways disease. Ch. 4 In: *Pulmonary Pathology* (Dail DH, Hammar SP, eds.), New York: Springer-Verlag, 1988, pp. 651–669.

131. Churg A: Current issues in the pathologic and mineralogic diagnosis of asbestos induced disease. *Chest* 84:275–280, 1983.

132. Cagle PT: Criteria for attributing lung cancer to asbestos exposure. *Am J Clin Pathol* 117:9–15, 2002.

8

Other Neoplasia

Raj Rolston and Tim D. Oury

Introduction

While the carcinogenic effect of asbestos in the etiology of mesothelioma and lung cancer is widely accepted today (see Chapters 5 and 7), conflicting opinion exists for cancer of other sites. This is partly because of the fact that methodological limitations and weaknesses may be found in most of the studies reported in the literature. Epidemiologic studies have suggested a relationship between asbestos exposure and malignancies of the gastrointestinal tract, larynx, kidney, liver, pancreas, ovary and hematopoietic systems.[1,2] One must bear in mind that, in any population studied for asbestos exposure, cigarette smoking, alcohol consumption, and diet remain confounding variables. Also, the route of asbestos exposure, inhalation versus ingestion, has its own implications. Despite evidence both for and against, one cannot ignore the possibility that the carcinogenicity of asbestos may extend to sites of the body other than the lung and pleura to which the carcinogenic fibers can gain access. The pathologic features of these malignant neoplasms do not differ from those occurring in individuals not exposed to asbestos. Therefore, the role of the pathologist includes the accurate diagnosis of these diseases and also the examination of the lungs and pleural cavities for evidence of other asbestos-related tissue injury (see Chapters 4 and 6).

This chapter reviews the evidence for the association of these various malignancies with exposure to asbestos, including relevant experimental studies where the data are available. Pathologic features will also be noted when they are of relevance to the interpretation of the available epidemiologic studies. Possible mechanisms of asbestos-induced carcinogenesis (reviewed in Chapter 10) are not included in this review.

Gastrointestinal Cancer

Historical Background

Selikoff et al.[3] in 1964 were the first to suggest there was an excess of cancers of the digestive tract among individuals exposed to asbestos.

This observation was based on an epidemiologic study of asbestos insulation workers, and the association was maintained in subsequent follow-up studies involving larger numbers of workers followed for longer periods of time.[1] The rationale for this observation relates to the fact that many asbestos fibers deposited in the airways are removed by the mucociliary escalator and can be recovered from the sputum of exposed workers (see Chapter 9). If this sputum is subsequently swallowed, then fibers may be transported to various sites in the gastrointestinal tract. Direct contact of asbestos with epithelial cells of the gastrointestinal tract could then result in malignant transformation, similar to that believed to occur from interaction of asbestos fibers with bronchial epithelial cells or mesothelial cells. These considerations have generated concern regarding possible risks not only among asbestos workers but also among populations exposed to asbestos in food, beverages and drinking water.[4]

Animal Studies

Relatively few studies have examined the occurrence of gastrointestinal neoplasms in experimental animals exposed to asbestos. In the classic inhalation studies of Wagner et al.[5] and Davis et al.,[6] no excess numbers of neoplasms were observed at sites other than the lung and serous cavities. Animal studies involving the ingestion of chrysotile[7,8] or amosite[7] asbestos in Fisher 344 rats resulted in increased incidence of intestinal tumors, but the increase did not reach statistical significance. Asbestos fibers were recovered from ashed colon specimens, and the colonic tissue level of cyclic AMP was significantly decreased in animals fed asbestos as compared to control diets, but there was no increase in colon cancer.[8] In another study, animals were exposed to both radiation of the colon followed by asbestos ingestion.[94] This study also failed to demonstrate increased colon cancers in animals exposed to asbestos. In a study of hamsters fed amosite asbestos in their drinking water, two squamous cell carcinomas of the forestomach were identified, though these could not be specifically attributed to asbestos.[9] In contrast, a study by Huff et al.,[10] found a fivefold increased incidence in adenomatous polyps of the large intestine in male rats exposed to asbestos (intermediate range chrysotile) compared to controls. In addition, a study by Corpet et al.[95] demonstrated increased aberrant crypts, thought to be a precursor of cancer, in the colon, but no increase in colon carcinoma in rats fed chrysotile or crocidolite. It is of interest that studies have demonstrated penetration of the intestinal mucosa by asbestos fibers,[11,12] and this migration of fibers to the peritoneal serosal tissues may be relevant to the pathogenesis of peritoneal mesothelioma.[11–13] However, in a study of a baboon gavaged with chrysotile and crocidolite asbestos, no significant intestinal penetration or migration of fibers to other tissue sites was demonstrated.[14] All in all, experimental animal studies do not support a role for inhaled or ingested asbestos fibers in the production of gastrointestinal neoplasms.[15]

Epidemiologic Studies

A number of studies have demonstrated an excess of gastrointestinal carcinomas among asbestos workers[1,3,16-21] and projections for the next 25 years have resulted in estimates of 33,000 excess deaths from gastrointestinal cancers among asbestos-exposed individuals.[22] However, a number of investigators have challenged the hypothesis that asbestos exposure is causally related to gastrointestinal carcinomas.[23-26,96] In a review of 32 independent cohorts of asbestos workers, Edelman[25] found no consistent evidence to indicate that exposure to asbestos increases the risk of gastrointestinal cancer. Furthermore, there was no apparent dose-response relationship between accumulated asbestos dose and the risk of gastrointestinal cancer.[25] On the other hand, not all of the cohorts in Edelman's review showed an increased standardized mortality ratio (SMR) for lung cancer, which is universally accepted as causally related to asbestos exposure (see Chapter 7). In this regard, a review of 18 studies by Doll and Peto[2] showed a statistically strong correlation between SMRs for lung cancer and SMRs for gastrointestinal cancer. These results imply that when sufficient asbestos exposure in a population has occurred to result in a detectable increase in lung cancer risk, then it is likely that that population will also demonstrate an increased risk of gastrointestinal cancers.

More recent studies continue to be varied as to the significance of asbestos in gastrointestinal tumors. Goodman et al.,[27] applying meta-analysis to existing asbestos-exposed occupational cohorts, found no evidence of association between gastrointestinal cancer and asbestos exposure and no evidence of a dose-response effect. Tsai et al.[28] studied 2504 maintenance employees who had a minimum of one year of potential exposure to asbestos-containing material, especially thermal insulation, and found that the total population had a decreased SMR for all causes and for all cancers. The only statistically significant excess of mortality found was a fourfold increase in mesothelioma. There was decreased mortality from cancers of the esophagus, stomach, large intestine, rectum, and pancreas.

In addition, an epidemiologic study by Garabrant et al.,[97] in which they controlled for a large number of confounding variables, demonstrated that there was no increase in colon cancer in asbestos exposed individuals. In fact, they found there was a trend for decreased colon cancer in the most heavily exposed individuals. This study by Garabrant et al. emphasizes the importance of controlling for the many confounding variables that have been shown to be important rusk factors in this disease.

In contrast, Szeszenia-Dabrowska et al.[29] reported a statistically significant increase in mortality for carcinoma of the large intestine as well as for pleural mesothelioma in male workers occupationally exposed to asbestos (chrysotile and crocidolite). In addition, Raffn et al.[20] reviewed cancer incidence and mortality in workers in the Danish asbestos cement industry and found a significantly increased risk among men for cancer of the lung, pleura, mediastinum and stomach. Kishimoto[30] in a study aimed at determining the relationship between malignancy and asbestos exposure, by estimating the number of asbestos bodies in wet lung tissue, reported that 37% of gastric cancers in his patient population occurred among patients exposed to asbestos.

One of the difficulties in these epidemiologic studies is the uncertainty regarding the diagnosis of gastrointestinal carcinomas.[2,31–33] Doll and Peto[2] believe that the excess risk of gastrointestinal carcinomas reported in some cohorts of asbestos workers could be explained on the basis of carcinomas of the lung or pleural or peritoneal mesotheliomas being misdiagnosed as gastrointestinal carcinomas. Although this could be the explanation for excess cases of carcinoma of the stomach, colon or rectum, it seems considerably less likely to be the case for esophageal carcinomas (Figure 8-1). Indeed, these authors state that the evidence relating esophageal cancer to asbestos exposure is suggestive of a causal relationship, but not conclusive.[2] This conclusion is tempered by the observation of Acheson and Gardner[23] that social factors are particularly important in regard to cancers of the upper alimentary tract, and differences between the workforces studied and the standard population with which they have been compared must be taken into account. The authors believe there is sufficient evidence to indicate that in individuals with esophageal carcinoma and substantial exposure to asbestos as well as evidence of other asbestos-related tissue injury, asbestos is a probable contributing factor to the carcinoma. However, for the reasons just noted, the relationship between asbestos exposure and colorectal or gastric carcinoma remains unconvincing.

Despite a number of epidemiologic studies investigating the association between asbestos ingestion and gastrointestinal cancer,[34–40] the existence of such an association has not been definitely established.[4] Only one study, which involved the population in the San Francisco Bay area, suggested a positive correlation, and that was weak.[35] The types of fibers present in drinking water are generally short, ultramicroscopic fibers of questionable carcinogenic potential (see Chapter 10). Overall, the evidence fails to indicate any increased risk of alimentary tract tumors following the direct ingestion of asbestos.[41]

Laryngeal Cancer

A number of investigators have reported an association between asbestos exposure and laryngeal carcinoma.[20,42–47] The rationale for such an association involves contact of the laryngeal mucosa both with aerosolized fibers breathed into the lung and with fibers in sputum cleared from the lung by the mucociliary escalator. Digestion studies of laryngeal tissues obtained from asbestos workers have demonstrated the presence of asbestos bodies[48] as well as uncoated asbestos fibers.[49] No information is available concerning the dose-response relationship with respect to asbestos and cancer of the larynx, nor is there clear evidence with regard to variation in risk by fiber type.[50]

Some investigators have challenged the relationship between asbestos exposure and laryngeal carcinoma.[24,51–53] Battista et al.[54] studied asbestos-related mortality in railway carriage construction and

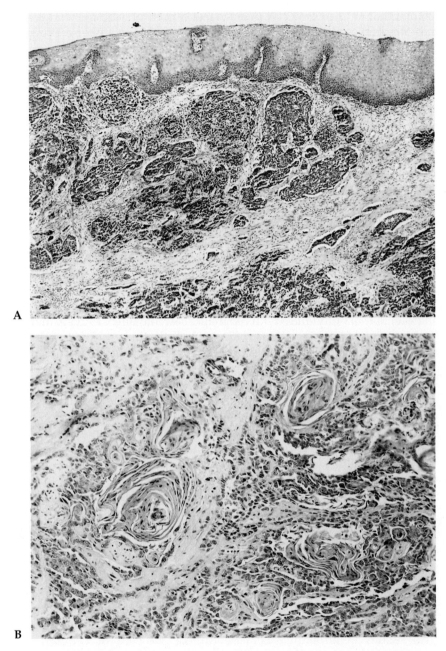

Figure 8-1. (A) Low-power view of esophageal carcinoma in a 63-year-old construction worker with bilateral parietal pleural plaques, showing esophageal mucosa (*above*) and infiltrating nests of carcinoma (*below*). **(B)** High-power view showing detail of squamous cell carcinoma with keratin pearls. H&E, (A) ×40, (B) ×100.

repair workers and could not establish a causal relationship between asbestos and laryngeal cancer. Experimental studies with rats exposed to aerosolized asbestos have not shown an excess of laryngeal tumors.[5,6] In a review of 13 cohort and eight case-control studies, Edelman[53] concluded that an increased risk of laryngeal cancer for asbestos workers has not been established. Other risk factors, such as cigarette smoking and alcohol consumption, have not been adequately accounted for in most of the reported studies. On the other hand, not all of the studies included in Edelman's review showed an increased SMR for lung cancer, either. Furthermore, the SMRs for laryngeal carcinoma exceeded 1.0 in at least some subgroups of workers examined in 10 of 13 cohort studies.[53] Edelman's review does not include references to three separate pathologic studies showing a strong relationship between laryngeal carcinoma and parietal pleural plaques.[55–57] Finally, Doll and Peto[2] and Smith et al.,[58] reviewing essentially the same cohort and case-control studies, concluded that asbestos should be regarded as one of the causes of laryngeal cancer. However, the relative risk is less than that for lung cancer and the absolute risk is much less.[2]

More recently, Saric and Vujovic[59] studied a Croatian population in an area with an asbestos processing plant where the number of primary malignant tumors of the pharynx and peritoneum were fewer than that of Croatia as a whole. Also, the incidence of lung cancer in this population was half that in Croatia. In contrast, they found the incidence of primary tumors of the pleura to be more than five times as high, and of laryngeal tumors more than twice as high in this group as in the country as a whole. Further studies[60–62] have also reported an increased risk of laryngeal/hypopharyngeal cancer related to asbestos exposure. The study by Murai et al.[62] compared autopsy cases with histologic evidence of asbestosis to those without asbestosis and found an increased risk of laryngeal cancer in patients with asbestosis. The authors agree with the position that asbestos, along with cigarette smoking and alcohol consumption, is a risk factor for laryngeal carcinoma, particularly in individuals with a substantial exposure to asbestos and evidence of other asbestos-related tissue injury.

The pathologic features of laryngeal carcinomas in asbestos workers are not different from those occurring in individuals with no known exposure to asbestos. Among the 35 cases reviewed by one of the editors (VLR), 33 have been squamous cell carcinomas (Figure 8-2), one pleomorphic spindle cell carcinoma, and one verrucous carcinoma. Asbestos bodies have never been described in histologic sections of laryngeal tissues, and normal ranges of asbestos fiber content have not been established for larynges from the general population. Thus there is at present no indication for performing digestion analysis of laryngeal tissues in an individual case. In the presence of neoplastic processes, uncontrolled replication of malignant cells will result in a dilutional effect on whatever fibers may have been present in the tissues prior to the initiation of the malignant process.

Renal Cell Carcinoma

Selikoff et al.[1] were the first to report an association between asbestos exposure and renal cell carcinoma. This observation was supported by the cohort study of Enterline et al. and others.[19,63–65] Smith et al.[65]

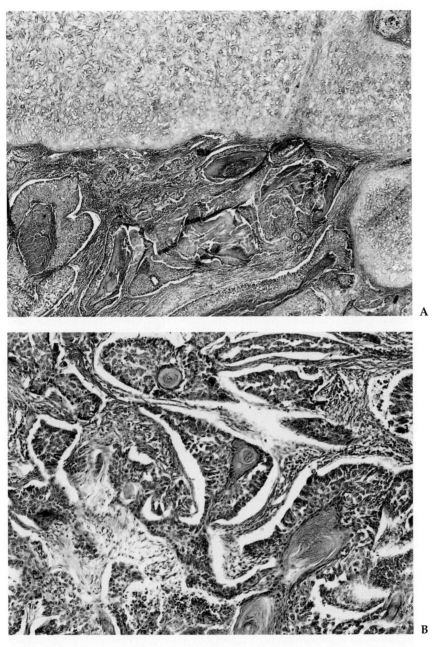

Figure 8-2. (A) Low-power view of laryngeal carcinoma in a 65-year-old patient with bilateral calcified parietal pleural plaques, showing laryngeal cartilages (*above and right*) and adjacent invasive carcinoma (*below*). **(B)** High-power view showing detail of squamous cell carcinoma with keratin pearls. H&E, (A) ×25, (B) ×100.

reviewed the cohort study of Enterline et al.[19] and two other large cohort studies of asbestos workers, including the study of Selikoff et al.,[1] and concluded that the available evidence supports a causal association between asbestos exposure and renal cell carcinoma. The rationale for this association involves the penetration of asbestos fibers into the lumen of capillaries, where they may then be transported to other organs, such as the kidneys.[66–67] Studies have identified the presence of asbestos fibers in human urine samples[68,69] and both amphibole and chrysotile fibers have been observed.

On the other hand, Acheson et al.[70] and Peto et al.[71] were unable to confirm an association between asbestos exposure and renal carcinoma in humans. In this regard, Smith et al.[65] argued that with the exception of the three large cohort studies noted earlier, none of the other studies in the literature had sufficient statistical power to detect an excess mortality from kidney cancer among workers exposed to asbestos. Experimental animal studies in which rats were chronically exposed to aerosolized asbestos fibers have failed to produce an excess of renal tumors,[5,6] although one study, in which rats were fed 50 mg/kg/body weight/day of a powdered filter material composed of 53% chrysotile, reported a statistically significant excess of renal malignancies.[72] Studies of urine samples from populations drinking water contaminated with asbestos[73] or from chrysotile asbestos cement workers,[74] failed to show a significant elevation of urinary asbestos fibers. In the latter study,[74] considerable precautions were taken to avoid sample contamination, a problem that has plagued some of the earlier studies.[69] In a study of a baboon gavaged with chrysotile and crocidolite asbestos, none of the urine samples from the test animal exceeded the level of background contamination for chrysotile, and only one crocidolite bundle was observed in a test sample.[14] Furthermore, virtually all fibers found in urine samples are shorter than 2.0 to 2.5 μm,[74] and the carcinogenic potential of such fibers is questionable (see Chapter 10). Overall, in the authors' opinion, the balance of the evidence available at present does not support an association between asbestos exposure and renal cell carcinoma.

Lymphoma/Leukemia

Ross et al.[75] reported in 1982 an excess of large cell lymphomas primary to the gastrointestinal tract and oral cavity in a case-control study of male patients with a substantial exposure to asbestos. Kagan and Jacobson[76] reported six cases of multiple myeloma, six cases of chronic lymphocytic leukemia, and one case of primary large cell lymphoma of the lung in patients with a history of asbestos exposure ranging from 3 to 37 years. Roggli et al.[77] referred to three patients with hematopoietic malignancies and parietal pleural plaques, including one patient with nodular poorly differentiated lymphocytic lymphoma, one with chronic granulocytic leukemia, and one with acute myelomonocytic leukemia. None had asbestosis histologically. Kishimoto et al.[78] reported two additional cases of acute myelocytic leukemia in individuals with a long history of exposure to asbestos. Asbestos bodies and crocidolite asbestos fibers were recovered from the bone marrow in both instances. More recently, in a study aimed at determining the relationship between malignancy and asbestos exposure by estimating the number of asbestos bodies in wet lung tissue, the same author reported that five out of ten cases of leukemia were related to asbestos exposure.[30] The rationale for the association between asbestos exposure and lymphoid neoplasms relates to the occurrence of asbestos bodies and fibers in lymph nodes[79] and to the variety of perturbations of the immune system observed in patients with exposure to asbestos.[80]

Other studies have failed to identify an increased incidence of leukemia or lymphoma among asbestos workers. These include two reports from Sweden[81,82] as well as the long-term follow-up of a large cohort of US–Canadian insulation workers by Selikoff et al.[1] In a study of 412 tumors other than lung tumors or mesotheliomas occurring in rats exposed to aerosolized asbestos or room air (controls), Wagner et al.[5] observed eight lymphomas/leukemias in asbestos-exposed rats versus two in controls. Davis et al.[6] also noted a single example of lymphoma/leukemia in a rat exposed to aerosolized chrysotile asbestos. None of these observations were considered to be statistically significant.[5,6] Overall, in the authors' opinion, the balance of the evidence available at present does not support an association between asbestos exposure and lymphoma or leukemia.

Ovarian Cancer

Several studies have reported an increased mortality from ovarian cancer among women exposed occupationally to amphibole asbestos.[83–85] Some peritoneal mesotheliomas were reported among women asbestos workers in each of these studies. In contrast, no increased mortality from ovarian cancer was reported among women working only with chrysotile asbestos[83] or among women involved with friction products manufacture.[86] In these two latter studies, no peritoneal mesotheliomas were reported either. In a case-control study of ovarian cancer, Cramer et al.[87] reported that women with ovarian cancer were about three times more likely to have used talcum powder for perineal dusting or sanitary napkins containing talc than matched control patients without ovarian neoplasms. Cosmetic talc is known to be contaminated with the noncommercial amphibole fibers, tremolite and anthophyllite (see Chapter 1). Wagner et al.[5] reported ten examples of ovarian cancer among more than 350 rats at risk that were exposed to aerosolized asbestos and none in controls. However, this difference did not reach statistical significance. Germani et al.[88] studied the cause-specific mortality of women compensated for asbestosis and reported significantly increased mortality for ovarian cancer as well as for lung and uterine cancer.

As noted by Doll and Peto,[2] peritoneal mesothelioma and ovarian carcinoma may have similar clinical presentations, and there is some overlap in histologic appearances as well (see Chapter 5). It seems at least as likely that the epidemiologic association of asbestos exposure and ovarian cancer is due to the misdiagnosis of peritoneal mesothelioma as that occupational asbestos exposure actually causes ovarian cancer.[2]

Pancreatic Carcinoma

Selikoff et al.[1] initially reported an excess of pancreatic carcinoma among asbestos insulation workers. However, their subsequent review of death certificate diagnoses of pancreatic cancer based on the best medical evidence available in individual cases led to the reclassification of 26 of 49 cases as peritoneal mesothelioma, metastatic lung cancer, metastatic colon cancer, or peritoneal carcinomatosis with unknown primary site.[89] This left 23 cases of pancreatic cancer with an expected number of 17.5, a difference that was not statistically significant. The available information does not support an association between pancreatic carcinoma and occupational exposure to asbestos.[28,54,89–92]

Additional associations between asbestos exposure and cancer that have been reported include an association with cancer of the eye[19] and with cancer of the penis.[93] More information is needed before definitive conclusions regarding these sites can be made.

References

1. Selikoff IJ, Hammond EC, Seidman H: Mortality experience of insulation workers in the United States and Canada, 1943–1976. *Ann NY Acad Sci* 330:91–116, 1979.
2. Doll R, Peto J: Other asbestos-related neoplasms. Ch. 4 In: *Asbestos-Related Malignancy.* (Antman K, Aisner J, eds.), Orlando, FL: Grune & Stratton, 1987, pp. 81–96.
3. Selikoff IJ, Churg J, Hammond EC: Asbestos exposure and neoplasia. *J Am Med Assoc* 188:22–26, 1964.
4. Working Group for the DHSS Committee to Coordinate Environmental and Related Programs: Report on cancer risks associated with the ingestion of asbestos. *Environ Health Perspect* 72:253–265, 1987.
5. Wagner JC, Berry G, Skidmore JW, Timbrell V: The effects of the inhalation of asbestos in rats. *Br J Cancer* 29:252–269, 1974.
6. Davis JMG, Beckett ST, Bolton RE, Collings P, Middleton AP: Mass and number of fibers in the pathogenesis of asbestos-related lung disease in rats. *Br J Cancer* 37:673–688, 1978.
7. Ward JM, Frank AL, Wenk M, Devor D, Tarone RE: Ingested asbestos and intestinal carcinogenesis in F344 rats. *J Environ Pathol Toxicol* 3:301–312, 1980.
8. Donham KJ, Berf JW, Will LA, Lehninger JR: The effects of long-term ingestion of asbestos on the colon of F344 rats. *Cancer* 45:1073–1084, 1980.
9. Smith WE, Hubert DD, Sobel HJ, Peters ET, Doerfler TE: Health of experimental animals drinking water with and without amosite asbestos and other mineral particles. *J Environ Pathol Toxicol* 3:277–300, 1980.
10. Huff JE, Eustis SL, Haseman JK: Occurrence and relevance of chemically induced benign neoplasms in long term carcinogenicity studies. *Cancer Metastasis Rev* 8:1–21, 1989.
11. Storeygard AR, Brown AL: Penetration of the small intestinal mucosa by asbestos fibers. *Mayo Clin Proc* 52:809–812, 1977.
12. Westlake GE, Spjut HJ, Smith MN: Penetration of colonic mucosa by asbestos particles: An electron microscopic study in rats fed asbestos dust. *Lab Invest* 14:2029–2033, 1965.

13. Winkler GC, Ruttner JR: Penetration of asbestos fibers in the visceral peritoneum of mice: A scanning electron microscopic study. *Exp Cell Biol* 50:187–194, 1982.
14. Hallenbeck WH, Markey DR, Dolan DG: Analysis of tissue, blood and urine samples from a baboon gavaged with chrysotile and crocidolite asbestos. *Environ Res* 25:349–360, 1981.
15. Condie LW: Review of published studies of orally administered asbestos. *Environ Health Perspect* 53:3–9, 1983.
16. McDonald JC, Liddell FDK, Gibbs GW, Eyssen GE, McDonald AD: Dust exposure and mortality in chrysotile mining, 1910–1975. *Br J Ind Med* 37:11–24, 1980.
17. Finkelstein MM: Mortality among employees of an Ontario asbestos-cement factory. *Am Rev Respir Dis* 129:754–761, 1984.
18. Botha JL, Irwig LM, Strebel PM: Excess mortality from stomach cancer, lung cancer and asbestosis and/or mesothelioma in crocidolite mining districts in South Africa. *Am J Epidemiol* 123:30–40, 1986.
19. Enterline PE, Hartley J, Henderson V: Asbestos and cancer: A cohort followed up to death. *Br J Ind Med* 44:396–401, 1987.
20. Raffn E, Lynge E, Juel K, Korsgaard B: Incidence of cancer and mortality among employees in the asbestos cement industry in Denmark. *Br J Ind Med* 46:90–96, 1989.
21. Jakobsson K, Albin M, Hagmar L: Asbestos, cement, and cancer in the right part of the colon. *Occup Environ Med* 51(2):95–101, 1994.
22. Lilienfeld DE, Mandel JS, Coin P, Schuman LM: Projection of asbestos-related diseases in the United States, 1985–2009. I Cancer. *Brit J Ind Med* 45:283–291, 1988.
23. Acheson ED, Gardner MJ: Asbestos: The control limit for asbestos. London: Health and Safety Commission, HMSO, 1983.
24. Levine DS: Does asbestos exposure cause gastrointestinal cancer? *Dig Dis Sci* 30:1189–1198, 1985.
25. Edelman DA: Exposure to asbestos and the risk of gastrointestinal cancer: A reassessment. *Br J Ind Med* 45:75–82, 1988.
26. Mossman BT, Gee JBL: Asbestos-related diseases. *N Eng J Med* 320:1721–1730, 1989.
27. Goodman M, Morgan RW, Ray R, Malloy CD, Zhao K: Cancer in asbestos-exposed occupational cohorts: a meta-analysis. *Cancer Causes Control* 10:453–465, 1999.
28. Tsai SP, Waddell LC, Gilstrap EL, Ransdell JD, Ross CE: Mortality among maintenance employees potentially exposed to asbestos in a refinery and petrochemical plant. *Am J Ind Med* 29:89–98, 1996.
29. Szeszenia-Dabrowska N, Wilczynska U, Szymczak W: Mortality of workers at two asbestos-cement plants in Poland. *Int J Occup Med Env Health* 13:121–130, 2000.
30. Kishimoto T: Cancer due to asbestos exposure. *Chest* 101:58–63, 1992.
31. Heasman MA, Lipworth L: Accuracy of certification of cause of death. GRO Studies on Medical and Population Subjects, No. 20, London: HMSO, 1966.
32. Newhouse ML, Wagner JC: Validation of death certificates in asbestos workers. *Br J Ind Med* 26:302–307, 1969.
33. Berry G, Newhouse ML, Wagner JC: Mortality from all cancers of asbestos factory workers in east London 1933–80. *Occup Environ Med* 57:782–785, 2000.
34. Meigs JW, Walter S, Hestbon J, Millette JR, Craun GG, Woodhall RS, Flannery JT: Asbestos-cement pipe and cancer in Connecticut, 1955–1974. *Environ Res* 42:187–197, 1980.

35. Conforti PM, Kanarek M, Jackson L, Cooper RC, Murchio JC: Asbestos in drinking water and cancer in the San Francisco Bay Area: 1969–1974 incidence. *J Chron Dis* 34:211–224, 1981.
36. Sadler TD, Rom WN, Lyon JL, Mason JO: The use of asbestos-cement pipe for public water supply and the incidence of cancer in selected communities in Utah, 1967–1976. Master's thesis, University of Utah, Salt Lake City, Utah, 1981.
37. Sigurdson EE: Observations of cancer incidence in Duluth, Minnesota. *Environ Health Perspect* 53:61–67, 1983.
38. Millette JR, Craun GF, Stober JA, Kraemer DF, Tousignant HD, Hildago E, Duboise RL, Benedict J: Epidemiology study of the use of asbestos-cement pipe for the distribution of drinking water in Escambia County, Florida. *Environ Health Perspect* 53:91–98, 1983.
39. Siemiatycki J: Health effects on the general population (mortality in the general population in asbestos mining areas), In: Proceedings of the World Symposium on Asbestos, Montreal, 25–27 May 1982, Asbestos Information Centre, Quebec, pp. 337–348, 1983.
40. Polissar L, Severson RK, Boatman ES: A case-control study of asbestos in drinking water and cancer risk. *Am J Epidemiol* 119:456–471, 1984.
41. Royal Commission on Matters of Health and Safety Arising from the Use of Asbestos in Ontario: Report of the Royal Commission on Matters of Health and Safety Arising from the use of asbestos in Ontario. Toronto: Ontario Ministry of the Attorney General, 1984.
42. Stell PM, McGill T: Asbestos and laryngeal carcinoma. *Lancet* 2:416–417, 1973.
43. Newhouse ML, Berry G: Asbestos and laryngeal carcinoma. *Lancet* 2:615, 1973.
44. Libshitz HI, Wershba MS, Atkinson GW, Southard ME: Asbestosis and carcinoma of the larynx: A possible association. *J Am Med Assoc* 228:1571–1572, 1974.
45. Stell PM, McGill T: Exposure to asbestos and laryngeal carcinoma. *J Laryngol Otol* 89:513–517, 1975.
46. Morgan RW, Shettigara PT: Occupational asbestos exposure, smoking and laryngeal carcinoma. *Ann NY Acad Sci* 271:309–310, 1976.
47. Becklake MD: Asbestos-related diseases of the lung and other organs: Their epidemiology and implications for clinical practice. *Am Rev Respir Dis* 114:187–227, 1976.
48. Roggli VL, Greenberg SD, McLarty JL, Hurst GA, Spivey CG, Hieger LR: Asbestos body content of the larynx in asbestos workers: A study of five cases. *Arch Otolaryngol* 106:533–535, 1980.
49. Hirsch A, Bignon J, Sebastien P, Gaudichet A: Asbestos fibers in laryngeal tissues: Findings in two patients with asbestosis associated with laryngeal tumors. *Chest* 76:697–699, 1979.
50. Huuskonen MS: Asbestos and cancer. *Eur J Respir Dis* 63(Suppl 123): 145–152, 1982.
51. Hinds MW, Thomas DB, O'Reilly HP: Asbestos, dental x-rays, tobacco, and alcohol in the epidemiology of laryngeal cancer. *Cancer* 44:1114–1120, 1979.
52. Chan CK, Gee JB: Asbestos exposure and laryngeal cancer: An analysis of the epidemiologic evidence. *J Occup Med* 30:23–27, 1988.
53. Edelman DA: Laryngeal cancer and occupational exposure to asbestos. *Int Arch Occup Environ Health* 61:223–227, 1989.
54. Battista G, Belli S, Comba P, Fiumalbi C, Grignoli M, Loi F, Orsi D, Paredes I: Mortality due to asbestos-related causes among railway carriage construction and repair workers. *Occup Med (Lond)* 49:536–539, 1999.

55. Hillerdal G: Pleural plaques and risks for cancer in the county of Uppsala. *Eur J Respir Dis* 61(Suppl 107):111–117, 1980.

56. Mollo F, Andrion A, Colombo A, Segnan N, Pira E: Pleural plaques and risk of cancer in Turin, Northwestern Italy: An autopsy study. *Cancer* 54:1418–1422, 1984.

57. Wain SL, Roggli VL, Foster WL: Parietal pleural plaques, asbestos bodies, and neoplasia: A clinical, pathologic and roentgenographic correlation of 25 consecutive cases. *Chest* 86:707–713, 1984.

58. Smith AH, Handley MA, Wood R: Epidemiological evidence indicates asbestos causes laryngeal cancer. *J Occup Med* 32:499–506, 1990.

59. Saric M, Vijovic M: Malignant tumors in an area with an asbestos processing plant. *Public Health Rev* 22:293–303, 1994.

60. Gustavsson P, Jakobsson R, Johansson H, Lewin F, Norell S, Rutkvist LE: Occupational exposures and squamous cell carcinoma of the oral cavity, pharynx, larynx, and oesophagus: a case-control study in Sweden. *Occup Environ Med* 55:393–400, 1998.

61. Marchand JL, Luce D, Leclerc A, Goldberg P, Orlowski E, Bugel I, Brugere J: Laryngeal and hypopharyngeal cancer and occupational exposure to asbestos and man-made vitreous fibers: Results of a case-control study. *Am J Ind Med* 37:581–589, 2000.

62. Murai Y, Masanobu K: Autopsy cases of asbestosis in Japan: A statistical analysis on registered cases. *Arch Env Health* 55:447–452, 2000.

63. Enterline PE, Henderson V: Asbestos and kidney cancer. *Am J Ind Med* 17:645–646, 1990.

64. Maclure M: Asbestos and renal adenocarcinoma: A case-control study. *Environ Res* 42:353–361, 1987.

65. Smith AH, Shearn VI, Wood R: Asbestos and kidney cancer: The evidence supports a causal association. *Am J Ind Med* 16:159–166, 1989.

66. Holt PF: Transport of inhaled dust to extrapulmonary sites. *J Pathol* 33:123–129, 1981.

67. Brody AR, Hill LH, Adkins B, O'Connor RW: Chrysotile asbestos inhalation in rats: Deposition pattern and reaction of alveolar epithelium and pulmonary macrophages. *Am Rev Respir Dis* 123:670–679, 1981.

68. Cook PM, Olson GF: Ingested mineral fibers: Elimination in human urine. *Science* 204:195–198, 1979.

69. Finn MB, Hallenbeck WH: Detection of chrysotile in workers' urine. *Ann Ind Hyg Assoc J* 46:162–169, 1985.

70. Acheson ED, Gardner MJ, Winter PD, Bennett C: Cancer in a factory using amosite asbestos. *Internat J Epidemiol* 13:3–10, 1984.

71. Peto J, Doll R, Hermon C, Binns W, Clayton R, Goffe T: Relationship of mortality to measures of environmental asbestos pollution in an asbestos textile factory. *Ann Occup Hyg* 29:305–335, 1985.

72. Gibel W, Lohs K, Horn K, Wildner G, Hoffman F: Animal experiments concerning cancerogenic effects of asbestos fiber material following oral administration. *Arch Geschwulstforsch* 46:437–442, 1976.

73. Boatman ES, Merrill T, O'Neill A, Polissar L, Millette JR: Use of quantitative analysis of urine to assess exposure to asbestos fibers in drinking water in the Puget Sound Region. *Environ Health Perspect* 53:131–141, 1983.

74. Guillemin MP, Litzistorf G, Buffat PA: Urinary fibres in occupational exposure to asbestos. *Ann Occup Hyg* 33:219–233, 1989.

75. Ross R, Nichols P, Wright W, Lukes R, Dworsky R, Paganini-Hill A, Koss M, Henderson B: Asbestos exposure and lymphomas of the gastrointestinal tract and oral cavity. *Lancet* 2:1118–1120, 1982.

76. Kagan E, Jacobson RJ: Lymphoid and plasma cell malignancies: Asbestos-related disorders of long latency. *Am J Clin Pathol* 80:14–20, 1983.

77. Roggli VL, Pratt PC, Brody AR: Asbestos content of lung tissue in asbestos-associated diseases: A study of 110 cases. *Br J Ind Med* 43:18–28, 1986.
78. Kishimoto T, Ono T, Okada K: Acute myelocytic leukemia after exposure to asbestos. *Cancer* 62:787–790, 1988.
79. Roggli VL, Benning TL: Asbestos bodies in pulmonary hilar lymph nodes. *Mod Pathol* 3:513–517, 1990.
80. Kagan E: Current perspectives in asbestosis. *Ann Allerg* 54:464–474, 1985.
81. Bengsston NO, Hardell L, Eriksson M: Asbestos exposure and non-Hodgkin's lymphoma. *Lancet* 2:1463, 1982.
82. Olsson H, Brandt L: Asbestos exposure and non-Hodgkin's lymphoma. *Lancet* 1:588, 1983.
83. Acheson ED, Gardner MJ, Pippard EC, Grime LP: Mortality of two groups of women who manufactured gas masks from chrysotile and crocidolite asbestos: A 40 year follow-up. *Br J Ind Med* 39:344–348, 1982.
84. Newhouse ML, Berry G, Wagner JC: Mortality of factory workers in East London, 1933–1980. *Br J Ind Med* 42:4–11, 1985.
85. Wignall BK, Fox AJ: Mortality of female gas-mask assemblers. *Br J Ind Med* 39:34–38, 1982.
86. Berry G, Newhouse ML: Mortality of workers manufacturing friction materials using asbestos. *Br J Ind Med* 40:1–7, 1983.
87. Cramer DW, Welch DR, Scully RE, Wojciechowski CA: Ovarian cancer and talc: A case-control study. *Cancer* 50:372–376, 1982.
88. Germani D, Belli S, Bruno C, Grignoli M, Nesti M, Pirastu R, Comba P: Cohort mortality study of women compensated for asbestosis in Italy. *Am J Ind Med* 36:129–134, 1999.
89. Selikoff IJ, Seidman H: Cancer of the pancreas among asbestos insulation workers. *Cancer* 47:1469–1473, 1981.
90. Ahlgren JD: Epidemiology and risk factors in pancreatic cancer. *Semin Oncol* 23:241–250, 1996.
91. Kauppinen T, Partanen T, Degerth R, Ojajarvi A: Pancreatic cancer and occupational exposures. *Epidemiology* 6:498–502, 1995.
92. Ojajarvi IA, et al. Occupational exposures and pancreatic cancer: a meta-analysis. *Occup Environ Med* 57:316–324, 2000.
93. Raffn E, Korsgaard B: Asbestos exposure and carcinoma of the penis. *Lancet* 2:1394, 1987.
94. Donham KJ, Will LA, Denman D, Leininger JR: The combined effects of asbestos ingestion and localized X-irradiation of the colon in rats. *J Environ Pathol Toxicol Oncol* 5:299–308, 1984.
95. Corpet DE, Pirot V, Goobet I: Asbestos induces aberrant crypt foci in the colon of rats. *Cancer Lett* 74:183–187, 1993.
96. Gamble JF: Asbestos and colon cancer: a weight-of-the-evidence review. *Environ Health Perspect* 102:1038–1050, 1994.
97. Garabrant DH, Peters RK, Homa DM: Asbestos and colon cancer: lack of association in a large case-control study. *Am J Epidemiol* 135:843–853, 1992.

9

Cytopathology of Asbestos-Associated Diseases

Thomas A. Sporn, Kelly J. Butnor, and Victor L. Roggli

Introduction

Following its distinction in 1971 as the first material to be regulated by the Occupational Safety and Health Administration (OSHA), asbestos has earned notoriety among commonly encountered compounds matched only by its ubiquity and industrial utility. A generic term for naturally occurring fibrous silicates, there are six types of asbestos: the serpentine chrysotile, and the amphiboles amosite, crocidolite, anthophyllite, tremolite and actinolite. A versatile industrial product as a result of its thermal and chemical stability, high flexibility, tensile strength, and low electrical conductivity, asbestos has been employed as insulation material in applications from heavy industry to hairdryers. In the United States in the year 2000, 5000 metric tons of asbestos were produced, all of it chrysotile, for usage in roofing, gaskets, and friction products.

Millions of people have been exposed to asbestos in the occupational and paraoccupational setting, with millions more exposed resulting from contamination of ambient air, albeit at a much lower intensity. As fibers enter the lung, they may undergo phagocytosis and become coated by alveolar macrophages, forming asbestos bodies[1] (Figure 9-1). Other fibers may escape such coating and become injurious to the lungs and serosal membranes, resulting in effusions, interstitial fibrosis (i.e., asbestosis, see Chapter 4), carcinoma of the lung (Chapter 7), and malignant mesothelioma (Chapter 5). Inhaled asbestos fibers are of varying lengths and widths, with deposition into the tracheobronchial tree and further occurring largely as a function of fiber diameter, rather than length. Those fibers longer than 100 microns are for the most part trapped within the nasal vibrissae and do not usually enter the tracheobronchial tree. Those fibers longer than 40 microns tend to impinge upon the walls of the trachea and larger bronchi and do not usually enter the peripheral airways or alveoli. Thus, most asbestos bodies are approximately 35 microns in length and 1 to 2 microns in diameter (Figure 9-2).[2] However, as the respirability of a particular fiber is chiefly determined by its diameter, some very long fibers may reach the

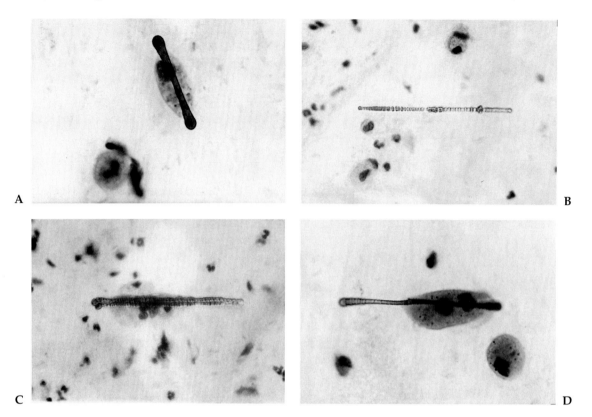

Figure 9-1. **(A)–(D)** Close view of single asbestos bodies in sputum. Several are partly within alveolar macrophages. Papanicolaou, ×700. (Reprinted from Ref. 1, with permission.)

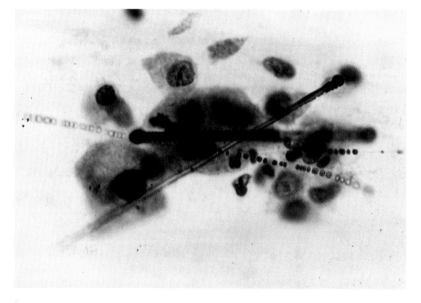

Figure 9-2. Photomicrograph showing numerous asbestos bodies within a thick covering of alveolar macrophages. Papanicolaou, ×600. (Reprinted from Ref. 54, with permission.)

peripheral lung. Animal models indicate that asbestos bodies may form in 4 to 6 months following implantation.

Cytopathology may be quite useful in the evaluation of patients with asbestos-related diseases. Its utility includes the diagnosis of malignancy in this setting as well as detection of excess tissue levels of asbestos. The advent of fine needle aspiration cytology and immuno-histochemical staining procedures has aided the clinician in this regard while decreasing the need for more invasive procedures. This chapter discusses in detail the uses and limitations of cytopathology in the evaluation of asbestos-associated diseases.

Historical Background

Stewart reported the presence of asbestos bodies, termed "curious bodies" in the sputa of asbestos miners in 1929.[3] The cytologic examination of specimens in those with asbestos-associated disease as a diagnostic tool was then largely ignored until the report of An and Koprowska in 1962. These authors described the first case of a concurrent cytologic diagnosis of asbestos bodies and squamous cell carcinoma of the lung in a cigarette smoker.[4] In 1978, Huuskonen examined the sputum cytology of asbestos workers, 114 with asbestosis, 59% of whom were chronic cigarette smokers. Although a range of squamous metaplasia, cytologic atypia, and dysplastic changes were detected, the study did not conclusively determine a role for the routine examination of sputum cytology in the early detection of bronchogenic carcinoma in this population.[5] In 1981, Gupta and Frost reported that sputum and bronchoscopy cytologies in people with asbestos exposure may demonstrate one or more of the following abnormalities: asbestos bodies, chronic inflammation, and epithelial atypia. They noted that people with known exposure to asbestos may not demonstrate asbestos bodies in cytologic preparations, while those without known exposure may show asbestos bodies (the latter likely with unrecognized exposure).[6] In 1982, Kotin and Paul reported on the results of a lung cancer detection program in an asbestos industry. They concluded that there was no evidence that early diagnosis will significantly improve the prognosis of lung cancer.[7]

Dodson et al. in 1983 reported on the ultrastructural study of sputa from former asbestos workers.[8] Their results were the first to confirm the presence of uncoated asbestos fibers, diatomaceous earth, and aluminum silicates in sputum. In 1984, Kobusch et al. reported on a study of sputum cytology in a cohort of Canadian chrysotile workers.[9] Finding significant cytologic abnormalities or malignancy in a distinct minority of 867 cases, they concluded that sputum cellular atypia increased with age and asbestos exposure. Unfortunately, no mention of asbestos bodies was included in this study, which could have provided insight as to the potential for chrysotile to form asbestos bodies.

The remainder of this chapter will discuss the findings of exfoliative and aspiration cytopathology in asbestos-associated disease.

Bronchial Epithelial Atypia

Exfoliative respiratory cytology to diagnose diseases of the tracheo-bronchial tree forms a "diagnostic triad," incorporating the complementary examinations of expectorated sputum, bronchial brushings, washings or lavages obtained during bronchoscopy, and postbronchoscopy sputum.[10] Perhaps the most crucial role for respiratory cytology in those with asbestos-associated pulmonary disease is in the detection and classification of lower respiratory tract malignancies alleged to be caused by an exposure to asbestos. Diagnostic sensitivity and specificity are affected by multiple factors, including the gross distribution and degree of differentiation of any particular tumor, as well as the technique of specimen procurement and processing. Interpretation of specimens may be hindered by regional inflammation or infection, leading to false positive diagnoses of malignancy. It is beyond the scope of this chapter to review exfoliative pulmonary cytopathology in its entirety, but important principles regarding those believed to be exposed to asbestos will be emphasized.

Bocking et al. report that three satisfactory sputum specimens may detect up to 60% of lung cancers.[11] Diagnostic yield is affected by location, size, and degree of differentiation of the tumor, with larger, central, and higher grade lesions detected more readily. Malignant mesothelioma does not produce exfoliated cells in sputum, and this type of specimen is not likely to be of much use excepting those cases that are complicated by direct extension of tumor into the lung parenchyma.[12] Well-differentiated squamous cell carcinomas and small cell carcinomas are the most accurately classified using sputum cytologies. Bronchoscopic specimens in general are more cellular with better preservation of cytologic features, and their procurement will aid in the detection of more peripheral tumors.

Squamous Cell Carcinoma

Epithelial cells may undergo a series of reactive and metaplastic changes in response to injury and irritation. Reactive changes include nuclear enlargement and hyperchromasia with the formation of visible nucleoli, but preservation of nuclear to cytoplasmic ratios. Squamous metaplasia, while not necessarily a preinvasive phenomenon, is associated with the development of invasive carcinoma. Squamous metaplastic cells are generally uniform in both size and shape, with abundant cyanophilic cytoplasm. These cells may develop small nucleoli if inflamed. Cytoplasmic orangophilia and nuclear pyknosis may supervene as degenerative changes. Following squamous metaplasia, injured or irritated epithelium may undergo the spectrum of dysplastic changes, leading to carcinoma. Mild dysplasia is evidenced by nuclear hyperchromasia and slight increase in nuclear to cytoplasmic ratio. Moderate to severe dysplasia shows progression in the nuclear abnormalities, with increase in granular and dispersed nuclear chromatin, nuclear membrane abnormalities, and further increase in nuclear to cytoplasmic ratio. Squamous cell carcinoma shows cellular

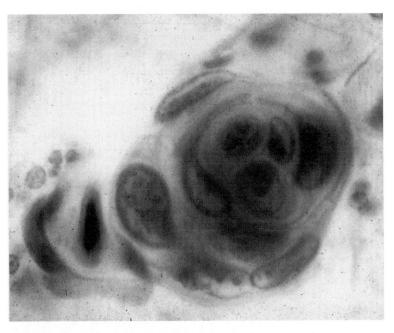

Figure 9-3. Cytologic specimen showing keratin pearl formation characteristic of squamous cell carcinoma. Note hyperchromatic, ink-drop nucleus at lower left. Papanicolaou stain, ×400.

pleomorphism with abnormal or bizarre shapes, dense cytoplasmic keratinization, and strikingly hyperchromatic "ink-drop" nuclei (Figure 9-3). The detection of single cells with malignant features is an important observation in the diagnosis of malignancy.[13]

Adenocarcinoma

Adenocarcinoma is the most common histologic subtype of bronchogenic carcinoma and is less strongly associated with cigarette smoking than squamous or small cell carcinoma. The typically peripheral location of adenocarcinoma makes it more difficult to diagnose in sputum specimens, but bronchial exfoliative cytologies and directed aspiration biopsies of peripheral lesions allow its detection in most cases. The cells may be arranged in abortive papillae, acinar units, or crowded into three-dimensional clusters. Cell size is typically large, with appreciable cytoplasm that may contain mucin vacuoles, large nuclei with polar orientation, vesicular chromatin, and prominent nucleoli (Figure 9-4).

Small Cell Carcinoma

The gross distribution and cytologic features of small cell carcinoma of the lung stand in contrast to squamous cell carcinoma and the other nonsmall cell variants and provide additional challenges to the cytopathologist. While typically arising in the major bronchi, small cell carcinoma often presents a submucosal infiltrative pattern and may

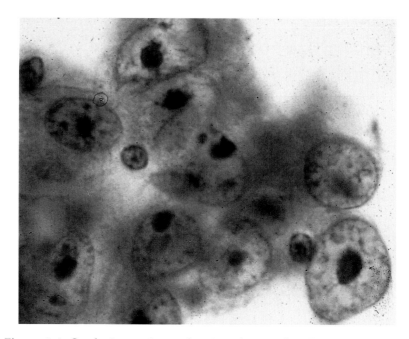

Figure 9-4. Cytologic specimen showing cluster of malignant cells, high nuclear to cytoplasmic ratio, and macronucleoli, characteristic of adenocarcinoma. Papanicolaou stain, ×400.

demonstrate only extrinsic compression of the airway to the bronchoscopist. This stands in contrast to the obstructing endobronchial tumor mass characteristic of squamous cell carcinoma. The exfoliated cells are generally small, 1.5 to 4 times the size of a small lymphocyte, with scant cytoplasm, hyperchromatic nuclei, and inconspicuous nuclei (Figure 9-5). The nuclei of neighboring cells appear to "mold" one another's shape and the cells often appear in a diathesis of cellular debris and necrosis.

Large Cell Carcinoma

Large cell carcinomas comprise a heterogeneous group of malignant epithelial tumors that lack the cytologic features of squamous or glandular differentiation, or the features of small cell carcinoma. In cytologic preparations, large cell carcinoma shows cell clusters as well as dispersed single cells with clearly malignant features. Cytoplasm is usually abundant, but lacks evidence of keratinization or mucin production (Figure 9-6). The nuclear features are also striking, with demonstration of thickened, irregular nuclear contours, coarse chromatin, and large, often multiple, nucleoli. Ultrastructural examination of these cells may occasionally show evidence of rudimentary squamous or glandular differentiation, suggesting that large cell carcinoma may be related to squamous cell or adenocarcinoma.[14] The differential diagnosis of large cell carcinoma includes metastatic melanoma, epithelioid sarcoma, and germ cell neoplasms. Cytologic atypia in benign cells following chemotherapy and/or radiation is often marked, and

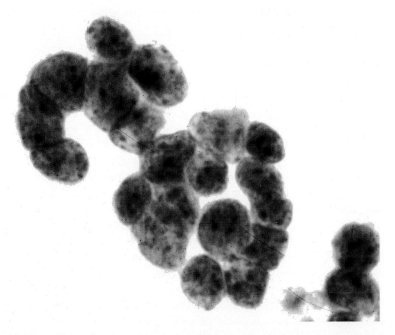

Figure 9-5. Cytologic specimen showing tumor cells with high nuclear to cytoplasmic ratio, salt and pepper chromatin, inconspicuous nucleoli, and nuclear molding, characteristic of small cell carcinoma. Papanicolaou stain, ×400.

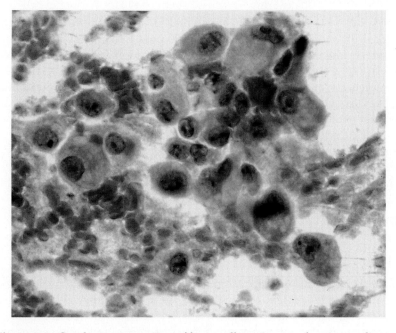

Figure 9-6. Cytologic preparation of large cell carcinoma, showing malignant nuclear features and nondescript cytoplasmic detail, characteristic of large cell carcinoma. Papanicolaou stain, ×125.

failure to distinguish such from large cell carcinoma may also constitute a diagnostic pitfall.

Effusion Cytologies

Effusions in the pleural or peritoneal spaces generally require significant accumulation before becoming clinically evident (300 cc in the pleural cavity, 1000 cc in the peritoneal cavity),[10] although much smaller effusions may be detected on radiologic studies. The development of pleural effusions in particular is an important clinical sequela of exposure to asbestos. In addition to the typical nonasbestos-related pathologies such as heart failure or parapneumonic effusions, those exposed to asbestos may develop benign asbestos pleural effusions (see Chapter 6), or effusions complicating asbestos-associated pleuropulmonary malignancy. Cytopathologic examination of exfoliated cells plays an important role in the evaluation of the broad differential diagnosis these effusions pose. Some 40% to 80% of pleural effusions are malignant, most commonly due to metastatic adenocarcinoma of the lung, followed by metastatic adenocarcinoma of the breast. Mesothelioma commonly results in malignant pleural effusions that present a special set of challenges to the cytopathologist. Ascites commonly results from hyponatremia, portal venous hypertension, or malignancy. Malignant ascites most commonly complicates ovarian or gastrointestinal malignancy, but may be associated with hepatobiliary carcinoma and peritoneal mesothelioma as well.

Benign Effusions

Benign asbestos pleural effusions (BAPE) are a common and dose-related phenomenon affecting those exposed to asbestos, with the shortest latency time of any of the common asbestos-associated diseases.[15] Often asymptomatic, BAPE may be attended by dyspnea and pleurisy, and may also accumulate in the pericardial and peritoneal spaces as well.[6] The effusions are typically exudative and may be serous or serosanguinous. An inflammatory pleocytosis is usual, often with a conspicuous population of eosinophils. Asbestos bodies have not been identified within the effusion specimen. Benign effusions may result in the exfoliation of mesothelial cells with striking cytologic atypia, including large size and nuclear abnormalities such as multinucleation. Misinterpretation of reactive changes in mesothelium as malignant mesothelioma or carcinoma constitutes a major pitfall in exfoliative cytology, and will be discussed in more detail below.

Malignant Effusions

Malignant pleural effusions are most commonly caused by involvement with adenocarcinoma, either in the form of direct extension of tumor, studding of the pleural surface, lymphovascular obstruction, or combinations thereof. Carcinomatous pleural effusions and ascites are characterized by tight, three-dimensional clusters of cells with high nuclear to cytoplasmic ratios, nuclear membrane irregularities, pleo-

morphism, and hyperchromasia, and prominent nucleoli. The demonstration of mucin in such cells is strongly suggestive of malignancy. On
cytologic grounds alone, it may be difficult or impossible to distinguish
metastatic adenocarcinoma from primary malignancies of the serosal
membranes (i.e., malignant mesothelioma). The cytologic distinction
between mesothelioma and reactive mesothelial hyperplasia may likewise be problematic (Figure 9-7).

Up to 90% of malignant mesotheliomas may present with serous
effusions.[16] Whitaker reports that the presence of diagnostically useful
cells in effusion cytology is predicted by the histologic subtype of
mesothelioma, with sarcomatoid and desmoplastic subtypes tending to
produce more paucicellular effusions.[17] The fibrotic component of the
tumor in these cases likely retards tumor cell exfoliation into the effusion. The general cytologic criteria for malignancy, namely, large cells
with large and hyperchromatic nuclei and nuclear membrane irregularities, macronucleoli, and high nuclear to cytoplasmic ratios, holds
true for malignant mesothelioma. No single cytologic feature is diagnostic of malignant mesothelioma. At low power, mesothelioma may
be suggested by the presence of cell aggregates, consisting of "more
and bigger cells" in "more and bigger clusters."[10,17,18] Benign proliferations may exfoliate as a monolayer, but papillary aggregates within
the cytology specimen may be seen in both pleural mesothelioma and
adenocarcinoma. They are rare in benign pleural effusions, but such
papillary aggregates have been described in benign effusions of

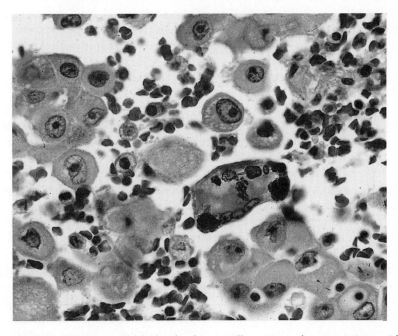

Figure 9-7. Cytology cell block of a fine needle aspirate from a patient with
malignant mesothelioma. Such specimens are difficult to distinguish from
metastatic adenocarcinoma on the one hand, and atypical reactive mesothelium on the other. Note the multinucleate giant cell (*center*) with phagocytosed
asbestos body. Hematoxylin and eosin, ×200.

the pericardial and peritoneal spaces.[19] The complexity and three dimensionality of the cell aggregates favors mesothelioma. A uniform population of exfoliated cells favors mesothelioma over adenocarcinoma, but this is also a feature of benign effusions.[19] Other findings suggestive of mesothelioma include peripheral cytoplasmic blebbing, cell-to-cell apposition with formation of intercellular windows, and cell cannibalism. Nuclear features suggestive of mesothelioma include paracentral location, macronucleoli, and multinucleation with atypia. Bizarre or anaplastic forms favor an alternative diagnosis.

Exceptions to these general observations exist and warrant caution in distinguishing malignant from reactive mesothelial processes. Zakowski reported that the cytologic features of benign mesothelial cells exfoliated into pericardial effusions of patients with the acquired immunodeficiency syndrome (AIDS) may have striking atypia beyond that normally encountered in pericardial effusions, and particular caution is warranted in the examination of fluids from this population.[20] The distinction between mesothelioma and adenocarcinoma therefore may not be possible on cytomorphologic grounds alone.

Ancillary studies may be of some use in this regard. Chief among such studies is immunocytochemistry. An extensive review of the histochemical and immunohistochemical profile of mesothelioma will be presented in Chapter 5. In brief, establishment of mesothelial differentiation has historically been based on negative staining patterns for mucin and adenocarcinoma-associated epitopes.[21] The development of antibodies highly, but not completely, specific to mesothelium have advanced the ability to distinguish mesothelioma from adenocarcinoma in histologic preparations. These antibodies include calretinin, HBME-1, and CK5/6, used in concert with antibodies directed against carcinoma-associated antigens such as CD15 (Leu M-1), BerEP4, carcinoembryonic antigen (CEA), and thyroid transcription factor 1 (TTF-1).[22–28]

The utility of such antibodies in cytologic preparations in distinguishing mesothelial differentiation among the constituent cells is less well established. Immunostains may be performed on formalin-fixed, paraffin-embedded cell block specimens of exfoliative material as well as material obtained by aspiration biopsy.[29] The monoclonal antibody HBME-1 was among the first developed with enhanced mesothelial specificity. However, calretinin has emerged as the antibody with the greatest specificity, especially with respect to nuclear staining.[24] Calretinin is a 29 kilodalton calcium binding protein, and member of the family of EF hand proteins to which S-100 belongs. It is expressed in normal, reactive, and neoplastic mesothelium, as well as some neural tissues. The distinction of mesothelioma from adenocarcinoma is typically undertaken using a panel of the above antibodies. Strongly positive staining for one or more of the carcinoma-associated antibodies renders the diagnosis of mesothelioma unlikely. Motherby reports that of the above epitopes, BerEP4 is the most useful in identifying neoplastic epithelial cells in effusions. It is most useful in discriminating between metastatic carcinoma and mesothelioma, positive staining for the latter detected in 0% of their cases.[28]

It is crucial to note that while antibodies such as calretinin are sensitive and specific markers for mesothelial differentiation, they are unable to discriminate between mesothelioma and reactive mesothelial proliferations. Some studies have employed antibodies such as desmin, E- and N-cadherin, and epithelial membrane antigen (EMA) to aid in the very difficult separation of reactive from neoplastic mesothelium.[30–32] While progress has been made in this regard, the separation of reactive from transformed mesothelium on cytologic grounds remains problematic, and consensus regarding a sensitive and reproducible immunophenotype to distinguish the two for usage in routine clinical practice has not yet been reached.[33]

Sakuma et al. examined the utility of electron microscopy in the diagnosis of malignant effusions. Their observations concerning exfoliated mesothelioma cells joins the body of ultrastructural literature which hold that mesothelioma is distinguishable from adenocarcinoma in tissue sections on the basis of long slender surface microvilli that characterize mesothelial cells. Such cells also have more abundant intermediate filaments and fewer free ribosomes. Reactive mesothelial cells, by contrast, contain fewer mitochondria than mesothelioma cells.[34]

In summary, cytologic differences among adenocarcinoma, epithelial and biphasic subtypes of malignant mesothelioma, and reactive mesothelial proliferations are subtle with overlapping features in some cases.[22–28,35,36] The broad application of immunohistochemistry and electron microscopy has rendered obsolete views expressed in older literature that the diagnosis of mesothelioma could not be made with certainty in the absence of an autopsy. Nonetheless, the diagnosis of mesothelioma based solely on examination of cytologic specimens, even with ancillary studies, remains fraught with hazards.[37] It is our practice to utilize the cytologic examination of pleural or ascites fluid as a screening test. Such cytologic examination, augmented by the application of immunohistochemical studies as described above, can allow one to become extremely suspicious of the diagnosis of mesothelioma. However, we advocate additional biopsy directed by CT, or guided by thoracoscopy or laparoscopy, to secure the diagnosis. Fine needle aspiration (FNA) has also been employed in the evaluation of mesothelioma,[38–42] but in our opinion the same caveats hold true for cytologic preparations obtained by aspiration biopsy as for exfoliative specimens. Core tissue specimens obtained by FNA in some cases may be sufficient for diagnosis.

Effusion cytologies have also provided a substrate for cytogenetic and DNA ploidy analyses to separate benign proliferations, mesothelioma, and carcinoma,[43,44] but to date such studies have not obviated the requirement for cytologic or tissue diagnoses of malignancy. The confirmation of positive cytologic findings with surgical biopsy is also advocated by other centers with extensive experience in the care of mesothelioma patients.[45] Such an approach seems only reasonable in view of the dire prognostic, therapeutic, and medicolegal ramifications following the diagnosis of mesothelioma.

Occurrence and Significance of Asbestos Bodies in Cytologic Preparations

Inhaled asbestos fibers are physical and mechanical irritants, injurious to the lung. They are deposited in alveolar ducts, and their sharp ends allow penetration across the alveolar walls and into adjacent units. Inhaled fibers undergo phagocytosis by alveolar macrophages, where they are coated by ferritin and glycoproteins, forming the asbestos body.[46] Asbestos body maturation has been studied using scanning electron microscopy, demonstrating progression from a membrane bound, smoothly coated fiber to the characteristic beaded form.[47] Changes in the morphology of the asbestos body may reflect physical forces imparted on the fibers during the inspiratory and expiratory phases of breathing.[47] Studies of macrophage viability following incubation with asbestos bodies confirm the minimal potential for cytoxicity of these coated fibers.[48] In histologic sections, asbestos bodies may be observed embedded within fibrotic pulmonary interstitium, or free within alveolar spaces. The latter may be mobilized onto the mucociliary apparatus, expectorated or swallowed, and otherwise rendered accessible to removal through the techniques of bronchoalveolar lavage or fine-needle aspiration. A similar fate also applies, obviously, to uncoated fibers within the lung.

Some degree of caution is advised in the interpretation of ferruginous bodies/asbestos bodies. Coated fibers resembling asbestos bodies, so-called pseudoasbestos bodies, have been described in end-users of refractory ceramic fibers (RCF). Dumortier found such bodies in the lavage fluid of 9 of 1800 such end-users (0.5%). Seventy percent of core fibers analyzed proved to be aluminum silicates typical of RCF and 30% were asbestos fibers.[49] The presence of asbestos bodies in lavage fluids is thus a valid marker for asbestos exposure and fiber retention. However, the possibility of pseudoasbestos bodies at least in this population merits consideration.

Sputum

Although asbestos bodies, the hallmark of asbestos exposure, are commonly identified using digestion techniques in the lung tissue of the general population,[50] their presence in the sputa of nonexposed individuals has not been reported, and their presence in bronchoalveolar lavage fluid (BALF) obtained from such populations is infrequent and of low concentration.[50] Modin reviewed 31,353 sputum and BALF specimens over a five-year period, finding asbestos bodies in five cases (3 sputa, 2 BALF). Further investigation determined that all five cases had significant exposure to asbestos, and asbestosis was identified in four of the five cases.[51] From these studies, it was concluded that asbestos bodies in sputum and bronchial washing specimens are highly specific markers for past asbestos exposure and reflect a significant asbestos fiber burden within the lung.

On the other hand, asbestos workers may frequently have asbestos bodies in sputum specimens (Figure 9-8). A study of asbestos workers

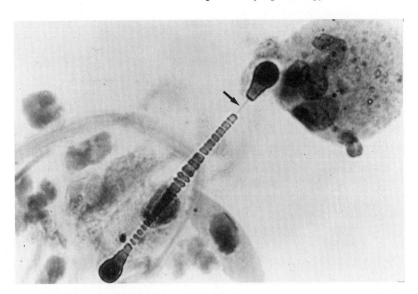

Figure 9-8. Asbestos body with an incomplete coating of iron and protein, found in the sputum of a Tyler, Texas, asbestos worker. *Arrow* points to the fiber forming the core of the body. Papanicolaou, ×700. (Reprinted from Ref. 55, with permission.)

in Tyler, Texas, demonstrated asbestos bodies in their sputa, statistically related to the age and duration of the worker's exposure (Figure 9-9). None of the control subjects studied showed asbestos bodies in their sputum.[52] Correlative studies of sputum and lung asbestos body content show that asbestos bodies do not appear in sputum until there is a substantial parenchymal asbestos fiber burden. Bignon et al.[53] showed that the presence of sputum asbestos bodies correlated with a lung asbestos burden of 1000 bodies or more per cubic centimeter of lung. Roggli et al. showed that asbestos bodies appear in sputum when the lung asbestos burden is 900 or more asbestos bodies per gram of wet lung tissue (Table 9-1).[54] Lack of better correlation between sputum and lung tissue digest may reflect a diminution in sputum clearance of asbestos bodies in those with high fiber burdens, with severely fibrotic lungs trapping fibers within the interstitium.

The demonstration of asbestos bodies in the sputum of occupationally exposed individuals may antedate radiographic changes, but is also a sensitive marker for pulmonary impairment. The Tyler Asbestos Workers Program examined the relationship between asbestos bodies in sputum and clinical findings in 674 former asbestos workers. Over a five-year study period, statistical analysis showed that asbestos bodies in the sputum were significantly related to radiographic findings of interstitial lung disease, pleural fibrosis, and restrictive ventilatory defects.[55] Thus, it appears that the detection of asbestos bodies in sputum is a rather insensitive but highly specific marker of occupational exposure, with a high likelihood of parenchymal lung disease.

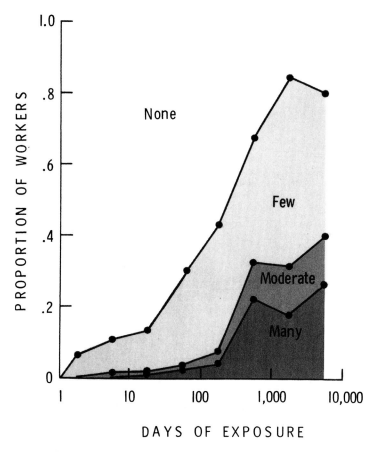

Figure 9-9. Graph demonstrating the proportion of asbestos workers with asbestos bodies in their sputum compared to the length of their employment (in days). (Reprinted from Ref. 52, with permission.)

Bronchoalveolar Lavage

Bronchoalveolar lavage fluid (BALF) provides another analytic medium for the detection, quantification, and mineralogic examination of asbestos fibers. Recovery of asbestos bodies may be influenced by areas sampled, with lavages of lower lung zones more likely to yield asbestos bodies in the exposed subject.[56] Unlike sputum, asbestos bodies may be detected in the lavage fluid of populations with no his-

Table 9-1. Correlation between asbestos bodies in cytological specimens and lung tissue digests*

Source	Cytologic Specimens	Lung Tissue
Sputum		
Bignon et al., 1974[53]	>1 AB	>1000 AB/cm^3
Roggli et al., 1980[54]	>1 AB	>900 AB/gm
BALF		
De Vuyst et al.[61]	1 AB/ml	1800 AB/gm
Sebastien et al.[62]	1 AB/ml	2200 AB/gm
Karjalainen et al.[60]	1 AB/ml	2500 AB/gm

*Sputum studies are reported as AB/cm^3 or AB/gm wet lung. BALF studies are reported as AB/gm dry lung. 1 AB/cm^3 ≅ 1 AB/gm wet lung ≅ 10 AB/gm dry lung.

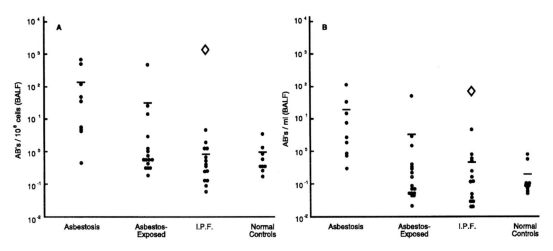

Figure 9-10. Distribution of asbestos body content per million cells recovered **(A)** or per ml BALF **(B)** for 50 cases as determined by light microscopy. Each dot represents one case, and a horizontal line indicates the median value for each group. Open diamond represents black-cored pseudoasbestos bodies isolated from one case that was excluded from the median calculation. Note the logarithmic scale. (Reprinted from Ref. 58, with permission.)

torical exposure to asbestos, although in low concentrations.[51,57] Similar to sputum, the presence of asbestos bodies in lavage fluid is best considered a marker of exposure to asbestos rather than disease. However, the actual properties of the lavage fluid allow for additional testing and formulation of opinions regarding their significance.

Roggli et al. provided qualitative and quantitative assessment of asbestos fibers, coated and uncoated, in BALF obtained from patients with asbestosis, those exposed to asbestos but without parenchymal lung disease, those with idiopathic pulmonary fibrosis, and non-exposed controls (Figures 9-10 and 9-11). They observed excessive

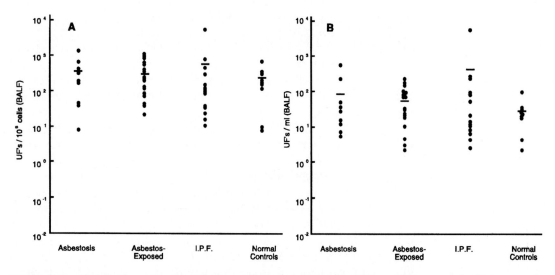

Figure 9-11. Distribution of uncoated fibers ≥5 μm in length per million cells recovered **(A)** or per ml BALF **(B)** for 50 cases as determined by scanning electron microscopy. Each dot represents one case, and a horizontal line indicates the median value for each group. Note the logarithmic scale. (Reprinted from Ref. 58, with permission.)

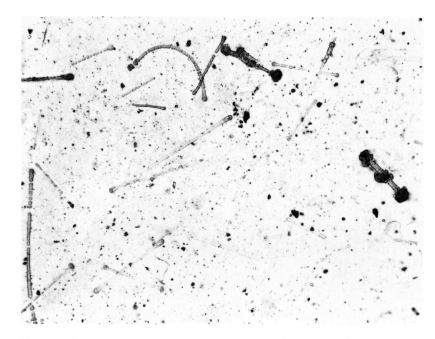

Figure 9-12. Asbestos bodies on Nuclepore filter isolated by digesting bronchoalveolar lavage fluid pellet in hypochlorite solution. Unstained, ×400. (Reprinted from Ref. 50, with permission.)

numbers of asbestos bodies only in highly exposed individuals (Figures 9-12 and 9-13), but noted that the uncoated fiber burden as determined by scanning electron microscopy (SEM) was similar in all groups. Commercial amphibole asbestos (amosite and crocidolite) fibers were detected more frequently in lavage fluid from patients with asbestosis than those from other groups. They concluded that the findings of >1 asbestos body per 10^6 cells, 1 asbestos body per ml of lavage fluid by light microscopy, or commercial amphibole fibers by SEM all were indicative of considerable exposure to asbestos in the majority of cases.[58] The concentration of one asbestos body per ml of lavage fluid has been corroborated by Karjalainen et al. as a threshold concentration, excesses of which are indicative of significant exposure in the majority of cases.[59]

A susbsequent study by Karjalainen[60] also compared concentrations of asbestos bodies in both lavage fluid and matched lung tissue specimens. Finnish usage of commercial asbestos, unlike most other industrialized nations, has historically included the employment of anthophyllite. This study found significant correlations between the concentrations of asbestos bodies in lavage fluid and in lung tissue, the concentrations of asbestos bodies and amphibole asbestos fibers in lung tissue, and the concentration of asbestos bodies in lavage fluid and amphibole asbestos fibers in lung tissue (Table 9-1). In those patients who had been exposed to predominantly commercial anthophyllite, significantly higher concentrations of asbestos bodies were observed relative to the total pulmonary amphibole burden. This observation is probably related to the greater likelihood of commercial anthophyllite fibers becoming coated. This study also supports prior observations that low or negative asbestos body counts in BALF do not exclude heavy exposure, and that bronchoalveolar lavage is an insensitive indicator of cumulative chrysotile exposure.[61–64]

Teschler et al. evaluated the lavage fluid profiles of 64 patients with diverse asbestos exposure histories and compared these to a control population of nonexposed patients. Ninety-nine percent of controls had less than 0.5 asbestos bodies per ml BALF. In this study, the demonstration of greater than one AB/ml BALF was associated with the high probability of tissue levels of more than 1000 asbestos bodies per cm^3 of lung tissue (Table 9-1).[65] In a subsequent study, Teschler et al. analyzed asbestos fiber counts in 23 individual sample pairs of BALF and lung tissue samples from patients with occupational asbestos exposure, using transmission electron microscopy.[66] Fiber type, size, and aspect ratio were compared. The study concluded that concentrations of both

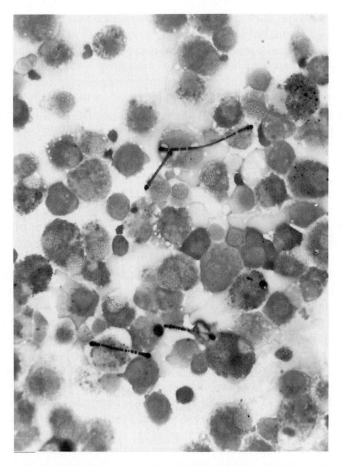

Figure 9-13. Cytocentrifuge preparation of bronchoalveolar lavage fluid in an individual with asbestosis. Typical asbestos bodies are present. Wright stain, ×400. (Reprinted from Ref. 50, with permission.)

coated and uncoated amphibole asbestos fibers in lavage fluid correlate with the degree of concentrations in lung tissue. The authors of this study had three cases where no asbestos bodies were detected in lavage fluid, yet were present in lung parenchyma, further supporting the notion that negative lavage results are not exclusionary of significant exposure. This study found no significant correlation between lavage fluid and lung tissue specimens for chrysotile, in keeping with the findings that bronchoalveolar lavage is not a reliable indicator of parenchymal chrysotile burden or exposure.[62,63]

Bronchoalveolar lavage has also been used to assess environmental asbestos exposure in areas of Turkey with a high incidence of disease attributable to asbestos in the soil. Compared to control populations in Belgium and Turkey without environmental exposure, BALF tremolite burdens were demonstrated in this study in the same range as commercial amphiboles in subjects occupationally exposed in Belgium.[67,68] In a study of American construction workers largely exposed to chrysotile, Schwartz et al. found that the concentration of asbestos bodies in BALF correlated poorly with measures both of exposure and clinical/radiographic hallmarks of asbestos-associated pulmonary disease, likely at least due in part to the diminished biopersistence of chrysotile in lung tissue.[63]

The reasonable conclusion from the balance of these numerous studies is that asbestos bodies, when present in BALF, are an accurate and reproducible predictor of asbestos exposure. However, their absence does not exclude significant exposure or necessarily exonerate asbestos in the causation of disease, particularly in those patients exposed to chrysotile asbestos.

Fine Needle Aspiration Biopsy

Aspiration biopsies of the lung are typically undertaken as part of the diagnostic workup of peripheral nodular lesions and, largely for this reason, are not likely to yield asbestos bodies as these are much less numerous in tumors than in adjacent sections of lung. Roggli et al. reported the first two instances of asbestos bodies identified in aspiration biopsies.[69] In one case aspiration biopsy of a peripheral infiltrate yielded asbestos bodies and fungal hyphae typical of aspergillus infections, highlighting the reported association between asbestosis and aspergillus infection (Figure 9-14). In the second case, aspiration biopsy of a peripheral adenocarcinoma also yielded asbestos bodies (Figures 9-15 and 9-16). Tissue asbestos analysis was performed in each case, confirming markedly elevated amphibole asbestos concentrations. Only one case had histologic evidence of asbestosis.

Leiman reviewed a series of 1256 thoracic aspiration biopsies, which yielded asbestos bodies in 52 cases. Significant occupational exposure was documented in all but eight patients. Malignant neoplasms were diagnosed in 30 of these cases, and required additional diagnostic studies for confirmation in 20% of the cases. The remaining 22 cases were benign lesions, typically abscesses or tuberculosis, and required additional confirmatory studies in 50% of cases. The author concluded

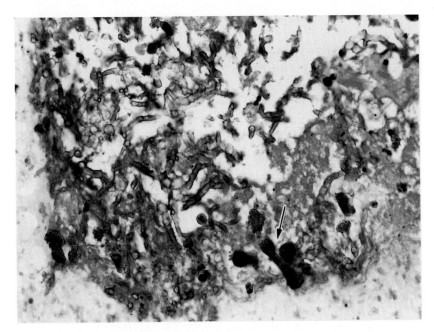

Figure 9-14. Hematoxylin and eosin-stained fine-needle aspirate cell block shows a clump of branching septate hyphae, compatible with Aspergillus sp., and a nearly dumbbell-shaped asbestos body (*arrow*), one of many identified in the aspirated material.

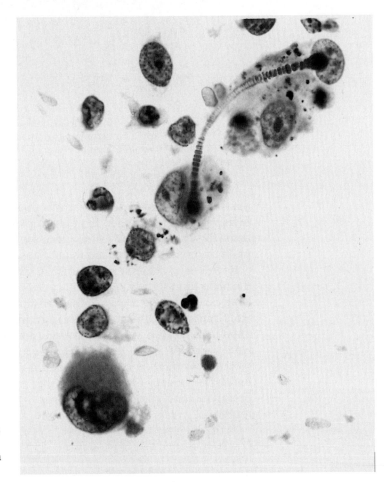

Figure 9-15. Papanicolaou-stained fine-needle aspirate smear demonstrates an asbestos body associated with several macrophages. Numerous asbestos bodies were identified in the specimen. A malignant cell is present at lower left. ×1000. (Reprinted from Ref. 69, with permission.)

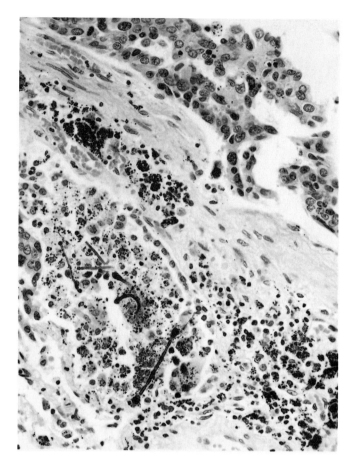

Figure 9-16. Sections of primary lung tumor at autopsy (same case as Figure 9-15) demonstrate sheets of malignant cells with ill-defined lumen formation and adjacent desmoplastic stroma. Several asbestos bodies are visible adjacent to the tumor at lower left. Hematoxylin and eosin, ×400. (Reprinted from Ref. 69, with permission.)

that the demonstration of asbestos bodies is highly associated with pulmonary pathology other than asbestosis, and the detection of such using aspiration biopsy technique is diminished, possibly the result of parenchymal fibrosis related to asbestos.[70]

Roggli et al. also reported a case of two asbestos bodies detected on the aspiration biopsy of a cavitary lesion. This patient was shown to have asbestos body counts within the normal range for our laboratory.[69] Such a chance occurrence is quite uncommon, and we have not encountered asbestos bodies in the several thousand aspiration biopsies that have followed. The demonstration of asbestos bodies in aspiration biopsy specimens is best considered a marker of significant exposure for that patient, and suggests that the radiographic lesion that prompted the aspiration biopsy has a high likelihood of being asbestos related.

Summary and Conclusions

The evaluation of patients with respiratory disease suspected or alleged to complicate exposure to asbestos requires the synthesis of clinical, radiographic, and laboratory data, as well as data gleaned from the inspection of pathologic specimens. The examination of cytologic materials including body cavity fluids, bronchial washings, and sputa (often obtained with a minimum of expense and attendant morbidity) may provide a wealth of information regarding the various disease states believed to be related to prior asbestos exposure. Moreover, these specimens may lend themselves to the application of special techniques discussed elsewhere in this book to identify and quantify asbestos fibers and thereby implicate them in the causation of disease.

References

1. Greenberg SD, Hurst GA, Matlage WT, Miller JM, Hurst IJ, Mabry LC: Tyler asbestos workers program. *Ann NY Acad Sci* 271:353–364, 1976.
2. Roggli VL, Greenberg SD, Seitzman LH, McGavran MH, Hurst GA, Spivey CG, Nelson KG, Hieger LR: Pulmonary fibrosis, carcinoma and asbestos body counts in amosite asbestos workers. *Am J Clin Pathol* 73:496–503, 1980.
3. Stewart MJ, Haddow AC: Demonstration of the peculiar bodies of pulmonary asbestosis in material obtained by lung puncture and in the sputum. *J Pathol Bacteriol* 32:172, 1929.
4. An SH, Koprowska I: Primary cytologic diagnosis of asbestosis associated with bronchogenic carcinoma: Case report and review of the literature. *Acta Cytol* 6:391–398, 1962.
5. Huuskonen MS, Taskinen E, Vaaranen V: Sputum cytology of asbestosis patients. *Scand J Work Environ Health* 4:284–294, 1978.
6. Gupta PK, Frost JK: Cytologic changes associated with asbestos exposure. *Sem Oncol* 8:283–289, 1981.
7. Kotin P, Paul W: Results of a lung cancer detection program in an asbestos industry. *Recent Results in Cancer Research* 82:131–137, 1982.
8. Dodson RF, Williams MG, McLarty JW, Hurst GA: Asbestos bodies and particulate matter in sputum from former asbestos workers: An ultrastructural study. *Acta Cytol* 27:635–40, 1983.
9. Kobusch AB, Simard A, Feldstein M, Vauclair R, Gibbs GW, Bergeron F, Morissette N, Davis R: Pulmonary cytology in chrysotile asbestos workers. *J Chron Dis* 37:599–607, 1984.
10. DeMay RM: Respiratory Cytology. Ch. 7 In: *The Art and Science of Cytopathology: Exfoliative Cytology*, Chicago: ASCP Press, 1996, pp. 207–256.
11. Bocking A, Biesterfeld S, Chatelain R: Diagnosis of bronchial carcinoma on sections of paraffin-embedded sputum: Sensitivity and specificity of an alternative to routine cytology. *Acta Cytol* 36:37–42, 1992.
12. Nakajima J, Manabe T, Yagi S: Appearance of mesothelioma cells in sputum: A case report. *Acta Cytol* 36:731–736, 1999.
13. Naryshkin S, Young NA: Respiratory cytology: A review of non-neoplastic mimics of malignancy. *Diag Cytopathol* 9:89–97, 1993.

14. Colby TV, Koss MN, Travis WT: Tumors of the Lower Respiratory Tract. *Atlas of Tumor Pathology*, Series 3, Fascicle 13, Washington, DC: Armed Forces Institute of Pathology, 1995, pp. 259–278.

15. Epler GR, McLoud TC, Gaensler EA: Prevalence and incidence of benign asbestos pleural effusion in a working population. *JAMA* 247:617–622, 1982.

16. Chahinian AP, Pajak TF, Holand JF: Diffuse malignant mesothelioma. Prospective evaluation of 69 patients. *Ann Intern Med* 96:746–775, 1982.

17. Whitaker D, Shilkin KB, Sterrett GF: Cytologic appearance of malignant mesothelioma, In: *Malignant Mesothelioma* (Henderson DW, Shilkin KB, Langlois SLP, eds.) New York: Hemisphere, 1991, pp. 167–182.

18. Leong ASY, Stevens MW, Mukherjee TM: Malignant mesothelioma: cytologic diagnosis with histologic, immunohistochemical and ultrastructural correlation. *Sem Diag Pathol* 9:141–150, 1992.

19. Stevens MW: Cytopathology of malignant mesothelioma: A stepwise logistic regression analysis. *Diag Cytopathol* 8:333–344, 1992.

20. Zakowski MF, Ianuale-Sherman A: Cytology of pericardial effusions in AIDS patients. *Diag Cytopathol* 9:266–269, 1993.

21. McCaughey WTE, Kannerstein M, Churg J: Tumors and pseudotumors of the serous membranes. In: *Atlas of Tumor Pathology*, Series 2, Fascicle 20, Washington, DC: Armed Forces Institute of Pathology, 1985, pp. 60–61.

22. Attanoos RL, Gibbs AR: Pathology of malignant mesothelioma. *Histopathol* 30:403–418, 1997.

23. Tickman RJ, Cohen CC, Varma VA, Fekete PS, Derose PB: Distinction between carcinoma cells and mesothelial cells in serous effusions—usefulness of immunohistochemistry. *Acta Cytol* 34:491–496, 1990.

24. Fetsch PA, Simsir A, Abati A: Comparison of antibodies to HBME-1 and calretinin for the detection of mesothelial cells in effusion cytology. *Diag Cytopathol* 25:158–161, 2001.

25. Lozano MD, Panizo A, Toledo GR, Sola JJ, Pardo-Mindan J: Immunocytochemistry in the differential diagnosis of serous effusions: a comparative evaluation of eight monoclonal antibodies in Papanicolaou stained smears. *Cancer* 93:68–72, 2001.

26. Barberis MC, Faleri M, Veronese S, Casadio C, Viale G: Calretinin. A selective marker of normal and neoplastic mesothelial cells in serous effusions. *Diag Cytopathol* 41:1757–1761, 1997.

27. Hecht JL, Pinkus JL, Weinstein LJ, Pinkus GS: The value of thyroid transcription factor 1 in cytologic preparations as a marker for metastatic adenocarcinoma of lung origin. *Am J Clin Pathol* 116:483–488, 2001.

28. Motherby H, Kube M, Friedrichs N, Jadjari B, et al.: Immunocytochemistry and DNA-image cytometry in diagnostic effusion cytology. Part 1. *Analyt Cell Pathol* 19:7–20, 1999.

29. Wieczorek TJ, Krane JF: Diagnostic utility of calretinin immunohistochemistry in cytologic cell block preparations. *Cancer* 90:312–319, 2000.

30. Kitazume H, Kitamura K, Mukai K, Inayama Y, Kawano N, Nakamura N, Sano J, Mitsui K, Yoshida S, Nakatani Y: Cytologic differential diagnosis among reactive mesothelial cells, malignant mesothelioma and adenocarcinoma: utility of combined E-cadherin and calretinin immunostaining. *Cancer* 90:55–60, 2000.

31. Davidson B, Nielsen S, Christensen J, Asschenfeldt P, Berner A, Risberg R, Johansen P: The role of desmin and N-cadherin in effusion cytology: A comparative study using established markers of mesothelial and epithelial cells. *Am J Surg Pathol* 25:1405–1412, 2001.

32. Simsir A, Fetsch P, Mehta D, Zakowski M, Abati A: E-cadherin, N-cadherin and calretinin in pleural effusions: the good, the bad, the worthless. *Diag Cytopathol* 20:125–130, 1999.

33. Lee A, Baloch ZW, Yu G, Gupta PK: Mesothelial hyperplasia with reactive atypia: diagnostic pitfalls and role of immunohistochemical studies—a case report. *Diag Cytopathol* 22:113–116, 2000.

34. Sakuma N, Toshiaki K, Ishihara T: Ultrastructure of pleural mesothelioma and pulmonary adenocarcinoma in malignant effusions as compared with reactive mesothelial cells. *Acta Cytol* 43:777–779, 1999.

35. DiBonito L, Falconieri G, Colautti I, Gori DB, Dudine S, Giarelli L: Cytopathology of malignant mesothelioma: a study of its patterns and histological bases. *Diag Cytopathol* 9:25–31, 1992.

36. Sherman ME, Mark EJ: Effusion cytology in the diagnosis of malignant epithelioid and biphasic pleural mesothelioma. *Arch Pathol Lab Med* 114:845–851, 1990.

37. Johnston WW: Cytologic correlations. Ch. 31 In: *Pulmonary Pathology* (Dail DH, Hammar SP, eds.) New York: Springer-Verlag, 1988, pp. 1029–1095.

38. Yu GH, Baloch ZW, Gupta PK: Cytopathology of metastatic mesothelioma in fine needle aspiration specimens. *Diag Cytopathol* 20:328–332, 1999.

39. Nguyen GK, Akin MR, Villanueva RR, Slatnik J: Cytopathlogy of malignant mesothelioma of the pleura in fine needle aspiration biopsy. *Diag Cytopathol* 21:253–259, 1999.

40. Yu GH, Soma L, Hahn S, Friedberg JS: Changing clinical course of patients with malignant mesothelioma: implications for FNA cytology and utility of immunocytochemical staining. *Diag Cytopathol* 24:322–327, 2001.

41. Obers VJ, Leiman G, Girdwood RW, Spiro FI: Primary malignant pleural tumors (mesotheliomas) presenting as localized masses: Fine needle aspiration cytologic findings, clinical and radiologic features and review of the literature. *Acta Cytol* 32:567–575, 1988.

42. Sterrett GF, Whitaker D, Shilkin KB, Walters MNI: Fine needle aspiration cytology of malignant mesothelioma. *Acta Cytol* 31:185–193, 1987.

43. Friedman MT, Gentile P, Tarectecan A, Fuchs A: Malignant mesothelioma: Immunohistochemistry and DNA ploidy analysis as methods to differentiate mesothelioma from benign reactive mesothelial cell proliferation and adenocarcinoma in pleural and peritoneal effusions. *Arch Pathol Lab Med* 120:959–966, 1996.

44. Granados R, Cibas ES, Fletcher JA: Cytogenetic analysis from effusions malignant mesothelioma—a diagnostic adjunct to cytology. *Acta Cytol* 38:711–717, 1994.

45. Renshaw AA, Dean BR, Antman KH, Sugarbaker DJ, Cibas ES: The role of cytologic evaluation of pleural fluid in the diagnosis of mesothelioma. *Chest* 111:106–109, 1997.

46. Greenberg SD: Asbestos lung disease. *Sem Resp Med* 4:130–136, 1982.

47. Mace ML, McLemore TL, Roggli VL, Brinkley BR, Greenberg SD: Scanning electron microscopic examination of human asbestos bodies. *Cancer Lett* 9:95–104, 1980.

48. McLemore TL, Mace ML, Roggli VL, Marshall MV, Lawrence EC, Wilson RK, Martin RR, Brinkley BR, Greenberg SD: Asbestos body phagocytosis by human free alveolar macrophages. *Cancer Lett* 9:85–93, 1980.

49. Dumortier P, Broucke I, De Vuyst P: Pseudoasbestos bodies and fibers in bronchoalveolar lavage of refractory ceramic fiber users. *Am J Respir Crit Care Med* 164:499–503, 2001.

50. Roggli VL, Piantadosi CA, Bell DY: Asbestos bodies in bronchoalveolar lavage fluid: A study of 20 asbestos-exposed individuals and comparison to patients with other chronic interstitial lung diseases. *Acta Cytol* 30: 470–476, 1986.

51. Modin BE, Greenberg SD, Buffler PA, Lockhart JA, Seitzman LH, Awe RJ: Asbestos bodies in a general hospital/clinic population. *Acta Cytol* 26: 667–670, 1982.

52. Farley ML, Greenberg SD, Shuford EH, Hurst GA, Spivey CG: Ferruginous bodies in sputa of former asbestos workers. *Acta Cytol* 21:693–700, 1977.

53. Bignon J, Sebastien P, Jaurand MC, Hem B: Microfiltration methods for quantitative study of fibrous particles in biologic specimens. *Environ Health Persp* 9:155–160, 1974.

54. Roggli VL, McLarty JW, Greenberg SD, Hurst GA, Hieger LR, Farley ML, Mabry LC: Comparison of sputum and lung asbestos body counts in former asbestos workers. *Am Rev Respir Dis* 122:941–945, 1980.

55. McLarty JW, Greenberg SD, Hurst GA, Spivey CG, Seitzman LH, Hieger LR, Farley ML, Mabry LC: The clinical significance of ferruginous bodies in sputa. *J Occup Med* 22:92–96, 1980.

56. Teschler H, Konietzko N, Schoenfeld B, Ramin C, Schraps T, Costabel U: Distribution of asbestos bodies in the human lung as determined by bronchoalveolar lavage. *Am Rev Respir Dis* 147:1211–1215, 1993.

57. De Vuyst P, Dumortier P, Moulin E, Yourassowsky N, Yernault JC: Diagnostic value of asbestos bodies in bronchoalveolar lavage fluid. *Am Rev Respir Dis* 136:1219–1224, 1987.

58. Roggli VL, Coin PG, McIntyre NR, Bell DY: Asbestos content of bronchoalveolar lavage fluid: a comparison of light and scanning electron microscopic analysis. *Acta Cytol* 38:502–510, 1994.

59. Karjalainen A, Anttila A, Mantyla T, Taskinen E, Kyyronen P, Tukianen P: Asbestos bodies in bronchoalveolar lavage fluid in relation to occupational history. *Am J Ind Med* 26:645–654, 1994.

60. Karjalainen A, Piipari R, Mantyla T, Monkkonen M, Numinen M, Tukianen P, Vanhala E, Anttila S: Asbestos bodies in bronchoalveolar lavage in relation to asbestos bodies and asbestos fibers in lung parenchyma. *Eur Respir J* 9:1000–1005, 1996.

61. De Vuyst P, Dumortier P, Moulin E: Asbestos bodies in bronchoalveolar lavage reflects lung asbestos body concentration. *Eur Resp J* 1:362–367, 1988.

62. Sebastien P, Armstrong B, Monchaux G, Bignon J: Asbestos bodies in bronchoalveolar lavage fluid and in lung parenchyma. *Am Rev Respir Dis* 137:75–78, 1988.

63. Schwartz DA, Galvin JR, Burmeister LF, Merchant RK, Dayton CS, Merchant JA, Hunninghake GW: The clinical utility and reliability of asbestos bodies in bronchoalveolar fluid. *Am Rev Respir Dis* 144:684–688, 1991.

64. Albin M, Johansson L, Pooley FD, Jakobsson K, Attewell R, Mitra R: Mineral fibres, fibrosis and asbestos bodies in lung tissue. *Br J Ind Med* 47:767–774, 1990.

65. Teschler H, Hoheisel G, Fischer M, Muller KM, Konietzko N, Costabel U: The content of asbestos bodies in the bronchoalveolar fluid as a parameter of an increased pulmonary asbestos load. *Deutsch Med Wochenschr* 118:1749–1754, 1993.

66. Teschler H, Friedrichs KH, Hoheisel GB, Wick G, Soltner U, Thompson AB, Konietzko N, Costabel U: Asbestos fibers in bronchoalveolar lavage and lung tissue of former asbestos workers. *Am J Respir Crit Care Med* 149:641–645, 1994.

67. Dumortier P, Coplu L, de Martier V, Emri S, Baris I, De Vuyst P: Assessment of environmental asbestos exposure in Turkey by bronchoalveolar lavage. *Am J Respir Crit Care Med* 158:1815–1824, 1998.
68. De Vuyst P, Dumortier P, Gevenois PA: Analysis of asbestos bodies in BAL from subjects with particulate exposures. *Am J Ind Med* 31:699–704, 1997.
69. Roggli VL, Johnston WW, Kaminsky DB: Asbestos bodies in fine needle aspirates of the lung. *Acta Cytol* 28:494–498, 1984.
70. Leiman G: Asbestos bodies in fine needle aspirates of lung masses. *Acta Cytol* 35:171–174, 1991.

10

Experimental Models of Asbestos-Related Diseases

Cheryl L. Fattman, Charleen T. Chu, and Tim D. Oury

Introduction

Much of our understanding of the mechanisms by which asbestos injures the lung has been derived from experimental animal studies. Such studies have confirmed the fibrogenic and carcinogenic properties of asbestos fibers that have been surmised from human observations and have provided insights into the ways in which asbestos fibers interact with biological systems. Information on asbestos-induced diseases has been obtained through experiments involving inhalation exposures, intratracheal instillations, and in vitro studies of various cellular systems. Each of these techniques has particular advantages and disadvantages. Inhalation studies, being more physiologic, more closely approximate the actual human situation. While more facilities are developing methods for performing these studies, they can be time-consuming and expensive. Conversely, experiments involving intratracheal instillation of asbestos fibers are simpler to perform and less expensive, but have the disadvantage that the normal defense mechanisms of the respiratory tract are bypassed and the distribution is not uniform. Hence, the results are not directly comparable to inhalation exposures. In vitro studies of cellular systems permit the investigation of the direct effects of asbestos and other particulates on cellular function under carefully controlled conditions. However, it is not always clear how the results apply to the more complex in vivo conditions or whether the particular mechanisms under investigation contribute significantly to the overall pathogenesis of asbestos-induced tissue damage. These limitations notwithstanding, each of these approaches has contributed substantially to our understanding of the mechanisms underlying asbestos-related disease.

This chapter reviews the current understanding of the pathogenesis of asbestos-related diseases as derived from experimental models. To understand asbestos-related tissue injury, it is first necessary to understand the patterns of deposition of asbestos fibers within the lung parenchyma and the subsequent clearance of fibers from the lung through the mucociliary escalator, the macrophage defense system, and the pulmonary lymphatics. Next, the factors influencing the production of pulmonary fibrosis and thoracic neoplasms in inhalation models will be reviewed. Finally, in vitro studies suggesting particular mechanisms by which asbestos produces its effects will be examined. Although asbestos-induced fibrogenesis and carcinogenesis share many common features and may involve similar molecular mechanisms of tissue injury, these two processes will be reviewed separately for the sake of clarity.

Historical Background

Experimental models of asbestos-induced tissue injury were established in the 1930s and '40s by the pioneering work of Gardner[1] and King et al.[2] In 1951, Vorwald et al.[3] published the results of the classic inhalation studies performed at Saranac Lake, New York. These investigators showed that inhalation (or intratracheal instillation) of chrysotile, crocidolite, and amosite asbestos produced interstitial fibrosis similar to that observed in human asbestosis. Long asbestos fibers were found to be more injurious than short fibers, and the duration of exposure required for disease to develop varied inversely with the concentration of long fibers in the atmosphere.[3] The development of a dependable and reproducible fiber aerosolization system by Timbrell[4] paved the way for the inhalation studies of Wagner et al.[5] reported in 1974. These studies performed with SPF Wistar rats showed that both amphibole and chrysotile forms of asbestos produced asbestosis in a dose-dependent fashion, and that the fibrosis continued to progress after removal from exposure. Furthermore, inhalation exposures to all forms of asbestos tested resulted in the production of thoracic neoplasms, including adenomas, carcinomas, and mesotheliomas.[5] There was a positive correlation between the severity of asbestosis and the development of pulmonary neoplasms. These early studies paved the way for subsequent investigations and provided the basis for more detailed analysis of pathogenic mechanisms at the cellular level.[6]

Deposition and Clearance of Asbestos Fibers

The mammalian respiratory system is equipped with a variety of defense mechanisms for protection against foreign matter, and these mechanisms in turn affect the size, shape, and number of particles that are deposited and that ultimately accumulate in the lower respiratory tract. These defense mechanisms include four major components: (a) the fine hairs, or vibrissae, in the nasal cavity that filter out most of the larger particles [>10 μm aerodynamic equivalent diameter (AED)] that are inhaled; (b) the mucociliary escalator of the tracheobronchial tree, which carries upward toward the mouth any particles that affect the surface of the airways; (c) the alveolar macrophages, which phagocytize particles that make their way past the first two levels of defenses and are deposited in the gas-exchange regions of the lung; (d) the pulmonary lymphatics, through which many particles deposited in the lung are transported to regional lymph nodes or the pleura.[7]

Particles that have the greatest probability of deposition and retention in the gas-exchange regions of the lung are in the size range of 1 to 5 μm AED. Particles less than 0.5 μm in maximum dimension are deposited by Brownian motion or diffusion. Deposition patterns may be influenced by such factors as tidal volume, respiratory rate, and pattern of breathing (nose vs. mouth). Similarly, subsequent clearance of particles deposited in the lung is dependent upon a number of factors, including the anatomic site of deposition, particle solubility, and the efficiency of the host's phagocytic system. In addition, cigarette smoking has been shown to interfere with particle clearance from the lower respiratory tract.[8]

A unique feature of fibrous dusts is that fibers of considerable length can be deposited in the lower respiratory tract, even though most particles 5 μm or greater in size are excluded. This is because of the tendency for fibrous dusts to line up along the direction of laminar airflow, so that the diameter of a fiber rather than its length is the primary determinant of respirability.[9,10] As a result, most fibers deposited in the lungs of humans or experimental animals are 1 μm or less in diameter, but may exceed 200 μm in length. In this respect, some important differences exist between the amphibole fibers and the serpentine chrysotile. Very long fibers of chrysotile tend to be curly and are thus more likely to lodge in the upper respiratory tract, where they are subsequently removed on the mucociliary escalator.[9,10] Even very long amphibole fibers tend to be straight, and thus they have a greater likelihood of penetrating into the gas-exchange regions of the lung. Differences between the accumulation of amphibole versus chrysotile fibers within the lungs of experimental animals following long-term inhalational exposure were noted by Wagner et al.[5] These observations have stimulated the investigation of the pulmonary deposition and clearance of asbestos fibers, with particular attention to differences between chrysotile and the amphiboles.

Fiber Deposition

The development of methods for producing radio-labeled asbestos fibers[11] has greatly facilitated the determination of total lung fiber burden after administration,[12] as well as the patterns of fiber deposition in the respiratory tract. Early studies using these techniques demonstrated a tendency for fiber deposition and concentration at bifurcation points in the conducting airways, with a relatively uniform distribution throughout the alveolar regions.[13,14] Studies using scanning electron microscopy have shown that this tendency for deposition at bifurcation points extends to the alveolar regions of the lungs.[15–18] In rats exposed to aerosolized chrysotile asbestos for a brief period of time, fibers in the distal anatomic regions of the lung were localized primarily at alveolar duct bifurcations (Figure 10-1). The greatest concentration of fibers occurs at bifurcations closest to the terminal bronchiole, and are less numerous at the more distant (e.g., second- and

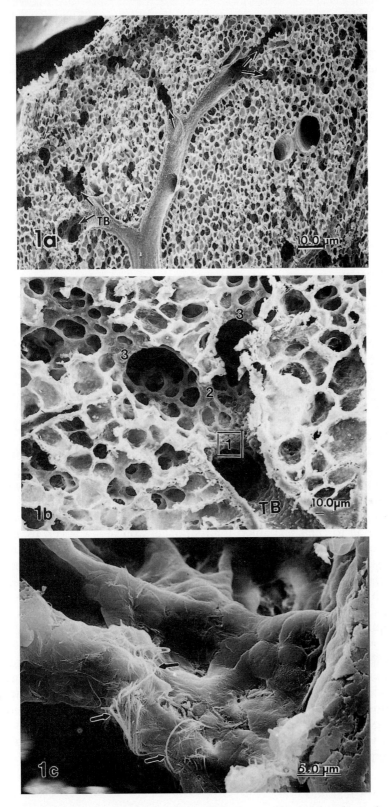

Figure 10-1. (A) Low-power scanning electron micrograph of rat lung parenchyma showing terminal bronchioles (TB) and alveolar ducts (*arrows*). **(B)** Higher magnification of a terminal bronchiole and its alveolar ducts exhibiting three bifurcations. **(C)** Detailed view of the first alveolar duct bifurcation, outlined in part **(B)**, showing large numbers of chrysotile asbestos fibers (*arrows*) littering the bifurcation surface. Few fibers are observed on the alveolar surfaces. (Reprinted from Ref. 18, with permission.)

third-order) alveolar duct bifurcations.[6,16,17] Very few fibers are observed on the surfaces of adjacent alveoli. A similar pattern is observed for chrysotile and amphibole asbestos fibers.[18]

These observations indicate that the geometry of the tracheo-bronchial tree is an important determining factor in the deposition of particulates in the lower respiratory tract.[19] Studies in which meticulous dissections of the tracheobronchial tree in asbestos-exposed rats were performed demonstrate that the quantity of asbestos deposited in the lung parenchyma is inversely related to airway path length and the number of airway bifurcations.[20] Variations in airway geometry among different species could result in different patterns of deposition, which in turn could account for some of the variation in species response to asbestos inhalation.[21] In this regard, it should be noted that marked differences in deposition pattern are obtained for dust administered by inhalation versus intratracheal instillation.[22] The distribution of dust resulting from instillation is much less homogeneous than that from inhalation, and penetration to the lung periphery is minimal. The resultant inflammatory responses are also quite different,[23] so that one must use caution in extrapolating results based on intratracheal instillation in experimental animals to human inhalation exposures.[6]

Opinions differ regarding the fractional deposition of chrysotile versus amphibole asbestos fibers in the lower respiratory tract. Morgan et al.,[14] in a study in which rats were exposed to three concentrations (4, 11, and 32 μg/l) of two different samples of radiolabeled chrysotile asbestos for 30 minutes in nose-only chambers, found that 12% and 15% of the respirable mass was deposited in the lower respiratory tract. Roggli and Brody,[24] in a study in which rats were exposed to 15 μg/l of Jeffery mine chrysotile asbestos (a standardized preparation) for one hour in nose-only chambers, found that 23% of the respirable mass was deposited in the lower respiratory tract. In studies in which rats were exposed to U.I.C.C. (Union Internationale Contre le Cancer) asbestos samples by inhalation for six weeks, Middleton et al.[25] found that the relative retention of chrysotile in the lungs decreases with increasing aerosolized concentrations. For the highest concentration employed in their study (7.8 μg/l), the fractional deposition of chrysotile in the lungs was 17%. Short-term inhalation studies result in a similar fractional deposition for crocidolite as compared to chrysotile asbestos: 16% of the respirable mass in the study by Morgan et al.[14] and 19% in the study by Roggli et al.[26] In contrast, Middleton et al.[25] determined that, for rats exposed to amphibole fibers for six weeks, the fractional deposition for amosite was 65% and for crocidolite approached 100%. These comparisons are summarized in Table 10-1. Although the reason for these discrepancies is unclear, it is apparent that, with durations of exposure of six weeks or longer, the relative retention of amphibole fibers in the lungs is considerably greater than that of chrysotile.[5,25]

Fiber Clearance

The fate of a fiber that has been deposited in the respiratory tract is dependent to some degree on the site of deposition. Fibers deposited

Table 10-1. Fractional deposition of chrysotile versus amphibole asbestos fibers in lungs of rats following inhalational exposure*

Authors	Exposure dose	Exposure duration	Fractional deposition	
			Chrysotile	Amphibole
Morgan et al.[14]	4, 11, & 32 µg/1	30 min	12–15%	16%
Roggli and Brody[24]	15 µg/l	1 h	23%	—
Roggli et al.[26]	3.5 µg/l	1 h	—	19%
Middleton et al.[25]	1, 5, & 10 µg/l	6 wks	17–36%	65–100%

*The studies by Morgan el al.,[14] Roggli and Brody,[24] and Roggli et al.[26] employed nose-only exposure chambers, whereas the studies by Middleton et al.[25] used open-chamber (i.e., whole animal) exposures.

on the surface of the large or small airways may become trapped in the mucous layer, where they will be transported upward by ciliary motion at a rate as high as several millimeters per minute.[9] Fibers deposited on the alveolar epithelium may be transported across the epithelium into the underlying interstitium via a mechanism that probably involves an actin-containing microfilament system.[6,27,28] Thus, within hours of a brief inhalational exposure, asbestos fibers are observed within the cytoplasm of Type I epithelial cells (Figure 10-2). Within 24 hours, fibers have been translocated into the interstitial compartment, including basement membrane, connective tissue, and cytoplasm of interstitial cells.[6] In addition, there is evidence that transepithelial transport occurs to some extent in the airways as well.[29,30] Once within the interstitium, fibers may then penetrate the cytoplasm of endothelial cells[16,17] and gain access to the vascular and lymphatic systems.[9]

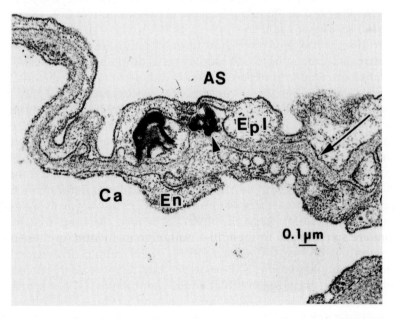

Figure 10-2. Transmission electron micrograph showing fibrils of chrysotile asbestos (*arrowhead*) adjacent to the alveolar capillary basement membrane (*arrow*). Five hours postexposure: capillary endothelium, En; Type I epithelium, EpI; alveolar spaces, AS. (Reprinted from Ref. 17, with permission.)

Fibers within lymphatic channels may then be carried to the visceral pleura[31] and hence gain access to the pleural space,[32] or be transported to hilar or mediastinal lymph nodes.[33,34] Also, within 24 hours of a brief inhalational exposure to asbestos, there is an influx of alveolar macrophages that proceed to phagocytize any free asbestos fibers on the alveolar surfaces. These macrophages accumulate at the site of initial fiber deposition, and are found on more than 90% of alveolar duct bifurcations by 48 hours postexposure.[35] Fibers that have been transported to the pulmonary interstitium may similarly be phagocytized by interstitial macrophages. Once ingested within the macrophage, fibers may remain for prolonged periods within alveoli or the interstitium. Alternatively, phagocytized fibers may be removed from the lung when macrophages enter onto the mucociliary escalator of the small airways or into the pulmonary lymphatics.[9]

A number of studies have demonstrated that the average length of fibers retained within the lung increases with time postexposure, and that this effect is observed for both chrysotile and amphibole asbestos.[24,26,36–40] The presumed mechanism of this effect is the more efficient clearance of short fibers, with preferential retention of longer fibers.[15,41] This phenomenon can be particularly well demonstrated by measuring the half-times for clearance of fibers in various size categories after a single exposure (Figure 10-3). In these studies, it can be seen that the residence time within the lung for fibers 10 μm or more in length is particularly prolonged.[37] More direct evidence for the more efficient clearance of shorter fibers comes from the studies of Kauffer et al.,[39] which showed a progressive decrease in mean length of fibers recovered by bronchoalveolar lavage following a brief inhalational exposure, with a concomitant increase in mean length of fibers remaining in the lungs.

With regard to fiber type, short-term inhalation studies have shown similar clearance rates for chrysotile versus amphibole asbestos fibers. Following a one-hour exposure period, the percentage of the original deposited mass remaining one month postexposure was 25% for crocidolite[26] and 19% for chrysotile asbestos.[24] Middleton et al.[25] also reported that the rate of clearance is similar for chrysotile and amphibole types of asbestos, and that the clearance could be expressed in terms of a three-compartment model with half-lives of 0.38, 8, and 118 days for each respective compartment. These observations are difficult to reconcile with the results of long-term inhalational studies, in which amphibole asbestos fibers accumulate within the lungs to a much greater extent than chrysotile fibers.[5,42] In fact, the lung content of chrysotile appears to level off and remain constant after two or three months of exposure, whereas amphibole fibers continue to accumulate progressively with continued exposure.[5] Middleton et al.[25,43] also noted substantially greater accumulation of amphiboles as compared to chrysotile following a six-week exposure, and attributed the difference to a greater fractional deposition of amphibole fibers (see Table 10-1). Substantial differences in the pulmonary content of crocidolite versus chrysotile asbestos in rats exposed to similar doses of the two fiber types for a three-month period have also been observed (Table 10-2).

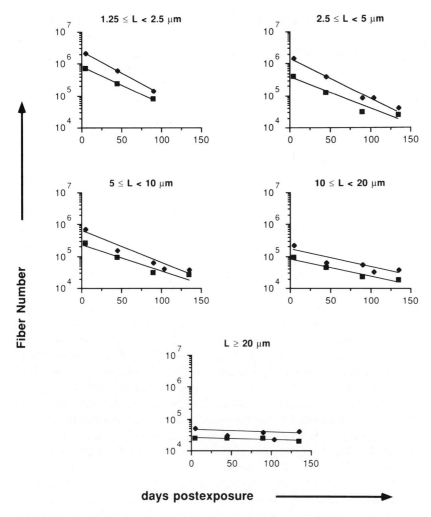

days postexposure ⟶

Figure 10-3. Washout curves (phase-contrast light microscopy). The points plotted are geometric means of fiber number in each length class. The lines shown are linear regressions of log (fiber number) for each animal vs. time (i.e., a one-compartment model). The slopes of all regression lines for fiber length <20 μm are significantly different from zero ($p < 0.00001$ in each case). Correlation coefficients range from 0.87–0.96. For length ≥20 μm, the slopes are not significantly different from zero ($p = 0.38$ for washout I, and $p = 0.25$ for washout II). (Reprinted from Ref. 37, with permission.)

Table 10-2. Accumulation of chrysotile versus crocidolite asbestos in rat lungs following inhalational exposure[a]

Fiber type	Fibers/gm[b]	Asbestos/rat (μg)[c]
Crocidolite	1.85×10^8 ($\pm 1.12 \times 10^8$)	814 ($\pm$435)
Chrysotile	2.50×10^7 ($\pm 8.4 \times 10^6$)	71.6 ($\pm$28.9)
Sham[d]	3.5×10^4 ($\pm 4.9 \times 10^4$)	0.045 ($\pm$0.025)

[a] Rats sacrificed following 3 months' exposure in inhalation chambers to 10.7 mg/m³ chrysotile or 11.2 mg/m³ crocidolite asbestos
[b] Fibers per gram of wet lung ±1 SE (4 animals in each group)
[c] Calculated mass of asbestos in both lungs ±1 SE
[d] Animals exposed to room air only

Observations using intratracheal instillation of asbestos have demonstrated more rapid clearance of chrysotile fibers as compared to amphibole beginning almost immediately after exposure.[44,45]

Although the reasons for the preferential retention of amphibole fibers are not entirely clear, one very important factor is undoubtedly the tendency for chrysotile to divide longitudinally into individual fibrils.[41] Roggli and Brody[24] reported a progressive decrease in mean fiber diameter following a one-hour inhalational exposure to chrysotile asbestos, and this observation has been confirmed by a number of investigators.[36,39,44,46] In comparison, no significant alteration in mean fiber diameter is observed for amphibole fibers.[26,36,44,46] The longitudinal splitting of chrysotile fiber bundles creates fibrils with a very fine diameter. Short fibrils created by this splitting process are readily cleared from the lung, whereas long, thin chrysotile fibrils are retained.[15,24,46] Kimizuka et al.[46] reported a further fragmentation of long, thin chrysotile fibers two years postexposure in hamsters, with a concomitant increase in the percentage of fibers less than $5\,\mu$m in length from 13% one year postexposure to 56% at two years. The decrease in mean fiber diameter of chrysotile has been associated with leaching of magnesium by some investigators[36,46] but not others.[44] No significant change in elemental composition is observed for amphibole fibers with increasing time postexposure.[36,46] Progressive leaching of magnesium from chrysotile fibers occurring in an acid environment could result in fiber dissolution, and some investigators believe that this may be an important mechanism of chrysotile clearance from the lung, especially for very small fibrils.[47–49] In this regard, in vitro studies with alveolar macrophages have shown a rate of magnesium leaching from chrysotile asbestos that is comparable to the leaching rate in an acid solution with a pH of 4.[50] Although the in vivo significance of magnesium leaching from chrysotile asbestos fibers is controversial, it is of potential importance, because the cytotoxicity and carcinogenicity of chrysotile asbestos is significantly reduced by in vitro depletion of magnesium.[51]

Additional factors may significantly influence the clearance of asbestos fibers from the lower respiratory tract. Bolton et al.[52] have shown that, once a critical pulmonary burden of asbestos has been reached, there is an overload of the clearance mechanism. This phenomenon occurs at relatively high lung burdens, and may be related to inhibition of clearance by alveolar macrophages. Other studies have shown that administration of a toxic dust such as asbestos or quartz can interfere with the subsequent clearance of a nontoxic dust such as titanium dioxide.[53,54] However, when looking at clearance of asbestos fibers (particularly chrysotile), titanium dioxide appeared to increase fiber retention while quartz reduced it.[55] In addition, there is evidence that cigarette smoke interferes with the clearance of asbestos fibers from the lower respiratory tract, largely by increasing the retention of short fibers.[56–58] Exposure to low levels of ozone also enhances pulmonary retention of inhaled asbestos fibers, apparently by interfering with fiber clearance.[59] Fiber clearance may play an important role in the development and severity of asbestosis following inhalation of asbestos fibers. Experimental studies have shown that high alveolar dust retention precedes the development of asbestosis and that individual variability in alveolar dust clearance capacity may be a major determinant in the development of asbestos-induced pulmonary fibrosis.[60]

Fibrogenesis

In Vivo Inhalation Studies

Inhalation studies in experimental animals have shown that asbestos produces interstitial pulmonary fibrosis. Three specific lesions have been identified:[3,5,42] (a) peribronchiolar accumulation of dust containing macrophages, giant cells, and fibrous tissue in association with respiratory bronchioles and alveolar ducts; (b) extension of bronchiolar epithelium into adjacent alveolar ducts and alveoli producing a pattern referred to as bronchiolar metaplasia (or the older term, pulmonary adenomatosis); and (c) diffuse stromal thickening of the alveolar septa associated with proliferation of Type II pneumocytes. Initially, the sites of dust deposition are rich in reticulin fibers, which become coarser over time and eventually stain strongly for collagen. The earliest lesion is in the vicinity of respiratory bronchioles, and with continuing exposure, appears to extend to involve alveolar ducts and adjacent alveoli.[3,5] All types of asbestos, including chrysotile,[3,5,42] amosite,[5,42] crocidolite,[5,42] anthophyllite,[5,42] and tremolite,[61] produce asbestosis in experimental animal models, and there appears to be a dose-response relationship for each of the fiber types tested.[5,42] Although there is a variation in species response to either intratracheal instillation or inhalation of asbestos,[3,6,21] asbestosis has been produced in a wide range of experimental animals, including baboons,[62] sheep,[63–66] mice,[67–69] guinea pigs,[3,57,70,71] hamsters,[46] and the white rat.[3,5,42]

The classic observations regarding experimental asbestos-induced lung injury[3,5,42] have been extended to the cellular level by means of ultrastructural morphometry of animals exposed to asbestos fibers by chronic inhalation.[6] Examination of the lungs of animals exposed to chrysotile asbestos for one week, three months, or one year has demonstrated that the most significant changes occur in the epithelial and interstitial compartments.[72–74] Within the epithelial compartment, an increase in cell number and average cell volume can be largely attributed to alveolar Type II pneumocyte hyperplasia. Similarly, the interstitial compartment shows an increase in cell number and average cell volume, most of which can be attributed to accumulation of interstitial macrophages.[74] Increases in smooth muscle cell numbers surrounding the arterioles and venules near alveolar duct bifurcations has also been noted.[75] In addition to morphometric analysis, several studies have looked at proliferation of specific subsets of cell populations by BrdU and ^{3}H-thymidine incorporation. Animals exposed to chrysotile and crocidolite asbestos had significantly increased incorporation of BrdU in the nuclei of epithelial and interstitial cells located in the bronchiolar/alveolar regions of the lung[76–78] and visceral pleural mesothelial cells.[76] Also, in models of both acute and chronic lung injury by asbestos, ^{3}H-thymidine incorporation by mesothelial cells, subpleural fibroblasts, and interstitial macrophages was demonstrated.[79,80]

Asbestos fibers may be identified, via transmission electron microscopy, within pulmonary epithelial cells and interstitial macrophages. A decrease in the ratio of magnesium to silicon in some of these fibers, as determined by energy-dispersive x-ray analysis, is indicative of some leaching of magnesium.[73] Microcalcifications also are identified within some interstitial cells. The endothelial and capillary compartments of the lung are for the most part unaffected. Fibers are gradually cleared from epithelial cells and macrophages following cessation of exposure, and these compartments then resolve toward unexposed-control levels. However, significant clearance of fibers from the pulmonary interstitium does not occur even one year following cessation of exposure (Figure 10-4). This persistence of fibers in the interstitial compartment is associated with continuing fibrogenesis.[72] Long-term studies following intratracheal instillation of chrysotile asbestos in rats have shown, by means of biochemical analysis, significantly increased collagen and elastin content per unit lung weight.[81]

Electron microscopic studies following brief (one-hour) inhalation exposures allow more detailed evaluation of the earliest events in asbestos-induced tissue injury.[6] Within 24 hours of a brief exposure to aerosolized asbestos fibers, the lung responds with an influx of alveolar macrophages at the site of initial fiber deposition.[35] This accumulation of macrophages persists for at least 30 days, and is associated with a significantly increased bifurcation tissue volume as assessed by morphometric studies (Figure 10-5).[82] In the interstitium adjacent to these alveolar duct bifurcations, asbestos fibers can readily be identified one month postexposure, both intracellularly and extracellularly, and are often associated with microcalcifications.[83] These microcalcifications consist of calcium and phosphate (Figure 10-6), and may be the consequence of fiber-induced membrane injury of interstitial cells.[83]

Transmission electron microscopy correlated with autoradiography shows that epithelial proliferation is associated with bronchiolar Clara cells and alveolar Type II cells, whereas interstitial proliferation is related to division of interstitial macrophages and fibroblasts.[84,85] Furthermore, blood vessels adjacent to alveolar duct bifurcations show increased labeling of both endothelial and smooth muscle cell nuclei by H[3]-TdR 19 to 72 hours following a brief inhalation exposure to chrysotile asbestos.[75] This mitogenic response may be the result of the release of diffusible growth factors derived from asbestos-stimulated alveolar macrophages. Ultrastructural examination of alveolar duct bifurcations of rats exposed to asbestos for one day has shown persistence of fibers at these sites as long as one year postexposure.[20]

Role of Fiber Dimensions

The importance of fiber length in asbestos-induced fibrogenesis has been addressed in a number of studies. The classic studies reported by Vorwald et al.[3] suggested that fibers greater than 20μm in length are

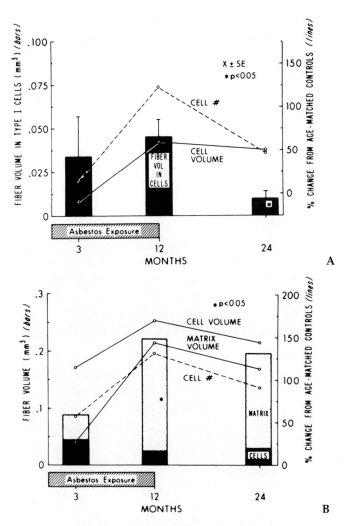

Figure 10-4. (A) Morphometrically determined total asbestos fiber volume within Type I alveolar epithelial cells for both lungs (*bars*), and the corresponding increase in cell number and cell volume (*lines*), in rats after prolonged inhalation of chrysotile asbestos. Changes in total cell number and tissue volume are expressed as percentage change from age-matched controls. **(B)** Total asbestos fiber volume present in interstitial cells (*solid portion of bars*) and extracellular matrix (*open portion of bars*), and corresponding increase in cell number, cell volume, and matrix volume (*lines*), in rats after chronic inhalation of chrysotile. (Reprinted from Ref. 72, with permission.)

the most fibrogenic, an opinion supported by the studies of Davis et al.[42] Other investigators have also concluded that long-fiber asbestos results in considerably more lung injury than short-fiber asbestos,[67,68,71,73,86–88] and that there is progression of injury after cessation of exposure only with the long-fiber inhalation.[73] It is difficult to determine a fiber length below which no significant fibrosis will occur regardless of intensity or duration of exposure, in part because of the problem of contamination of "short fiber" samples with a small

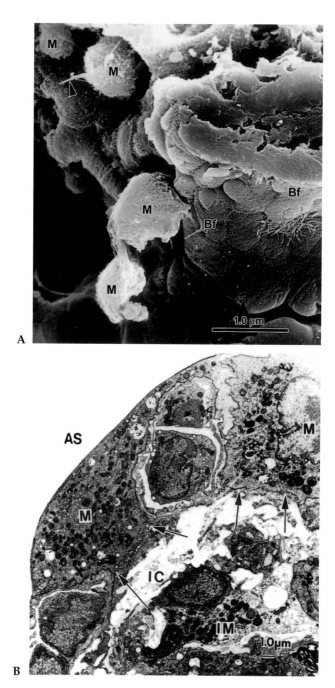

Figure 10-5. (A) Scanning electron micrograph of an alveolar duct bifurcation (Bf) 48 hours after a 1-hour exposure to chrysotile asbestos. Alveolar macrophages (M) are accumulating at sites of fiber deposition and phagocytizing some fibers (*arrowheads*). **(B)** Transmission electron micrograph of asbestos containing macrophages (M) at an alveolar duct bifurcation. The macrophages are tightly adherent to the underlying Type I epithelial cells (*arrows*). Alveolar spaces, AS; interstitial connective tissue, IC; interstitial macrophages, IM. (Reprinted from Ref. 35, with permission.)

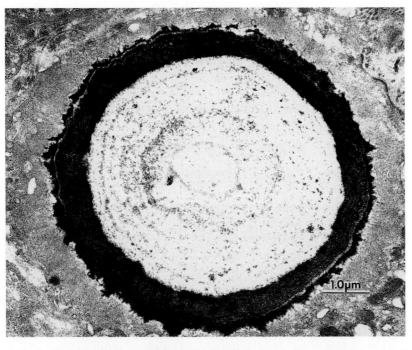

A

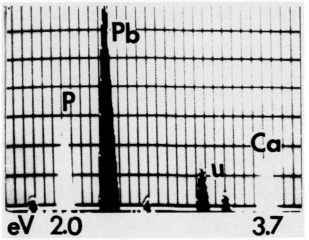

B

Figure 10-6. **(A)** Transmission electron micrograph of an intracellular micro-calcification within the pulmonary interstitium showing a laminated central portion and a dark outer rim. **(B)** Energy dispersive spectrum from the micro-calcification showing peaks for calcium (Ca) and phosphorus (P). Peaks for uranium (U) and lead (Pb) are due to staining with lead citrate and uranyl acetate. (Reprinted from Ref. 83, with permission.)

percentage of "long fibers."[87] However, LeMaire et al.[89] studied rats injected intratracheally with 5 mg of a preparation of very short chrysotile fibers (100% < 8 μm) and found an alveolitis 60 days postexposure but no apparent fibrosis.

Platek et al.[90] exposed rats by inhalation of short chrysotile asbestos with a mean concentration of fibers in the chamber of 1.0 mg/m^3 and only 0.79 fibers/ml with length exceeding five microns. These investigators showed that a concentration of 23×10^6 chrysotile fibers >5 μm in length per gram of dry lung or 272×10^6 chrysotile fibers <5 μm in length per gram of dry lung or a combination of the two is insufficient to produce pulmonary fibrosis in the rat 18 to 24 months after initiation of exposure.[90] Adamson and Bowden found no appreciable fibrosis in the lungs of mice following intratracheal instillation of 0.1 mg of short crocidolite asbestos fibers (mean length 0.6 μm, with 98.8% of fibers less than 2.5 μm in length),[67] whereas peribronchiolar fibrosis and significantly increased collagen levels were observed following instillation of 0.1 mg of long crocidolite asbestos fibers (mean length 24.4 μm, with 88% of fibers greater than 2.5 μm in length).[68] Contrary to the findings of most other investigators, Fasske[91] reported the production of interstitial fibrosis following intratracheal instillation of ultrashort-fiber chrysotile asbestos (fiber length between 0.05 and 0.2 μm). However, the one published light micrograph shows dense fibrosis at too high a magnification to determine whether the pattern is typical for that observed with asbestosis.[6]

In contrast to fiber length, relatively few studies have examined the role of fiber diameter in the pathogenesis of asbestos-induced tissue injury. The major importance of fiber diameter appears to be its role as a limiting factor for fiber deposition. For fibers with an aspect ratio between 10 and 100, the aerodynamic equivalent diameter is approximately three to four times the actual fiber diameter.[9] Hence, for fibers with an aspect ratio of 10 or more, 2 μm is about the maximum diameter of a fiber that may be deposited in the lower respiratory tract of the rat.[9] Other physical parameters of fibers are also potentially important. Some studies have indicated that fiber surface area is the most important determinant of the severity of pulmonary fibrosis.[92] In this regard, the progressive decrease in mean fiber diameter of chrysotile may be an important feature in its pathogenicity. This decrease in fiber diameter is believed to be due to longitudinal splitting of chrysotile fibers in vivo, which would result in both increased fiber number and increased surface area.[93] Each of these factors has been shown to correlate positively with the severity of fibrosis. Finally, another physical feature of importance is fiber charge, with highly charged fibers being more likely to be deposited in lung tissue.[94] This effect is probably greatest for long fibers, and electrostatically charged chrysotile asbestos produces more fibrosis than a similar level of asbestos that has been charge neutralized.[94]

Mechanisms of Asbestos-Induced Fibrogenesis

There is abundant evidence both in vitro and in vivo that asbestos is directly cytotoxic to a variety of cells and tissues.[95,96] The mechanisms of asbestos-induced cytotoxicity were first explored in red blood cells[97–99] and later in cell and tissue cultures.[29,30,100,101] Photoelectron spectrometry analysis demonstrated that phospholipid membranes are adsorbed as a bilayer onto the surface of chrysotile asbestos fibers.[99] Scanning electron microscopic examination of red blood cells treated with chrysotile asbestos showed distortion of the cells, and this effect was almost totally ablated by pretreatment of the cells with neuraminidase.[97] Similar observations have been reported for the binding of chrysotile fibers to alveolar macrophages in vitro.[102] These studies suggest that chrysotile binds to sialic acid residues of membrane surfaces. In contrast, neuraminidase treatment had no demonstrable effect on crocidolite binding. Other investigators using cell cultures of rat tracheal epithelium concluded that membrane damage was only a minor component of fiber-induced toxicity, and that a sequence of fiber binding, phagocytosis, nuclear damage, disruption of mitosis, and inhibition of proliferation or cell death is an important alternative pathway of fiber toxicity.[103]

One mechanism by which asbestos can injure cells is through generation of reactive oxygen species,[104] which can produce alterations in membrane fluidity, lipid peroxidation,[104,105] breakage of DNA, and induction of programmed cell death.[106] Asbestos fibers have been shown to catalyze the production of hydroxyl radicals and superoxide anions from hydrogen peroxide in cell-free systems as well as in animal models,[107] which may occur by a modified Haber-Weiss (Fenton-like) reaction.[108-110] These iron-catalyzed reactions may play key roles in the pathogenesis of asbestos-induced tissue damage. For example, in rat tracheal explants treated with asbestos fibers that were increasingly loaded with Fe^{++}/Fe^{+++}, increases in procollagen gene expression were evident after 7 days of treatment. Increased iron loading also resulted in increased expression of mitogenic and fibrogenic cytokines such as PDGF-α and TGF-β but did not affect the expression of other cytokines such as PDGF-β, TNF-α or TGF-α.[111] Phytic acid, an iron chelator, reduces asbestos-induced hydroxyl radical generation, DNA strand breaks, and injury to pulmonary epithelial cells.[112] When asbestos fibers were pretreated with phytic acid, fewer alveolar macrophages (AM) and polymorphonuclear leukocytes (PMN) accumulated in the BAL fluid of treated rats.[112] In addition, pretreatment of asbestos fibers with another iron chelator, deferoxamine, prevented AM-induced superoxide release[113] and asbestos-induced cell death of alveolar type I and II cells.[106] Notably, some flavinoid compounds such as quercetin and dihydroquercetin can also protect rat peritoneal macrophages against oxidative cellular injury both through their ability to scavenge superoxide and their ability to chelate iron.[114]

As discussed above, ROS may play an integral part in the pathogenesis of asbestos-mediated disease. Studies exploring the effectiveness of both enzymatic and nonenzymatic antioxidant scavengers on the cytotoxic effects of asbestos can shed significant light on the mechanisms involved in the development of asbestosis.[115] Under pathologic conditions, significant depletion of glutathione (GSH) and alterations in other GSH redox system enzymes were observed in both the alveolar macrophages and lung tissue of chrysotile-exposed animals.[116] In addition, both short- and long-term exposure of Wistar rats to asbestos fibers resulted in decreased levels of antioxidants (ascorbic acid, retinol, α-tocopherol, glutathione peroxidase) and increases in markers of lung injury (lipid peroxidation, total protein, alkaline phosphatase).[117]

However, studies examining rats exposed to crocidolite asbestos demonstrated increased mRNA expression of several antioxidant enzymes including Mn- and Cu/Zn-superoxide dismutases, glutathione peroxidase, and catalase.[119,120,121] Protein levels and enzymatic activity of these antioxidants after similar exposures were also found to increase,[119,121,122] suggesting a compensatory mechanism for tissues under oxidative stress.

The potential importance of ROS is well illustrated by the prevention of asbestos-induced cell death in rat lung fibroblasts and alveolar macrophages by catalase, Mn- and Cu/Zn-superoxide dismutase, glutathione peroxidase and dimethylthiourea—all scavengers of reactive oxygen species.[113,115,118] In an in vivo model of crocidolite-induced pulmonary interstitial fibrosis, continuous administration of polyethylene glycol-conjugated catalase significantly reduced the inflammatory response and severity of fibrosis secondary to inhalation of aerosolized asbestos fibers.[95]

Recently a second pathway for ROS generation independent of the metal-catalyzed pathways has been described.[123] In response to inflammatory stimuli such as asbestos, lung endothelial, alveolar and airway epithelial cells, as well as macrophages produce both nitric oxide (NO)[124] and superoxide anion (O^{-2}).[113] These two radicals can react with one another at diffusion-limited rates to produce the highly toxic peroxynitrite anion $(ONOO^-)$, which can oxidize or nitrate specific amino acids in key lung proteins and inhibit their function.[304] In inhalation and intratracheal instillation studies, rats exposed for 2 weeks to chrysotile or crocidolite asbestos showed significant increases in inducible nitric oxide synthase protein levels[125] and activity[124] as well as strong nitrotyrosine staining.[125] In addition, macrophages also show an increase in iNOS mRNA in response to asbestos.[126] Alveolar macrophages from these rats generated increased levels of nitrite/nitrate[124–126] which was inhibited by NG-monomethyl-L-arginine (NMMA), an inhibitor of nitric oxide synthase.[126] These finding suggest that asbestos inhalation can induce nitric oxide synthesis and peroxynitrite formation in vivo.

Although all forms of asbestos have been shown to be cytotoxic in vitro, results have varied as to which fiber type is the most cytotoxic. Early studies indicated that the order of cytotoxicity is chrysotile > crocidolite > amosite.[101] Other studies indicated that the order of cytotoxicity depends on the target cell type.[100] Most of these studies compared fiber toxicity on an equal-mass basis. However, when cytotoxicity in a cultured fibroblast cell line is compared on an equal-number basis (i.e., equal numbers of fibers per dish), it is found that crocidolite is more potent in causing cell death than chrysotile.[127] Of particular interest is the observation that erionite, a fibrous zeolite that is a potent cause of mesotheliomas in humans, is several orders of magnitude more potent on an equal-number basis in causing cell death than either crocidolite or chrysotile.[127] Fiber size is also an important factor, with longer and thinner fibers having the greatest cytotoxic effect.[100] Fibers with lengths greater than 8 to 10 μm and diameters less than 0.25 μm result in greater induction of ornithine decarboxylase activity in tracheal epithelial cells[128] and greater generation of reactive oxygen species in alveolar macrophages[129] than is observed with shorter, blunter fibers.

The Role of the Macrophage

In addition to the direct cytotoxicity of asbestos fibers, the inflammatory response to asbestos exposure is an extremely important mechanism of asbestos-induced tissue injury. Aerosolized chrysotile asbestos exposure produces a dose-related bronchiolitis and fibrosis associated with significantly elevated numbers of alveolar macrophages, neutrophils, and lymphocytes in bronchoalveolar lavage fluid.[130] Much of the in vitro work in this area has focused on the role of the alveolar macrophage as a mediator of asbestos-induced injury. Asbestos activates complement through the alternative pathway, resulting in the production of C_{5a} from C_5 and the subsequent accumulation of macrophages at first alveolar duct bifurcations.[131–133] This chemoattraction of macrophages is reduced or abolished by depletion of circulating complement, as shown by decreased numbers of macrophages at alveolar duct bifurcations in asbestos-exposed, complement-depleted rats.[132,134] Alterations in macrophage cytoplasmic and surface morphology are observed in animals exposed either briefly or chronically to aerosolized asbestos fibers.[35,135–138] These cells demonstrate diminished phagocytic capacity as assessed by carbonyl iron bead uptake[35,131] (Figure 10-7).

Alveolar macrophages can produce a wide variety of substances that are potential mediators of asbestos-induced tissue injury and repair (Table 10-3). It has been shown that phagocytosis of asbestos fibers by macrophages can result in the generation of reactive oxygen species,[129,139–142] which can in turn produce alterations in membrane fluidity, lipid peroxidation, and breakage of DNA. As mentioned above, alveolar macrophages produce nitric oxide, which can react to generate $ONOO^-$. Alveolar macrophages also secrete a number of hydrolytic enzymes, including aminopeptidase, acid phosphatase, esterase, lysozyme, cathepsing, RNase, lipase, phospholipase A_1 and A_2, elastase, hyaluronidase, β-glucuonidase, and catalase,[139,143–150] which could enhance tissue breakdown and destruction. In addition, alveolar macrophages may be stimulated to produce a broad spectrum of regulatory molecules that could in turn modulate the activity of other cells within the lung. These include the arachidonic acid metabolites, leukotriene B_4, prostaglandin E_2, and prostaglandin $F_{2\alpha}$,[151,152] as well as certain growth factors, such as platelet-derived growth factor, interleukin-1, fibroblast growth factor, and tumor necrosis factor.[153–155] Asbestos exposure in vitro[154] and in vivo[151] stimulates the release by alveolar macrophages of leukotriene B_4, a potent chemotaxin for neutrophils and eosinophils. Furthermore, both in vitro[154] and in vivo[156] exposure of alveolar macrophages to asbestos results in release of tumor necrosis factor, which can augment neutrophil and eosinophil functional activity as well as stimulate fibroblast growth. In vivo studies have also shown increased replication of interstitial fibroblasts in asbestos-exposed animals, as determined by autoradiography.[85,157]

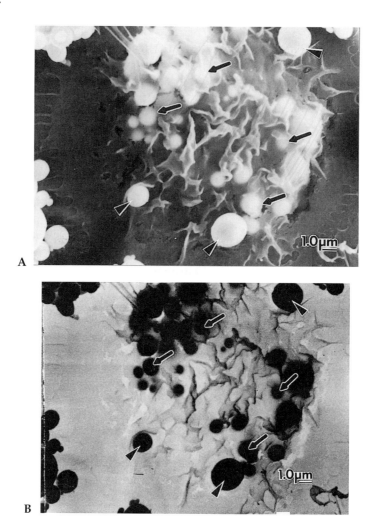

Figure 10-7. **(A)** Scanning electron micrograph of an alveolar macrophage showing carbonyl iron beads with sharp margins on the cell surface (*arrowheads*). **(B)** Back-scattered electron image of the same macrophage showing internalized beads (*arrows*). These same beads visualized in **(A)** have fuzzy borders. (Reprinted from Ref. 35, with permission.)

This latter effect is probably modulated by the release of fibroblast growth factor,[158,159] tumor necrosis factor,[153,154] interleukin-1,[152,160–163] prostaglandin $F_{2\alpha}$[152] and/or fibronectin[156] by asbestos-activated macrophages.

Much progress has been made with regard to the effect of soluble mediators produced and secreted by macrophages on the proliferation of other lung cells. It is now known that several cytokines including TNF-α, TGF-β, PDGF, and IL-1 are involved in triggering both the initial inflammatory reaction and the later formation of fibrotic lesions. A summary of the importance of several of these mediators is provided below.

TNF-α

In intratracheal instillation studies in rats, alveolar and pleural macrophages isolated from animals exposed to asbestos show increased production of the cytokine tumor necrosis factor alpha (TNF-α).[160,161] TNF-α production by macrophages can be stimulated by a variety of asbestos fibers and can initiate a cascade of responses involving adhesion molecule expression and production of chemotactic cytokines which ultimately result in the infiltration of inflammatory cells into sites of tissue injury in the respiratory tract.[164,165] Several studies have shown that TNF-α can stimulate chemokine expression in both immune and nonimmune cells. It appears that TNF-α production by alveolar macrophages is biphasic, because studies examining the effects of intratracheal injection of chrysotile asbestos in rats demonstrated a significant decrease in both TNF-α mRNA and protein levels at 1 and 3 weeks postexposure, but higher levels of TNF-α by 6 weeks postexposure.[166] Similar results were obtained for TNF-α production in pleural macrophages as well.[167] Since TNF-α seems to increase over time postexposure, investigators have hypothesized that this cytokine is primarily important for the development of chronic inflammation and fibrosis.[161,168]

Table 10-3. Potential mediators of asbestos-induced tissue injury and repair produced by alveolar macrophages

Mediator	References
Reactive oxygen species	
Superoxide anion	115, 118, 129, 140, 141
Hydroxyl radical	141, 142
Nitric Oxide/Peroxynitrite	124–126
Hydrolytic enzymes	
Aminopeptidase	144
Acid phosphatase	143, 144, 150
Esterase	144
Lysozyme	143
Cathepsin	143, 150
Ribonuclease	143
Lipase	143
Phospholipase A_1 and A_2	145
Elastase	148
Hyaluronidase	147
Beta-glucuronidase	143
Catalase	146, 149
Arachidonic acid metabolites	
Leukotriene B_4	151, 154
Prostaglandin E_2	152
Prostaglandin $F_{2\alpha}$	152
Growth Factors	
Platelet-derived growth factor	111, 155, 169, 178, 179
Interleukin-1	152–155, 160–163
Fibroblast growth factor	155, 158, 159
Tumor necrosis factor	153–155, 160, 161, 166–168, 170–172
Transforming growth factor	171, 173, 174, 177

TNF-α may play a key role in modulating the expression of other inflammatory and fibroproliferative cytokines. Studies involving TNF-α receptor knockout mice have shown that these mice fail to develop fibroproliferative disease in response to asbestos exposure, even though the levels of TNF-α gene expression and protein production increase on exposure of the knockout animals to asbestos. In situ hybridization studies on lung tissue from the knockout mice demonstrate reduced TGF-α, TGF-β and PDGF expression upon asbestos treatment.[169] It is thought that TNF-α may mediate its effects through induction and activation of other growth factors which, in turn, control cell growth and matrix production.[170,171] TNF-α may also regulate other cytokines and chemokines such as MCP-1[172] and may act synergistically with IL-1β to promote pulmonary inflammation and fibrosis.[168,172]

TGF-α, TGF-β and PDGF

Studies have demonstrated that TGF-α and TGF-β are rapidly upregulated specifically at sites of asbestos fiber deposition (particularly bronchiolar-alveolar duct regions) in the lungs of rats exposed to asbestos and remain elevated for extended periods of time.[173] In situ hybridization studies have demonstrated mRNA for both TGF-α and TGF-β is rapidly expressed in bronchiolar-alveolar epithelial cells, fibroblasts and alveolar macrophages in exposed rats and mice.[171,174] TGF-α is a potent mitogen for epithelial cells, while TGF-β, although inhibitory for fibroblast growth, stimulates extracellular matrix production.[171,175,176] Studies examining lungs of sheep treated intratracheally with chrysotile asbestos showed increased immunohistochemical staining for all three TGF-β isoforms in fibrotic lesions, associated with areas of extracellular matrix deposition and little staining of the interstitial cells. This study also demonstrated prominent IGF-1 staining in macrophages and proliferating epithelial cells, but not in the extracellular matrix. It is believed that TGF-β and IGF-1 have complementary roles in stimulating interstitial fibroblast proliferation and new collagen deposition in active fibrotic lesions.[177]

As mentioned above, platelet derived growth factor (PDGF) may also contribute to the development of asbestos-induced lung disease. Alveolar and pleural macrophages are known to secrete growth factors, including PDGF, that stimulate proliferation of fibroblasts.[178] PDGF-α and its matching receptor (PDGF-Rα) are upregulated in rat lung fibroblasts after exposure to chrysotile asbestos in vitro, which leads to fibroblast proliferation. There is also increased expression of PDGF-Rα mRNA and protein in asbestos-exposed rat lungs in vivo. Immunohistochemistry studies have shown that the receptor is located in the interstitial and subpleural regions of the lung. This suggests that a potent lung cell mitogen, PDGF-α and its receptor, are upregulated prior to the development of a fibroproliferative lesion, and may play a key role in asbestos-induced lung fibrosis.[179]

Other Signaling Pathways

Asbestos fibers can trigger alterations in gene expression in the lung by initiating signaling events upstream of gene transactivation. There have been at least two signaling cascades linked to activation of transcription factors that are stimulated after exposure of lung cells to asbestos fibers in vitro and in vivo. These include the NF-kB pathway and the MAPK signaling cascade, which ultimately leads to activation of the transcription factor AP-1. Both NF-kB and AP-1 bind to specific DNA sequences within the regulatory or promoter regions of genes that are critical to cell proliferation and inflammation.[180] The murine chemokine MIP-2 is expressed in response to inflammation induced by asbestos fibers in both epithelial cells and macrophages in the rodent lung. Notably, MIP-2 is regulated by NF-kB.[164] Crocidolite exposure causes a dose- and time-dependent induction of AP-1 activity both in vitro and in vivo. Initial activity was noted at 2 days postexposure and was increased 10-fold over control by day 3. AP-1 upregulation appeared to be mediated through the activation of MAPK family members including Erk-1 and Erk-2.[181] Activation of ERK has been associated with asbestos-induced apoptosis and proliferation in mesothelial and alveolar epithelial cells. ERK phosphorylation increases with the accumulation of inflammatory cells in the lung and in areas of fibrosis.[182]

Other Inflammatory Cells
Granulocytes (including neutrophils and eosinophils) have been shown to be present in increased numbers in bronchoalveolar lavage fluid obtained from patients with asbestosis.[151] Granulocytes are also increased in lavage fluid from experimental animals exposed to an asbestos aerosol.[130] Alveolar macrophages may play a key role in this influx of granulocytes[183] through the production and release of leukotriene B$_4$.[151,154] Neutrophils can then amplify asbestos-induced tissue injury by release of potent hydrolytic enzymes as well as reactive oxygen species. In vitro studies have shown that asbestos fibers have both a cytotoxic and an activating effect on neutrophils.[184,185] In the presence of extracellular calcium, asbestos fibers stimulate the release of granule-associated enzymes by exocytosis.[185] Incubation of asbestos fibers with normal human neutrophils also results in generation of reactive oxygen species as measured by chemilumenescence.[184] Furthermore, asbestos fibers and neutrophils interact to injure cultured human pulmonary epithelial cells in vitro through a mechanism that probably involves hydrogen peroxide production.[186] Fiber dimensions are once again an important factor, with long fibers producing greater neutrophil recruitment than short fibers.[187]

It is also possible that asbestos fibers may exert a direct effect on fibroblasts through the transport of fibers to the interstitium, where they may persist for prolonged periods.[72] In vitro studies in which a normal fibroblast cell line derived from rat lung was exposed to various concentrations of crocidolite asbestos, showed enhanced synthesis of total cellular collagen per ng of DNA.[157] These results were later confirmed in vivo, where exposure of rats to crocidolite asbestos resulted in elevated amounts of collagen deposition as assessed by hydroxyproline content.[78] In addition to increased synthesis, collagen turnover may also be an important contributor to fibrosis.[188]

Immunologic mechanisms may also contribute to the pathogenesis of asbestos-induced tissue injury.[189] A number of immune derangements have been described in individuals with asbestosis, as well as in in vitro studies of lymphocyte function.[189,190,191,192,193,194] However, the bulk of the immunologic abnormalities seen correlate poorly with clinical and radiographic parameters of asbestosis, and may thus represent epiphenomena unrelated to the pathogenesis of asbestos-induced lung disease.[190] Moreover, low-dose cyclophosphamide treatment in a sheep model of experimental asbestosis accelerated, rather than suppressed, the fibrotic process.[195] These results suggest that some of the immune responses which occur as a result of asbestosis may be adaptive rather than a direct contributer to fibrogenesis. While the dysregulation of the adaptive immune response may not contribute directly to fibrogenesis, the impaired cell mediated immunity that develops in patients with asbestosis undoubtedly contributes to the increased susceptibility to neoplasia seen in these individuals (see below).

Summary of Asbestos-Induced Fibrogenesis

Based on the foregoing discussion, a hypothetical scheme can be proposed for the mechanism of asbestos-induced fibrogenesis (Figure 10-8).[196–198] According to this scheme, asbestos is deposited on the alveolar surfaces, especially on first alveolar duct bifurcations, where transport

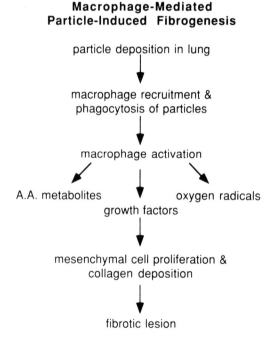

Figure 10-8. Hypothetical schema illustrating the pathogenesis of asbestos-induced pulmonary interstitial fibrosis. Fibers deposited on the surfaces of alveolar duct bifurcation stimulate the release of chemoattractants for alveolar macrophages. These cells phagocytize the fibers and become activated, releasing active oxygen species, arachidonic acid (A.A.) metabolites, and various growth factors. These various mediators then stimulate fibroblast replication and collagen synthesis, which eventuate in pulmonary interstitial fibrosis (i.e., asbestosis). (Courtesy Dr. Jamie Bonner, NIEHS, Research Triangle Park, NC.)

across the epithelium begins almost immediately. Asbestos initiates the conversion of C_5 to C_{5a} through the alternative pathway, which results in chemoattraction of alveolar macrophages to the site of asbestos deposition. These alveolar macrophages proceed to phagocytize the asbestos fibers, stimulating the release of reactive oxygen species and various hydrolytic enzymes. Also released are factors that amplify the inflammatory response through the attraction of granulocytes. In addition, activated macrophages release growth factors that stimulate the replication of interstitial macrophages and fibroblasts. Asbestos fibers translocated to the interstitium produce tissue injury by a combination of generating reactive oxygen species and direct interaction with cellular membranes of interstitial macrophages and fibroblasts. As a result of some combination of soluble growth factor release from alveolar (and perhaps interstitial) macrophages and direct tissue injury by translocated asbestos fibers, fibroblasts are stimulated to replicate and to synthesize collagen and other extracellular matrix components in increased amounts. Ongoing release of growth factors by activated macrophages and persistence of asbestos fibers within the interstitium would result in continuing fibrogenesis long after cessation of exposure.

Carcinogenesis

In Vivo Inhalation Studies

Inhalation studies in experimental animals have shown that asbestos produces neoplasms of the lung and pleura.[305] These include pulmonary adenoma, adenocarcinoma, squamous cell carcinoma,[5,42,86,87] and malignant mesotheliomas of the pleura and peritoneum.[5,42,87] These tumors have a prolonged latency period (300 days or more in the rat)[305] and there is some evidence of a dose-response relationship, with a greater incidence of tumors in rats exposed for 12 months as compared to six months, but no further increase in incidence from 12 to 24 months of exposure.[5] All types of asbestos, including chrysotile,[5,42,86,87] amosite,[5,86,88,199] crocidolite,[5] anthophyllite,[5] and tremolite[61] produce pulmonary and pleural neoplasms in experimental animals. In the classic studies of Wagner et al.,[5] chrysotile was as potent as crocidolite in the production of mesotheliomas by dust inhalation, with four mesotheliomas developing in 137 animals at risk with chrysotile exposure and four in 141 animals at risk due to crocidolite. Two animals developed mesotheliomas after only one day of exposure, one following exposure to crocidolite and the other, to amosite asbestos.[5] The mesotheliomas occurring in experimental animals exposed to asbestos are histologically, histochemically and ultrastructurally similar to those occurring in humans (Figure 10-9).[200,201] In addition, experimental pulmonary adenocarcinomas and squamous cell carcinomas are similar histologically to those occurring in humans.[5,88,201] However, one should always be cautious in extrapolating animal models to human risk assessments. Several studies have shown, for example, that humans suffer a tumor risk at approximately 100–1000 times lower

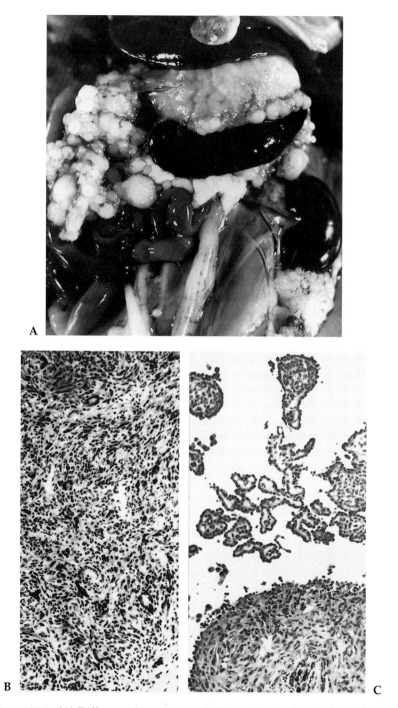

Figure 10-9. **(A)** Diffuse malignant mesothelioma developing in the abdomen of an asbestos-inoculated rat. These lesions exhibit a mixture of epithelial and fibrosarcomatous patterns **(B)** and **(C)**. (Reprinted from Ref. 31, with permission.)

concentration of asbestos fibers than those needed to produce the same risk in a rat inhalation model.[202,203]

The studies reported by Wagner et al.[5] and by Davis et al.[42] both showed a close association between the severity of interstitial fibrosis (i.e., asbestosis) and the development of pulmonary neoplasms. This finding suggests that pulmonary parenchymal tumors in asbestos-exposed animals derive from a metaplastic and hyperplastic epithelial response in areas of interstitial fibrosis that in some instances progressed to neoplasia. More recently, Davis and Cowie[204] have addressed this question in greater detail. These authors note that when adenomas or very early carcinomas are found, they are frequently in the center of areas of advanced asbestosis with exuberant epithelial metaplasia/hyperplasia. In studies comparing the pathological effects of various mineral fibers, there has also been a close association between the severity of pulmonary fibrosis and tumor development.[130,205,206] In an analysis of data from several different studies,[42,86,87] a strong correlation was observed between the percentage of lung occupied by fibrosis and the occurrence of pulmonary tumors ($p < 0.001$).[204] Tumors which developed in association with low-recorded levels of fibrosis (involving less than 4% of the lung area), were either advanced tumors occupying a single lung lobe or early tumors originating from the center of areas of interstitial fibrosis (Figure 10-10). While these studies support a role for fibrosis in the development of asbestos-associated tumors, these studies do not definitively answer the question as to whether fibrosis is an absolute prerequisite for the development of pulmonary tumors in experimental animals, which would require examination of a rela-

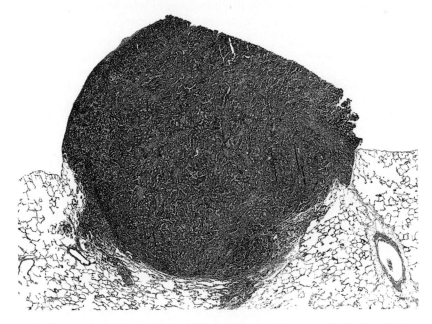

Figure 10-10. Pulmonary adenocarcinoma induced in a male Fischer 344 rat exposed to chrysotile asbestos. H&E, ×22. (Courtesy Dr. Gene McConnell, Raleigh, NC.)

tively large population of rats during the period of early tumor development.[204] Furthermore, the results may not be relevant to the great majority of lung cancers occurring in asbestos workers, in which cigarette smoke is an important cofactor.[207,208]

Role of Immune Function

The role of fibrosis in the deveopment of asbestos-associated pulmonary tumors is further supported by observations that individuals with asbestosis have been shown to have a number of immune derangements, including impaired cell-mediated immunity and hyperactive B-cell function.[189,190] Impaired cell-mediated immunity may manifest as cutaneous anergy, defective mitogen-induced lymphocyte blastogenesis and cytotoxic effector function, defective production of migration inhibitory factor, defective natural killer cell function, lymphopenia, and elevated T-helper suppressor ratio in blood and lavage fluid.[189] Hyperactive B-cell function is indicated by polyclonal hypergammaglobulinemia, elevated levels of secretory IgA, high frequency of autoantibodies and circulating immune complexes, enhanced spontaneous immunoglobulin production, and lymphoid neoplasms of B-cell lineage.[189] Derangements in immune response are known to be important in tumorogenesis because of changes in tumor surveillance. Thus, the changes in immune function seen in asbestosis patients may contribute to asbestos-induced pulmonary neoplasia.

A number of interesting observations have also been reported regarding asbestos effects on lymphocyte function. In vitro studies have shown that asbestos has a direct depressive effect on human lymphocyte mitogen response to phytohemagglutinin (PHA).[191] Asbestos inhalation is also associated with enhanced attachment of lymphocytes to alveolar macrophages,[192] which is followed by a vigorous lymphoproliferative response.[193] As noted earlier, asbestos exposure stimulates alveolar macrophages to release interleukin-1,[152] which can modulate T-cell function and lymphocyte proliferation.[189] In addition, IgG specifically enhances the production of superoxide anion by alveolar macrophages stimulated by chrysotile (but not crocidolite) asbestos.[194]

Role of Fiber Dimensions

Inhalation studies have indicated that in an analogous fashion to fibrogenic potential, long fibers have the greatest carcinogenic potential in experimental animal models.[5] Davis et al.,[86] using an amosite preparation with extremely few fibers greater than 5μm in length, reported no tumors in rats following long-term inhalation, whereas a clear excess of lung carcinomas and pleural mesotheliomas developed in rats breathing an amosite cloud containing considerable numbers of fibers 5μm or greater in length. Similar but less clear-cut results were obtained in a study of long and short preparations of chrysotile asbestos.[87] In this latter study, some longer fibers were still present in the "short fiber" chrysotile preparation, although the "long fiber" preparation (on an equal-mass basis) had five times as many fibers 5μm or greater in length and 80 times as many fibers 30 μm or greater in length. Both long and short chrysotile preparations produced mesotheliomas in more than 90% of rats following intraperitoneal injection of 25 mg. However, at a dose level of 2.5 mg, the short-fiber preparation produced only one-third as many mesotheliomas as the long fiber preparation, which still produced mesotheliomas in more than 90% of the animals injected. At a dose of 0.25 mg, the long-fiber preparation still produced tumors in 66% of rats.[87] The dose of short-fiber chrysotile that resulted in no mesothelial tumors in 24 rats (injected intraperitoneally) was calculated to contain 57 million fibers greater than 8 μm in length.[87] Studies using mineral fibers other than asbestos have also shown a strong association between fiber length and carcinogenicity.[87,206,209-211] Fasske[212] reported the development of pulmonary carcinomas or malignant pleural mesotheliomas in 24% of 70 rats treated by intratracheal instillation of 1 mg of chrysotile asbestos fibers 0.05 to 0.2 μm in length. However, the author did not specify details regarding how it was ascertained that there were no long fibers in the samples injected.

The classic studies of Stanton et al.[213,214] showed that, in addition to fiber length, fiber diameter is also an important determinant of carcinogenic potential. The "Stanton hypothesis" has emphasized the dimension and durability of fibers with regard to carcinogenicity, and states that, irrespective of chemical composition, the probability of developing mesotheliomas following implantation of mineral fibers into the pleural cavity correlates best with the numbers of fibers 8 μm or greater in length and 0.25 μm or less in diameter.[214] Hesterberg and Barrett[215] reported that in vitro studies with cultured Syrian hamster embryo cells showed the transforming potency to be greatest for long, thin fibers. Furthermore, in organ cultures of rodent tracheobronchial epithelial cells, long fibers (≥8 μm) cause enhanced incorporation of tritiated thymidine, increased biosynthesis of polyamines, and increased amounts of squamous metaplasia and keratinization.[95] These effects are only observed with short fibers (≤2 μm) at several-fold higher concentrations. In a review of asbestos exposure indices, Lippmann proposed, on the basis of the available data, that fibers 5 μm or greater in length and 0.1 μm or less in diameter are the most important in the production of mesotheliomas. In contrast, fibers 10 μm or greater in length and 0.15 μm or greater in diameter are the most important in the production of pulmonary carcinomas.[92]

Although fiber dimensions may be the most well-characterized determinant of carcinogenic potential, several other fiber characteristics may contribute to the overall incidence of tumor formation. It has been suggested that surface properties of mineral fibers may be an additional contributing factor to carcinogenic potency.[216,217] For example, fibrous erionite, which appears to have many times greater potential for mesothelioma induction than asbestos, has an internal surface area (due to "pores" in the crystal lattice) of 200 m^2/g, as compared to a total surface area of 8 to 10 m^2/g for crocidolite asbestos.[218] The mechanism by which this increased surface area enhances the carcinogenic potential of a fiber is unknown. Chemical composition of the fibers may also determine carcinogenic potential. Rats treated with amphibole asbestos fibers coated with either magnesium or cobalt had increased incidence of pleural mesotheliomas when compared to animals treated with uncoated fibers.[219]

In addition to the above-mentioned asbestos studies, there have been recent reports on the carcinogenic effects of various man-made mineral fibers, some commonly used as substitutes for asbestos. Some of these fibers, such as basic magnesium sulfate fiber[220] and kaolin refractory ceramic fibers (RCF),[221] produced significantly higher numbers of mesotheliomas and lung tumors in hamsters than chrysotile asbestos. On the other hand, other synthetic vitreous fibers, such as fibrous glass or other insulation wools, produced few if any tumors in these animals. These studies have shown that the fibers with the greatest biopersistence (i.e., least solubility) in vivo have the greatest carcinogenic potential.

Mechanisms of Asbestos-Induced Carcinogenicity

A great deal has been learned regarding the mechanisms by which fibers interact with cells and produce heritable alterations in cellular genetic material. Asbestos differs from most chemical carcinogens in that it tests negative in bacterial mutation assays[222–224] and is not mutagenic in liver epithelial cells[225] or Syrian hamster embryo fibroblasts.[226] A potential breakthrough in our understanding of asbestos-induced carcinogenicity is the development of methods for growing mesothelial cells in culture.[227–230] Cultured mesothelial cells have been shown to phagocytize chrysotile asbestos fibers in vitro,[231] which results in a slow leaching of magnesium from the chrysotile at a rate comparable to that which occurs in solution at pH 7.[50] Chrysotile asbestos produces intense vacuolization of cultured mesothelial cells[232] and also induces morphologically transformed colonies.[233] Incubation of mesothelial cells with either chrysotile or crocidolite asbestos fibers prolonged the doubling time in culture, although this effect occurred at lower doses of chrysotile as compared to crocidolite. With either fiber type, asbestos fibers were often observed within dividing cells.[232] Wang et al.[234] used scanning electron microscopy to demonstrate the interaction between asbestos fibers and metaphase chromosomes of rat pleural mesothelial cells. Chromosomes were frequently entangled with, adherent to severed or pierced by long curvilinear fibers, and this effect was more pronounced for chrysotile than for crocidolite asbestos.[234]

These observations are intriguing, considering that nonrandom chromosomal abnormalities, including translocations, rearrangements and marker chromosomes, have been identified in both experimental (asbestos-induced)[235–237] and human malignant pleural mesotheliomas.[238–240] Furthermore, studies with nonneoplastic human pleural mesothelial cells in culture have shown aneuploidy with consistent specific chromosomal losses in mesothelial cells surviving two cytotoxic exposures with amosite fibers.[235,241] These aneuploid cells exhibited altered growth control properties as well as a population doubling potential beyond the culture life span of control cells. Other studies using crocidolite, chrysotile, or amosite asbestos reported significant increases in numerical and/or structural chromosomal abnormalities in short-term cultured normal human mesothelial cells.[242] Also, crocidolite asbestos has been shown to induce sister chromatid exchanges in rat pleural mesothelial cells in vitro.[243] Specific DNA mutations, such as the formation of hydrophobic DNA adducts, have also been reported.[244,245]

Other in vitro approaches have also provided interesting information with respect to asbestos-induced carcinogenicity. Asbestos fibers have been shown to mediate the transfection of exogenous DNA into a variety of mammalian cells in vitro.[246,247] Exposure of Chinese hamster ovary cells to crocidolite asbestos fibers in cell culture resulted in an increased frequency of multinucleated cells, and various mitotic abnormalities were observed in cells containing fibers $20\,\mu m$ or greater in length.[248] Some studies have shown a strong correlation between fiber-induced cytotoxicity in a macrophage-like cell line and the probability of fiber-induced mesotheliomas,[249] whereas others have reported no direct relationship between cytotoxicity and carcinogenic potency.[250]

Oncogenes and growth factors might also play a role,[235,306] as suggested by the enhanced expression of the c-sis (PDGF-α) oncogene and the platelet-derived growth factor (PDGF) α-chain gene in 10 human malignant mesothelioma cell lines.[251] In addition, murine mesothelial cells that contain a point mutation in the p53 gene have shown increased sensitivity to asbestos-induced DNA damage.[252] Growth factors might also be implicated in the individual susceptibility for mesotheliomas that has been observed, since a significant interindividual variation in growth rates and response to various growth factors has been reported for normal cultured human mesothelial cells derived from different donors.[253] Also cytokines from tumor infiltrating macrophages and lymphocytes such as TGF-β, interleukin-6, interleukin-1 and TNF may contribute to malignant growth[254] and could provide possible therapeutic targets.[255,256]

In vitro models have provided useful information regarding the early events of asbestos interaction with the mesothelium. Studies by Moalli et al.[257] using stereomicroscopy and scanning electron microscopy demonstrated the rapid clearance of short asbestos fibers through the opening of diaphragmatic stomata, whereas long fibers ($60\% \geq 2\,\mu m$ in length) were trapped on the peritoneal surface, invoking an intense inflammatory reaction. This was associated with mesothelial cytotoxicity and regeneration at the periphery of asbestos fiber clusters. Maximal incorporation of tritiated-thymidine by mesothelial cells occurred seven days after exposure, and it was hypothesized that repeated episodes of injury and regeneration might promote the development of mesotheliomas.[257] Furthermore, asbestos fiber clusters on the peritoneal surface induce angiogenesis in the form of a capillary network radiating toward the center of the lesion, first notable 14 days after injection.[258] Recent studies detailing the early changes in the mesothelium following in vivo exposures to mineral fibers have been performed. Studies by Fraire et al.[302–303] suggest that there may be a gradual progression from mesothelial hyperplasia/dysplasia to mesothelioma, with intermediate stages characterized by the presence of fibrous adhesions and gross pleural nodular lesions.[302] The capability of growing mesotheliomas as xenographs in athymic rodents[259–261] should enhance the opportunity for investigators to study the properties of malignant mesothelial cells.

Much of the foregoing discussion has focused on the carcinogenic effects of asbestos fibers on mesothelial cells. However, asbestos is also carcinogenic for the respiratory epithelium and much knowledge has been gained by the study of the effects of asbestos on tracheal explants and organ cultures.[29,30] Crocidolite asbestos causes necrosis and desquamation of surface epithelial cells, with subsequent basal cell hyperplasia and squamous metaplasia.[29,262] Furthermore, asbestos-induced squamous metaplasia is inhibited by retinoids (retinyl methyl ether)[263] and vitamin C (ascorbic acid).[264] These studies may have implications regarding the prevention and prophylaxis of respiratory tract malignancies in workers who have been heavily exposed to asbestos in the past.

Asbestos as Promoter versus Initiator

In the previous discussion, mechanisms by which asbestos fibers might interact directly with DNA and chromosomes, and thus as an initiator of carcinogenesis, were emphasized. However, there is considerable epidemiologic data indicating that, with respect to carcinoma of the lung, asbestos interacts in a multiplicative fashion with cigarette smoke to enhance greatly the rate of neoplastic transformation. In this sense, asbestos behaves as a classic promoter of carcinogenesis. Numerous studies have explored various mechanisms by which asbestos could interact with cigarette smoke components in the process of carcinogenesis.[265]

One mechanism of interaction might be the adsorption of polycyclic aromatic hydrocarbons or other carcinogenic compounds within cigarette smoke onto the surface of the asbestos fiber, which then could act as a carrier particle, providing prolonged and intimate contact of the adsorbed carcinogens with respiratory epithelial cells. In vitro studies have demonstrated the adsorption of benzo[a]pyrene, nitrosonornicotine, and N-acetyl-2-aminofluorene onto the surface of all types of asbestos as well as other mineral fibers, with chrysotile binding significantly more carcinogen than the other mineral fibers tested.[266] It has also been shown that intratracheal instillation of either chrysotile or amosite asbestos concomitantly with benzo[a]pyrene over a six-week period significantly increased the number of tumors in hamsters as compared to any of these treatments alone.[267] Carcinogen binding is greatly enhanced by the prior adsorption of phospholipids (such as occur in surfactant) onto the asbestos fibers.[268] Studies using cell and organ cultures of tracheobronchial epithelium exposed to asbestos with and without adsorbed 3-methyl-cholanthrene (3-MC) show increased aryl hydrocarbon hydroxylase activity in cells treated with both asbestos and 3-MC as compared to 3-MC alone.[269] Furthermore, asbestos fibers and adsorbed carcinogens display a synergistic effect in the production of cell transformation in BALB/3T3 cells in vitro[270] and in the formation of malignant tumors from treated tracheal explants that were subsequently implanted into syngeneic animals.[271] Intratracheal instillation studies using chrysotile administered concomitantly with subcutaneously injected N-nitrosoheptamethyleneimine have also demonstrated a synergistic effect between these two agents in the induction of pulmonary neoplasms in rats.[272] Although cigarette smoking is not thought to be a cofactor in the production of malignant mesotheliomas in humans, the administration of 3-MC, along with chrysotile asbestos by intrapleural or intraperitoneal injection in rats, greatly enhances the production of mesotheliomas over that observed by chrysotile injection alone.[273]

Additional mechanisms whereby asbestos might interact with cigarette smoke or other environmental agents have also been explored. A novel hypothesis regarding the synergistic effect between asbestos fibers and polycyclic aromatic hydrocarbons suggests that the adsorption of lung surfactant phospholipids onto asbestos fibers[98,268] provides the opportunity for lipophilic carcinogens to diffuse within an all-lipid environment, with the asbestos fiber behaving like a chemical and physical bridge across the $5\mu m$-thick aqueous regions of the bronchial lining layer.[274] Others have reported results indicating that cigarette smoke and asbestos synergistically increase DNA damage and cell proliferation,[275,276] possibly by means of reactive oxygen species, such as hydroxyl radical formation.[142,275] Furthermore, cigarette smoke potentiates the uptake of asbestos fibers by the tracheobronchial epithelium.[57] This latter effect is blocked by prior treatment with superoxide dismutase, catalase, and deferoxamine, which are inhibitors of reactive oxygen species.[277] Studies have also suggested that asbestos might interact with ionizing radiation in the process of oncogenic transformation.[278] In this regard, ionizing radiation has been reported to augment the production of mesotheliomas in rats injected with chrysotile asbestos as compared to animals treated with chrysotile alone.[273]

Man-Made Mineral Fibers (MMMF) as Asbestos Substitutes

Since man-made mineral fibers are being used as substitutes for asbestos in a wide range of commercial products, the toxicity of these fibers with regard to fibrotic and carcinogenic potential deserves mention here. Like the earlier studies with various asbestos fibers, the most relevant animal model for the determination of pathogenicity and biopersistence of MMMF is the inhalation model.[279] Both acute and chronic studies involving a variety of fiber types such as refractory ceramic fibers (RCF), fibrous glass (FG), rock wool, and slag wool have been performed using a variety of animal models.[280–282,307–309] Like their asbestos counterparts, toxicity of these fibers is influenced primarily by fiber dimension, patterns of deposition, and solubility, all of which define the overall biopersistence of a particular fiber.[283]

Pathological responses to MMMF for the most part are similar to those of asbestos fibers, although some studies have shown that

MMMF have a lesser proliferative effect on bronchial epithelial cells than asbestos fibers.[284] MMMF have similar deposition patterns as asbestos fibers, are found lodged in the alveoli and small airways (especially at airway bifurcations), and can be found engulfed by macrophages.[285] As with asbestos, severity of lung and pleural lesions generally correlated with the cumulative fiber burden (especially for fibers >20 μm).[307–309] The faster the dissolution of the fibers, the lower the lung burden, and the less severe the effect. Many MMMF have been shown to induce inflammatory and fibrotic responses in a variety of cell and animal models. For example, an inhalation model using both RCF and rock wool produces an initial inflammatory response, followed by fibrosis (at 3 months and 12 months postexposure, respectively). RCF have been shown to also induce rare lung neoplasms.[286] In a second study, intratracheal injection of 1 mg of milled fibrous glass into mice resulted in epithelial injury and inflammatory cell response at bronchiolar alveolar ducts at 2–8 weeks postexposure, followed by proliferation of pulmonary epithelial cells and fibrosis. These results are similar to the fibrotic response typically observed upon exposure to crocidolite asbestos, although a 10-fold increase in MMMF concentration is required.[287]

Inhalation studies in animals also showed increases in tumor incidence with RCF and asbestos.[307–309] With regard to the various insulation wools, the results are still controversial but a significant increase in tumor formation was found upon intraperitoneal injection of rock wool, glass wool, glass microfibers and RCF.[288] The relationship between fiber dimension and carcinogenicity are similar for asbestos fibers, but other characteristics, such as overall biopersistence may also be important (see below).[288]

Biopersistence of MMMF is an important factor in determining the fibrogenic and carcinogenic potential of a particular fiber.[283,289] For all durable mineral fibers, critical length limits must be exceeded to warrant concern about chronic toxicity. For example, inhalation studies of ceramic fibers in rats and hamsters demonstrated that long ceramic fibers are retained in the rat lung to a greater extent than shorter glass fibers and thus produce an increase in tumor incidence.[281] However, fiber dimensions are only one indicator, since different fiber types of similar dimensions can vary substantially in biological activity.[290,291]

Many synthetic mineral fibers are much less biopersistent than asbestos fibers, most likely due to the more rapid dissolution of the fibers.[292] Several studies examining clearance rates of MMMF have demonstrated an inverse correlation between the rate at which a particular fiber type is cleared from the pulmonary interstitium and the severity of the resulting lesion.[293–296] For example, Bellman et al. compared intratracheal injections of stone wool or crocidolite in rats, and found that the number of stone wool fibers decreased exponentially with a half-life of 90 days for the short fibers and 120 days for the long fibers. However, clearance of the crocidolite fibers was significantly prolonged. Clearance of the stone wool fibers by macrophages was the most efficient clearance method for fibers <2.5 μm in length, and breakage and dissolution were responsible for clearance of fibers >5 μm.[280] In a similar study, wollastonite (a natural silicate) and xonotolite (a synthetic calcium silicate) administered to rats intratracheally showed half-lives of 15–21 days and 2 days, respectively, compared to 240 days for crocidolite.[280] In addition, a sheep inhalation model demonstrated that clearance rates of MMMF (via dissolution and phagocytosis) have a slow and fast component but are overall faster than clearance of crocidolite asbestos.[282]

As mentioned above, criteria other than fiber burden may be important in determining the pathogenicity of certain fiber types. Chronic inhalation studies in rats involving FG and RCF were performed to determine if fiber characteristics other than biopersistence of these fibers were important in the formation of lung fibrosis or lung neoplasms. In one study, rats were initially exposed to FG, RCF and asbestos and analyzed 2 years postexposure. After a two-year recovery period, the number of fibers of each type was comparable. In this experiment, fibrous glass did not induce lung fibrosis or result in increased incidence of lung tumors or mesotheliomas.[297] RCF exposure, on the other hand, resulted in an increase in both lung fibrosis and the incidence of lung tumors and mesotheliomas.[297,307–309] The authors suggest that changes in chemical composition of the fibers may be an important determinant of chronic toxicity of MMMF.[297] A later study by the same group demonstrated that similar lung burdens of fibrous glass or slag wool result in inflammatory responses, but did not induce neoplasms. Comparable numbers of rock wool fibers induced minimal fibrosis and no tumors. All fibers examined had similar clearance rates.[298] Finally, a study comparing biopersistence of MMMF (FG, RW, SW) to crocidolite asbestos, after 1 year postexposure, demonstrated that >95% of long MMMF had disappeared from the lung as compared to 17% of long crocidolite fibers. In addition, the mean diameter of MMMF decreased over time while crocidolite stayed the same. It was observed that various oxides were leached from the MMMF, which resulted in morphological changes to the fibers, and may serve to explain the noncarcinogenic nature of the fibers.[299]

Summary of Carcinogenesis

It appears that asbestos is a complete carcinogen, possessing both initiating and promoting properties.[222,300] The carcinogenic process is complex, and there are multiple ways in which asbestos can interact with the individual cell during the process of neoplastic transformation (Figure 10-11). In addition, suppression of cell mediated immune function may contribute to decreased capacity for tumor surveillance.

In the tracheobronchial tree, asbestos acts primarily as a promoter agent. Important steps in this process include epithelial cell injury, with subsequent basal cell hyperplasia and squamous metaplasia, cocarcinogenic effect of asbestos as a carrier for polycyclic aromatic hydrocarbons, and stimulation of DNA synthesis.[269] Squamous metaplasia interferes with mucociliary clearance mechanisms, and thus may encourage the transepithelial uptake of fibers otherwise cleared from the lung. This uptake in turn would bring fibers in contact with basal

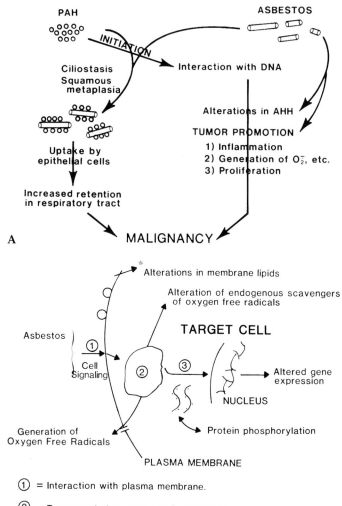

Figure 10-11. (A) Hypothetical schema illustrating several mechanisms of synergism between asbestos and polycyclic aromatic hydrocarbons in the induction of bronchogenic carcinoma. (Reprinted from Mossman BT and Craighead JE: Mechanisms of asbestos associated bronchogenic carcinoma. In: *Asbestos-Related Malignancy* (Antman K, Aisner J, eds.), Orlando, FL: Grune & Stratton, 1987, pp. 137–150, with permission.) **(B)** Direct interaction of asbestos fibers with target cell nuclear macromolecules (DNA, RNA, and proteins) could lead to altered gene expression and possible malignant transformation. (Courtesy of Dr. Brooke Mossman, University of Vermont, Burlington, VT.)

epithelium, where these cells would then be exposed to any carcinogens adsorbed to the surface of the asbestos fibers.[301] Asbestos exposure alone may also produce carcinomas in the lung periphery through the poorly understood mechanism of interstitial fibrosis with bronchiolar and alveolar cell hyperplasia proceeding to neoplastic transformation.[204,300]

In the pleural and peritoneal cavities, asbestos acts like a complete carcinogen, exhibiting both initiating and promoting activities.[300] A critical step appears to be the transport of durable fibers of appropriate dimensions to the pleura, through either the air spaces or the interstitial lymphatics (or both).[31] Peritoneal transport mechanisms include direct penetration of the intestinal wall by swallowed fibers, diaphragmatic penetration, or lymphatic pathways. Once fibers have come into contact with mesothelial cells, these cells seem to be particularly susceptible to asbestos-mediated cellular injury, as compared, for example, to bronchial epithelial cells or fibroblasts.[241]

Important steps in the neoplastic transformation of mesothelial cells probably include cellular injury with subsequent regeneration and hyperplasia, new blood vessel formation (angiogenesis), and chromosomal alterations. The latter occur as a result of either direct interaction of asbestos fibers with mesothelial cells during cellular division or indirectly through the generation of reactive oxygen species by asbestos fibers or inflammatory cells. The role of growth factors and oncogenes is an important area of active investigation,[222] and variable response of mesothelial cells to growth factors may be an important determinant of individual susceptibility to the development of fiber-induced mesotheliomas.[253]

References

1. Gardner LU: Experimental pneumoconiosis, In: *Silicosis and Asbestosis*, (Lanza AJ, ed.) New York: Oxford University Press, 1938, pp. 282–283.
2. King EJ, Clegg JW, Rae VM: The effect of asbestos and of aluminum on the lungs of rabbits. *Thorax* 1:188–195, 1946.
3. Vorwald AJ, Durkan TM, Pratt PC: Experimental studies of asbestosis. *Arch Ind Hyg Occup Med* 3:1–43, 1951.
4. Timbrell V: Human exposure to asbestos: dust controls and standards. The inhalation of fibrous dusts. *Ann N Y Acad Sci* 132:255–273, 1965.
5. Wagner JC, Berry G, Skidmore JW, Timbrell V: The effects of the inhalation of asbestos in rats. *Br J Cancer* 29:252–269, 1974.
6. Roggli VL, Brody AR: The role of electron microscopy in experimental models of pneumoconiosis, in *Electron Microscopy of the Lung* (Schraufnagel D, ed.), New York: Marcel Dekker, 1990, pp. 315–343.
7. Green GM, Jakab GJ, Low RB, Davis GS: Defense mechanisms of the respiratory membrane. *Am Rev Respir Dis* 115:479–514, 1977.
8. Raabe OG: Deposition and clearance of inhaled particles, In *Occupational Lung Disease* (Gee JBL, Morgan WKC, Brooks SM, eds.) New York: Raven Press, 1984, pp. 1–37.
9. Lee KP: Lung response to particulates with emphasis on asbestos and other fibrous dusts. *Crit Rev Toxicol* 14:33–86, 1985.
10. Timbrell V: *Aerodynamic considerations and other aspects of glass fiber.* Washington, DC: HEW, 1976, pp. 33–53.
11. Turnock AC, Bryks S, Bertalanffy FD: The synthesis of tritium-labeled asbestos for use in biological research. *Environ Res* 4:86–94, 1971.
12. Morgan A, Collier CG, Morris KJ, Launder KA: A radioactive tracer technique to determine in vivo the number of fibers in the lungs of rats following their administration by intratracheal instillation. *Environ Res* 63:182–190, 1993.

13. Evans JC, Evans RJ, Holmes A, Hounam RF, Jones DM, Morgan A, Walsh M: Studies on the deposition of inhaled fibrous material in the respiratory tract of the rat and its subsequent clearance using radioactive tracer techniques. 1. UICC crocidolite asbestos. *Environ Res* 6:180–201, 1973.

14. Morgan A, Evans JC, Evans RJ, Hounam RF, Holmes A, Doyle SG: Studies on the deposition of inhaled fibrous material in the respiratory tract of the rat and its subsequent clearance using radioactive tracer techniques. *Environ Res* 10:196–207, 1975.

15. Coin PG, Roggli VL, Brody AR: Persistence of long, thin chrysotile asbestos fibers in the lungs of rats. *Environ Health Perspect* 102 [Suppl 5]:197–199, 1994.

16. Brody AR, Hill LH: Deposition pattern and clearance pathways of inhaled chrysotile asbestos. *Chest* 80:64–67, 1981.

17. Brody AR, Hill LH, Adkins B, O'Connor RW: Chrysotile asbestos inhalation in rats: deposition pattern and reaction of alveolar epithelium and pulmonary macrophages. *Am Rev Respir Dis* 123:670–679, 1981.

18. Brody AR, Roe MW: Deposition pattern of inorganic particles at the alveolar level in the lungs of rats and mice. *Am Rev Respir Dis* 128:724–729, 1983.

19. Schlesinger RB: Particle deposition in model systems of human and experimental animal airways, In: *Generation of aerosols and facilities for exposure experiments* (Willeke K, ed.) Ann Arbor, MI: Ann Arbor Science, 1980, pp. 553–575.

20. Pinkerton KE, Plopper CG, Mercer RR, Roggli VL, Patra AL, Brody AR, Crapo JD: Airway branching patterns influence asbestos fiber location and the extent of tissue injury in the pulmonary parenchyma. *Lab Invest* 55:688–695, 1986.

21. Brain JD, Mensah GA: Comparative toxicology of the respiratory tract. *Am Rev Respir Dis* 128:S87–90, 1983.

22. Pritchard JN, Holmes A, Evans JC, Evans N, Evans RJ, Morgan A: The distribution of dust in the rat lung following administration by inhalation and by single intratracheal instillation. *Environ Res* 36:268–297, 1985.

23. Brain JD, Knudson DE, Sorokin SP, Davis MA: Pulmonary distribution of particles given by intratracheal instillation or by aerosol inhalation. *Environ Res* 11:13–33, 1976.

24. Roggli VL, Brody AR: Changes in numbers and dimensions of chrysotile asbestos fibers in lungs of rats following short-term exposure. *Exp Lung Res* 7:133–147, 1984.

25. Middleton AP, Beckett ST, Davis JM: Further observations on the short-term retention and clearance of asbestos by rats, using UICC reference samples. *Ann Occup Hyg* 22:141–152, 1979.

26. Roggli VL, George MH, Brody AR: Clearance and dimensional changes of crocidolite asbestos fibers isolated from lungs of rats following short-term exposure. *Environ Res* 42:94–105, 1987.

27. Brody AR, Hill LH, Stirewalt WS, Adler KB: Actin-containing microfilaments of pulmonary epithelial cells provide a mechanism for translocating asbestos to the interstitium. *Chest* 83:11S–12S, 1983.

28. Brody AR, Hill LH, Hesterberg TW, Barrett JC, Adler KB: Intracellular transport of inorganic particles, In: *The Cytoskeleton: A Target for Toxic Agents* (Clarkson TW, Sager PR, Syverson TL, eds.) New York: Plenum Publishing, 1986, pp. 221–227.

29. Mossman BT, Kessler JB, Ley BW, Craighead JE: Interaction of crocidolite asbestos with hamster respiratory mucosa in organ culture. *Lab Invest* 36:131–139, 1977.

30. Topping DC, Nettesheim P, Martin DH: Toxic and tumorigenic effects of asbestos on tracheal mucosa. *J Environ Pathol Toxicol* 3:261–275, 1980.
31. Craighead JE: Current pathogenetic concepts of diffuse malignant mesothelioma. *Hum Pathol* 18:544–557, 1987.
32. Viallat JR, Raybuad F, Passarel M, Boutin C: Pleural migration of chrysotile fibers after intratracheal injection in rats. *Arch Environ Health* 41:282–286, 1986.
33. Holt PF: Transport of inhaled dust to extrapulmonary sites. *J Pathol* 133:123–129, 1981.
34. Vincent JH, Jones AD, Johnston AM, McMillan C, Bolton RE, Cowie H: Accumulation of inhaled mineral dust in the lung and associated lymph nodes: implications for exposure and dose in occupational lung disease. *Ann Occup Hyg* 31:375–393, 1987.
35. Warheit DB, Chang LY, Hill LH, Hook GE, Crapo JD, Brody AR: Pulmonary macrophage accumulation and asbestos-induced lesions at sites of fiber deposition. *Am Rev Respir Dis* 129:301–310, 1984.
36. Bellmann B, Muhle H, Pott F, Konig H, Kloppel H, Spurny K: Persistence of man-made mineral fibres (MMMF) and asbestos in rat lungs. *Ann Occup Hyg* 31:693–709, 1987.
37. Coin P: *Pulmonary clearance of asbestos fibers*. Minneapolis, MN: University of Minnesota, 1989.
38. Holmes A, Morgan A: Clearance of anthophyllite fibers from the rat lung and the formation of asbestos bodies. *Environ Res* 22:13–21, 1980.
39. Kauffer E, Vigneron JC, Hesbert A, Lemonnier M: A study of the length and diameter of fibres, in lung and in broncho-alveolar lavage fluid, following exposure of rats to chrysotile asbestos. *Ann Occup Hyg* 31:233–240, 1987.
40. Morgan A, Talbot RJ, Holmes A: Significance of fibre length in the clearance of asbestos fibres from the lung. *Br J Ind Med* 35:146–153, 1978.
41. Churg A: Deposition and clearance of chrysotile asbestos. *Ann Occup Hyg* 38:625–633, 424–425, 1994.
42. Davis JM, Beckett ST, Bolton RE, Collings P, Middleton AP: Mass and number of fibres in the pathogenesis of asbestos-related lung disease in rats. *Br J Cancer* 37:673–688, 1978.
43. Middleton AP, Beckett ST, Davis JMG, A study of the short-term retention and clearance of inhaled asbestos by rats, using U.I.C.C. standard reference samples, In: *Inhaled Particles* (Walton WH, ed.) Oxford: Pergamon Press, 1977, pp. 247–257.
44. Churg A, Wright JL, Gilks B, DePaoli L: Rapid short-term clearance of chrysotile compared with amosite asbestos in the guinea pig. *Am Rev Respir Dis* 139:885–890, 1989.
45. Sebastien P, Armstrong B, Monchaux G, Bignon J: Asbestos bodies in bronchoalveolar lavage fluid and in lung parenchyma. *Am Rev Respir Dis* 137:75–78, 1988.
46. Kimizuka G, Wang NS, Hayashi Y: Physical and microchemical alterations of chrysotile and amosite asbestos in the hamster lung. *J Toxicol Environ Health* 21:251–264, 1987.
47. Hiroshima K, Suzuki Y: Characterization of asbestos bodies and uncoated fibers in lungs of hamsters. *J Electron Microsc (Tokyo)* 42:41–47, 1993.
48. Morgan A, Holmes A, Gold C: Studies of the solubility of constituents of chrysotile asbestos in vivo using radioactive tracer techniques. *Environ Res* 4:558–570, 1971.
49. Parry WT: Calculated solubility of chrysotile asbestos in physiological systems. *Environ Res* 37:410–418, 1985.

50. Jaurand MC, Gaudichet A, Halpern S, Bignon J: In vitro biodegradation of chrysotile fibres by alveolar macrophages and mesothelial cells in culture: comparison with a pH effect. *Br J Ind Med* 41:389–395, 1984.

51. Morgan A, Davies P, Wagner JC, Berry G, Holmes A: The biological effects of magnesium-leached chrysotile asbestos. *Br J Exp Pathol* 58:465–473, 1977.

52. Bolton RE, Vincent JH, Jones AD, Addison J, Beckett ST: An overload hypothesis for pulmonary clearance of UICC amosite fibres inhaled by rats. *Br J Ind Med* 40:264–272, 1983.

53. Ferin J, Leach LJ: The effect of amosite and chrysotile asbestos on the clearance of TiO$_2$ particles from the lung. *Environ Res* 12:250–254, 1976.

54. McMillan CH, Jones AD, Vincent JH, Johnston AM, Douglas AN, Cowie H: Accumulation of mixed mineral dusts in the lungs of rats during chronic inhalation exposure. *Environ Res* 48:218–237, 1989.

55. Davis JM, Jones AD, Miller BG: Experimental studies in rats on the effects of asbestos inhalation coupled with the inhalation of titanium dioxide or quartz. *Int J Exp Pathol* 72:501–525, 1991.

56. Churg A, Wright JL, Hobson J, Stevens B: Effects of cigarette smoke on the clearance of short asbestos fibres from the lung and a comparison with the clearance of long asbestos fibres. *Int J Exp Pathol* 73:287–297, 1992.

57. McFadden D, Wright J, Wiggs B, Churg A: Cigarette smoke increases the penetration of asbestos fibers into airway walls. *Am J Pathol* 123:95–99, 1986.

58. McFadden D, Wright JL, Wiggs B, Churg A: Smoking inhibits asbestos clearance. *Am Rev Respir Dis* 133:372–374, 1986.

59. Pinkerton KE, Brody AR, Miller FJ, Crapo JD: Exposure to low levels of ozone results in enhanced pulmonary retention of inhaled asbestos fibers. *Am Rev Respir Dis* 140:1075–1081, 1989.

60. Begin R, Sebastien P: Excessive accumulation of asbestos fibre in the bronchoalveolar space may be a marker of individual susceptibility to developing asbestosis: experimental evidence. *Br J Ind Med* 46:853–855, 1989.

61. Davis JM, Addison J, Bolton RE, Donaldson K, Jones AD, Miller BG: Inhalation studies on the effects of tremolite and brucite dust in rats. *Carcinogenesis* 6:667–674, 1985.

62. Hiroshima K, Murai Y, Suzuki Y, Goldstein B, Webster I: Characterization of asbestos fibers in lungs and mesotheliomatous tissues of baboons following long-term inhalation. *Am J Ind Med* 23:883–901, 1993.

63. Sebastien P, Begin R, Masse S: Mass, number and size of lung fibres in the pathogenesis of asbestosis in sheep. *J Exp Pathol* 71:1–10, 1990.

64. Begin R, Cantin A, Sebastien P: Chrysotile asbestos exposures can produce an alveolitis with limited fibrosing activity in a subset of high fibre retainer sheep. *Eur Respir J* 3:81–90, 1990.

65. Begin R, Cantin A, Masse S: Influence of continued asbestos exposure on the outcome of asbestosis in sheep. *Exp Lung Res* 17:971–984, 1991.

66. Begin R, Rola-Pleszczynski M, Masse S, Lemaire I, Sirois P, Boctor M, Nadeau D, Drapeau G, Bureau MA: Asbestos-induced lung injury in the sheep model: the initial alveolitis. *Environ Res* 30:195–210, 1983.

67. Adamson IY, Bowden DH: Response of mouse lung to crocidolite asbestos. 1. Minimal fibrotic reaction to short fibres. *J Pathol* 152:99–107, 1987.

68. Adamson IY, Bowden DH: Response of mouse lung to crocidolite asbestos. 2. Pulmonary fibrosis after long fibres. *J Pathol* 152:109–117, 1987.

69. Bozelka BE, Sestini P, Gaumer HR, Hammad Y, Heather CJ, Salvaggio JE: A murine model of asbestosis. *Am J Pathol* 112:326–337, 1983.

70. Filipenko D, Wright JL, Churg A: Pathologic changes in the small airways of the guinea pig after amosite asbestos exposure. *Am J Pathol* 119:273–278, 1985.

71. Wright GW, Kuschner M, The influence of varying lengths of glass and asbestos fibres on tissue response in guinea pigs, In: *Inhaled particles* (Walton WH, ed.) Oxford: Pergamon Press, 1977, pp. 455–474.

72. Pinkerton KE, Pratt PC, Brody AR, Crapo JD: Fiber localization and its relationship to lung reaction in rats after chronic inhalation of chrysotile asbestos. *Am J Pathol* 117:484–498, 1984.

73. Crapo JD, Barry BE, Brody AR, O'Neill JJ: Morphological, morphometric, and x-ray microanalytical studies on lung tissue of rats exposed to chrysotile asbestos in inhalation chambers, In: *Biological Effects of Mineral Fibers* (Wagner JC, ed.) IARC Scientific Publication, Lyon, 1980, pp. 273–283.

74. Barry BE, Wong KC, Brody AR, Crapo JD: Reaction of rat lungs to inhaled chrysotile asbestos following acute and subchronic exposures. *Exp Lung Res* 5:1–21, 1983.

75. McGavran PD, Moore LB, Brody AR: Inhalation of chrysotile asbestos induces rapid cellular proliferation in small pulmonary vessels of mice and rats. *Am J Pathol* 136:695–705,1990.

76. BeruBe KA, Quinlan TR, Moulton G, Hemenway D, O'Shaughnessy P, Vacek P, Mossman BT: Comparative proliferative and histopathologic changes in rat lungs after inhalation of chrysotile or crocidolite asbestos. *Toxicol Appl Pharmacol* 137:67–74, 1996.

77. Dixon D, Bowser AD, Badgett A, Haseman JK, Brody AR: Incorporation of bromodeoxyuridine (BrdU) in the bronchiolar-alveolar regions of the lungs following two inhalation exposures to chrysotile asbestos in strain A/J mice. *J Environ Pathol Toxicol Oncol* 14:205–213, 1995.

78. Mossman BT, Janssen YM, Marsh JP, Sesko A, Shatos MA, Doherty J, Adler KB, Hemenway D, Mickey R: Development and characterization of a rapid-onset rodent inhalation model of asbestosis for disease prevention. *Toxicol Pathol* 19:412–418, 1991.

79. Adamson IY, Bakowska J, Bowden DH: Mesothelial cell proliferation after instillation of long or short asbestos fibers into mouse lung. *Am J Pathol* 142:1209–1216, 1993.

80. Adamson IY, Bakowska J, Bowden DH: Mesothelial cell proliferation: a nonspecific response to lung injury associated with fibrosis. *Am J Respir Cell Mol Biol* 10:253–258, 1994.

81. Hirano S, Ono M, Aimoto A: Functional and biochemical effects on rat lung following instillation of crocidolite and chrysotile asbestos. *J Toxicol Environ Health* 24:27–39, 1988.

82. Chang LY, Overby LH, Brody AR, Crapo JD: Progressive lung cell reactions and extracellular matrix production after a brief exposure to asbestos. *Am J Pathol* 131:156–170, 1988.

83. Brody AR, Hill LH: Interstitial accumulation of inhaled chrysotile asbestos fibers and consequent formation of microcalcifications. *Am J Pathol* 109:107–114, 1982.

84. McGavran PD, Brody AR: Chrysotile asbestos inhalation induces tritiated thymidine incorporation by epithelial cells of distal bronchioles. *Am J Respir Cell Mol Biol* 1:231–235, 1989.

85. Brody AR, Overby LH: Incorporation of tritiated thymidine by epithelial and interstitial cells in bronchiolar-alveolar regions of asbestos-exposed rats. *Am J Pathol* 134:133–140, 1989.

86. Davis JM, Addison J, Bolton RE, Donaldson K, Jones AD, Smith T: The pathogenicity of long versus short fibre samples of amosite asbestos

administered to rats by inhalation and intraperitoneal injection. *Br J Exp Pathol* 67:415–430, 1986.

87. Davis JM, Jones AD: Comparisons of the pathogenicity of long and short fibres of chrysotile asbestos in rats. *Br J Exp Pathol* 69:717–737, 1988.
88. Lee KP, Barras CE, Griffith FD, Waritz RS, Lapin CA: Comparative pulmonary responses to inhaled inorganic fibers with asbestos and fiberglass. *Environ Res* 24:167–191, 1981.
89. Lemaire I, Nadeau D, Dunnigan J, Masse S: An assessment of the fibrogenic potential of very short 4T30 chrysotile by intratracheal instillation in rats. *Environ Res* 36:314–326, 1985.
90. Platek SF, Groth DH, Ulrich CE, Stettler LE, Finnell MS, Stoll M: Chronic inhalation of short asbestos fibers. *Fundam Appl Toxicol* 5:327–340, 1985.
91. Fasske E: Pathogenesis of pulmonary fibrosis induced by chrysotile asbestos. Longitudinal light and electron microscopic studies on the rat model. *Virchows Arch A Pathol Anat Histopathol* 408:329–346, 1986.
92. Lippmann M: Asbestos exposure indices. *Environ Res* 46:86–106, 1988.
93. Davis JM, Addison J, Bolton RE, Donaldson K, Jones AD: Inhalation and injection studies in rats using dust samples from chrysotile asbestos prepared by a wet dispersion process. *Br J Exp Pathol* 67:113–129, 1986.
94. Davis JM, Bolton RE, Douglas AN, Jones AD, Smith T: Effects of electrostatic charge on the pathogenicity of chrysotile asbestos. *Br J Ind Med* 45:292–299, 1988.
95. Mossman BT: In vitro studies on the biologic effects of fibers: correlation with in vivo bioassays. *Environ Health Perspect* 88:319–322, 1990.
96. *Asbestos toxicity*, ed. Fisher GL and Gallo MA. 1987, New York: Marcel Dekker.
97. Brody AR, George G, Hill LH: Interactions of chrysotile and crocidolite asbestos with red blood cell membranes. Chrysotile binds to sialic acid. *Lab Invest* 49:468–475, 1983.
98. Harington JS, Miller K, Macnab G: Hemolysis by asbestos. *Environ Res* 4:95–117, 1971.
99. Jaurand MC, Thomassin JH, Baillif P, Magne L, Touray JC, Bignon J: Chemical and photoelectron spectrometry analysis of the adsorption of phospholipid model membranes and red blood cell membranes on to chrysotile fibres. *Br J Ind Med* 37:169–174, 1980.
100. Reiss B, Solomon S, Weisburger JH, Williams GM: Comparative toxicities of different forms of asbestos in a cell culture assay. *Environ Res* 22:109–129, 1980.
101. Chamberlain M, Brown RC: The cytotoxic effects of asbestos and other mineral dust in tissue culture cell lines. *Br J Exp Pathol* 59:183–189, 1978.
102. Gallagher JE, George G, Brody AR: Sialic acid mediates the initial binding of positively charged inorganic particles to alveolar macrophage membranes. *Am Rev Respir Dis* 135:1345–1352, 1987.
103. Hesterberg TW, Ririe DG, Barrett JC, Nettesheim P: Mechanisms of cytotoxicity of asbestos fibers in rat tracheal epithelial cells in culture. *Toxicol In Vitro* 1:59–65, 1987.
104. Ghio AJ, Kadiiska MB, Xiang QH, Mason RP: In vivo evidence of free radical formation after asbestos instillation: an ESR spin trapping investigation. *Free Radic Biol Med* 24:11–17, 1998.
105. Petruska JM, Leslie KO, Mossman BT: Enhanced lipid peroxidation in lung lavage of rats after inhalation of asbestos. *Free Radic Biol Med* 11:425–432, 1991.
106. Aljandali A, Pollack H, Yeldandi A, Li Y, Weitzman SA, Kamp DW: Asbestos causes apoptosis in alveolar epithelial cells: role of iron- induced free radicals. *J Lab Clin Med* 137:330–339, 2001.

107. Schapira RM, Ghio AJ, Effros RM, Morrisey J, Dawson CA, Hacker AD: Hydroxyl radicals are formed in the rat lung after asbestos instillation in vivo. *Am J Respir Cell Mol Biol* 10:573–579, 1994.

108. Eberhardt MK, Roman-Franco AA, Quiles MR: Asbestos-induced decomposition of hydrogen peroxide. *Environ Res* 37:287–292, 1985.

109. Weitzman SA, Graceffa P: Asbestos catalyzes hydroxyl and superoxide radical generation from hydrogen peroxide. *Arch Biochem Biophys* 228:373–376, 1984.

110. Zalma R, Bonneau L, Jaurand MC, Guignard J, Pezerat H: Formation of oxy-radicals by oxygen reduction arising from the surface activity of asbestos. *Can J Chem* 65:2338–2341, 1987.

111. Dai J, Churg A: Relationship of fiber surface iron and active oxygen species to expression of procollagen, PDGF-A, TGF-beta(1) in tracheal explants exposed to amosite asbestos. *Am J Respir Cell Mol Biol* 24:427–435, 2001.

112. Kamp DW, Israbian VA, Yeldandi AV, Panos RJ, Graceffa P, Weitzman SA: Phytic acid, an iron chelator, attenuates pulmonary inflammation and fibrosis in rats after intratracheal instillation of asbestos. *Toxicol Pathol* 23:689–695, 1995.

113. Goodglick LA, Kane AB: Cytotoxicity of long and short crocidolite asbestos fibers in vitro and in vivo. *Cancer Res* 50:5153–5163, 1990.

114. Kostyuk VA, Potapovich AI: Antiradical and chelating effects in flavonoid protection against silica-induced cell injury. *Arch Biochem Biophys* 355:43–48, 1998.

115. Quinlan TR, Marsh JP, Janssen YM, Borm PA, Mossman BT: Oxygen radicals and asbestos-mediated disease. *Environ Health Perspect* 102 [Suppl 10]:107–110, 1994.

116. Abidi P, Afaq F, Arif JM, Lohani M, Rahman Q: Chrysotile-mediated imbalance in the glutathione redox system in the development of pulmonary injury. *Toxicol Lett* 106:31–39, 1999.

117. Kaiglova A, Kovacikova Z, Hurbankova M: Impact of acute and subchronic asbestos exposure on some parameters of antioxidant defense system and lung tissue injury. *Ind Health* 37:348–351, 1999.

118. Shatos MA, Doherty JM, Marsh JP, Mossman BT: Prevention of asbestos-induced cell death in rat lung fibroblasts and alveolar macrophages by scavengers of active oxygen species. *Environ Res* 44:103–116, 1987.

119. Janssen YM, Marsh JP, Absher MP, Hemenway D, Vacek PM, Leslie KO, Borm PJ, Mossman BT: Expression of antioxidant enzymes in rat lungs after inhalation of asbestos or silica. *J Biol Chem* 267:10625–10630, 1992.

120. Quinlan TR, Marsh JP, Janssen YM, Leslie KO, Hemenway D, Vacek P, Mossman BT: Dose-responsive increases in pulmonary fibrosis after inhalation of asbestos. *Am J Respir Crit Care Med* 150:200–206, 1994.

121. Holley JA, Janssen YM, Mossman BT, Taatjes DJ: Increased manganese superoxide dismutase protein in type II epithelial cells of rat lungs after inhalation of crocidolite asbestos or cristobalite silica. *Am J Pathol* 141:475–485, 1992.

122. Janssen YM, Marsh JP, Absher M, Borm PJ, Mossman BT: Increases in endogenous antioxidant enzymes during asbestos inhalation in rats. *Free Radic Res Commun* 11:53–58, 1990.

123. Zhu S, Manuel M, Tanaka S, Choe N, Kagan E, Matalon S: Contribution of reactive oxygen and nitrogen species to particulate-induced lung injury. *Environ Health Perspect* 106 [Suppl 5]:1157–1163, 1998.

124. Iguchi H, Kojo S, Ikeda M: Nitric oxide (NO) synthase activity in the lung and NO synthesis in alveolar macrophages of rats increased on exposure to asbestos. *J Appl Toxicol* 16:309–315, 1996.

125. Tanaka S, Choe N, Hemenway DR, Zhu S, Matalon S, Kagan E: Asbestos inhalation induces reactive nitrogen species and nitrotyrosine formation in the lungs and pleura of the rat. *J Clin Invest* 102:445–454, 1998.

126. Quinlan TR, BeruBe KA, Hacker MP, Taatjes DJ, Timblin CR, Goldberg J, Kimberley P, O'Shaughnessy P, Hemenway D, Torino J, Jimenez LA, Mossman BT: Mechanisms of asbestos-induced nitric oxide production by rat alveolar macrophages in inhalation and in vitro models. *Free Radic Biol Med* 24:778–788, 1998.

127. Palekar LD, Brown BG, Coffin DL: Correlation between in vitro tumorigenesis, in vitro CHO cytotoxicity and in vitro V79 cytotoxicity after exposure to mineral fibers, In: *Short-term bioassay in the analysis of the complex environmental Mixtures IV*, (Waters MD, Sandu SF, Lewtas J, Claxton J, Strauss G, Nesnow S, eds.) New York: Plenum Press, 1985, pp. 155–169.

128. Marsh JP, Mossman BT: Mechanisms of induction of ornithine decarboxylase activity in tracheal epithelial cells by asbestiform minerals. *Cancer Res* 48:709–714, 1988.

129. Hansen K, Mossman BT: Generation of superoxide (O2-.) from alveolar macrophages exposed to asbestiform and nonfibrous particles. *Cancer Res* 47:1681–1686, 1987.

130. Smith CM, Batcher S, Catanzaro A, Abraham JL, Phalen R: Sequence of bronchoalveolar lavage and histopathologic findings in rat lungs early in inhalation asbestos exposure. *J Toxicol Environ Health* 20:147–161, 1987.

131. Warheit DB, Hill LH, Brody AR: In vitro effects of crocidolite asbestos and wollastonite on pulmonary macrophages and serum complement. *Scan Electron Microsc* II:919–926, 1984.

132. Warheit DB, George G, Hill LH, Snyderman R, Brody AR: Inhaled asbestos activates a complement-dependent chemoattractant for macrophages. *Lab Invest* 52:505–514, 1985.

133. Wilson MR, Gaumer HR, Salvaggio JE: Activation of the alternative complement pathway and generation of chemotactic factors by asbestos. *J Allerg Clin Immunol* 60:218–222, 1977.

134. Warheit DB, Hill LH, George G, Brody AR: Time course of chemotactic factor generation and the corresponding macrophage response to asbestos inhalation. *Am Rev Respir Dis* 134:128–133, 1986.

135. Kagan E, Oghiso Y, Hartmann DP: The effects of chrysotile and crocidolite asbestos on the lower respiratory tract: analysis of bronchoalveolar lavage constituents. *Environ Res* 32:382–397, 1983.

136. Miller K: Alterations in the surface-related phenomena of alveolar macrophages following inhalation of crocidolite asbestos and quartz dusts: an overview. *Environ Res* 20:162–182, 1979.

137. Warheit DB, Hill LH, Brody AR: Surface morphology and correlated phagocytic capacity of pulmonary macrophages lavaged from the lungs of rats. *Exp Lung Res* 6:71–82, 1984.

138. Warheit DB, Hartsky MA: Assessments of pulmonary macrophage clearance responses to inhaled particulates. *Scanning Microsc* 2:1069–1078, 1988.

139. Afaq F, Abidi P, Matin R, Rahman Q: Activation of alveolar macrophages and peripheral red blood cells in rats exposed to fibers/particles. *Toxicol Lett* 99:175–182, 1998.

140. Case BW, Ip MP, Padilla M, Kleinerman J: Asbestos effects on superoxide production. An in vitro study of hamster alveolar macrophages. *Environ Res* 39:299–306, 1986.

141. Goodglick LA, Kane AB: Role of reactive oxygen metabolites in crocidolite asbestos toxicity to mouse macrophages. *Cancer Res* 46:5558–5566, 1986.

142. Jackson JH, Schraufstatter IU, Hyslop PA, Vosbeck K, Sauerheber R, Weitzman SA, Cochrane CG: Role of oxidants in DNA damage. Hydroxyl radical mediates the synergistic DNA damaging effects of asbestos and cigarette smoke. *J Clin Invest* 80:1090–1095, 1987.

143. Cohn ZA, Wiener E: The particulate hydrolase of macrophages I. Comparative enzymology, isolation, properties. *J Exp Med* 118:991–1008, 1963.

144. Dannenberg AM, Burstone MS, Walter PC, Kinsley JW: A histochemical study of phagocytic and enzymatic functions of rabbit mononuclear and polymorphonuclear exudate cells and alveolar macrophages. I. Survey and quantitation of enzymes, and states of cellular activation. *J Cell Biol* 17:465–486, 1963.

145. Franson R, Beckerdite S, Wang P, Waite M, Elsbach P: Some properties of phospholipases of alveolar macrophages. *Biochim Biophys Acta* 296: 365–373, 1973.

146. Gee JB, Vassallo CL, Bell P, Kaskin J, Basford RE, Field JB: Catalase-dependent peroxidative metabolism in the alveolar macrophage during phagocytosis. *J Clin Invest* 49:1280–1287, 1970.

147. Goggins JF, Lazarus GS, Fullmer HM: Hyaluronidase activity of alveolar macrophages. *J Histochem Cytochem* 16:688–692, 1968.

148. Janoff A: Elastase-like protease of human granulocytes and alveolar macrophages, In: *Pulmonary Emphysema and Proteolysis*, (Mittman C, ed.) New York: Academic Press, 1972, pp. 205–224.

149. Paul BB, Strauss RR, Selvaraj RJ, Sbarra AJ: Peroxidase mediated antimicrobial activities of alveolar macrophage granules. *Science* 181:849–850, 1973.

150. Sjostrand M, Rylander R, Bergstrom R: Lung cell reactions in guinea pigs after inhalation of asbestos (amosite). *Toxicology* 57:1–14, 1989.

151. Garcia JG, Griffith DE, Cohen AB, Callahan KS: Alveolar macrophages from patients with asbestos exposure release increased levels of leukotriene B$_4$. *Am Rev Respir Dis*, 139:1494–1501, 1989.

152. Sestini P, Tagliabue A, Bartalini M, Boraschi D: Asbestos-induced modulation of release of regulatory molecules from alveolar and peritoneal macrophages. *Chest* 89:161S–162S, 1986.

153. Bissonnette E, Rola-Pleszczynski M: Pulmonary inflammation and fibrosis in a murine model of asbestosis and silicosis. Possible role of tumor necrosis factor. *Inflammation* 13:329–339, 1989.

154. Dubois CM, Bissonnette E, Rola-Pleszczynski M: Asbestos fibers and silica particles stimulate rat alveolar macrophages to release tumor necrosis factor. Autoregulatory role of leukotriene B$_4$. *Am Rev Respir Dis* 139:1257–1264, 1989.

155. Kumar RK, Bennett RA, Brody AR: A homologue of platelet-derived growth factor produced by rat alveolar macrophages. *FASEB J* 2:2272–2277, 1988.

156. Davies R, Erdogdu G: Secretion of fibronectin by mineral dust-derived alveolar macrophages and activated peritoneal macrophages. *Exp Lung Res* 15:285–297, 1989.

157. Mossman BT, Gilbert R, Doherty J, Shatos MA, Marsh J, Cutroneo K: Cellular and molecular mechanisms of asbestosis. *Chest* 89:160S–161S, 1986.

158. Lemaire I, Beaudoin H, Masse S, Grondin C: Alveolar macrophage stimulation of lung fibroblast growth in asbestos-induced pulmonary fibrosis. *Am J Pathol* 122:205–211, 1986.

159. Lemaire I, Beaudoin H, Dubois C: Cytokine regulation of lung fibroblast proliferation. Pulmonary and systemic changes in asbestos-induced pulmonary fibrosis. *Am Rev Respir Dis* 134:653–658, 1986.

160. Lemaire I, Ouellet S: Distinctive profile of alveolar macrophage-derived cytokine release induced by fibrogenic and nonfibrogenic mineral dusts. *J Toxicol Environ Health* 47:465–478, 1996.

161. Li XY, Lamb D, Donaldson K: The production of TNF-alpha and IL-1-like activity by bronchoalveolar leucocytes after intratracheal instillation of crocidolite asbestos. *Int J Exp Pathol* 74:403–410, 1993.

162. Li XY, Lamb D, Donaldson K: Production of interleukin 1 by rat pleural leucocytes in culture after intratracheal instillation of crocidolite asbestos. *Br J Ind Med* 50:90–94, 1993.

163. Li XY, Lamb D, Donaldson K: Mesothelial cell injury caused by pleural leukocytes from rats treated with intratracheal instillation of crocidolite asbestos or Corynebacterium parvum. *Environ Res* 64:181–191, 1994.

164. Driscoll KE: TNF-alpha and MIP-2: role in particle-induced inflammation and regulation by oxidative stress. *Toxicol Lett* 112–113:177–183, 2000.

165. Fisher CE, Rossi AG, Shaw J, Beswick PH, Donaldson K: Release of TNF-alpha in response to SiC fibres: differential effects in rodent and human primary macrophages, and in macrophage-like cell lines. *Toxicol In Vitro* 14:25–31, 2000.

166. Ouellet S, Yang H, Aubin RA, Hawley RG, Wenckebach GF, Lemaire I: Bidirectional modulation of TNF-alpha production by alveolar macrophages in asbestos-induced pulmonary fibrosis. *J Leukoc Biol* 53:279–286, 1993.

167. Li XY, Lamb D, Donaldson K: Intratracheal injection of crocidolite asbestos depresses the secretion of tumor necrosis factor by pleural leukocytes in vitro. *Exp Lung Res* 18:359–372, 1992.

168. Driscoll KE, Maurer JK, Higgins J, Poynter J: Alveolar macrophage cytokine and growth factor production in a rat model of crocidolite-induced pulmonary inflammation and fibrosis. *J Toxicol Environ Health* 46:155–169, 1995.

169. Brass DM, Hoyle GW, Poovey HG, Liu JY, Brody AR: Reduced tumor necrosis factor-alpha and transforming growth factor-beta 1 expression in the lungs of inbred mice that fail to develop fibroproliferative lesions consequent to asbestos exposure. *Am J Pathol* 154:853–862, 1999.

170. Liu JY, Brass DM, Hoyle GW, Brody AR: TNF-alpha receptor knockout mice are protected from the fibroproliferative effects of inhaled asbestos fibers. *Am J Pathol* 153:1839–1847, 1998.

171. Liu JY, Brody AR: Increased TGF-beta 1 in the lungs of asbestos-exposed rats and mice: reduced expression in TNF-alpha receptor knockout mice. *J Environ Pathol Toxicol Oncol* 20:97–108, 2001.

172. Tanaka S, Choe N, Iwagaki A, Hemenway DR, Kagan E: Asbestos exposure induces MCP-1 secretion by pleural mesothelial cells. *Exp Lung Res* 26:241–255, 2000.

173. Liu JY, Morris GF, Lei WH, Corti M, Brody AR: Up-regulated expression of transforming growth factor-alpha in the bronchiolar-alveolar duct regions of asbestos-exposed rats. *Am J Pathol* 149:205–217, 1996.

174. Perdue TD, Brody AR: Distribution of transforming growth factor-beta 1, fibronectin, and smooth muscle actin in asbestos-induced pulmonary fibrosis in rats. *J Histochem Cytochem* 42:1061–1070, 1994.

175. Brody AR: Occupational lung disease and the role of peptide growth factors. *Curr Opin Pulm Med* 3:203–208, 1997.

176. Brody AR, Liu JY, Brass D, Corti M: Analyzing the genes and peptide growth factors expressed in lung cells in vivo consequent to asbestos exposure and in vitro. *Environ Health Perspect* 105[Suppl 5]:1165–1171, 1997.

177. Lee TC, Gold LI, Reibman J, Aston C, Begin R, Rom WN, Jagirdar J: Immunohistochemical localization of transforming growth factor-beta and insulin-like growth factor-I in asbestosis in the sheep model. *Int Arch Occup Environ Health* 69:157–164, 1997.

178. Adamson IY, Prieditis H, Young L: Lung mesothelial cell and fibroblast responses to pleural and alveolar macrophage supernatants and to lavage fluids from crocidolite-exposed rats. *Am J Respir Cell Mol Biol* 16:650–656, 1997.

179. Lasky JA, Tonthat B, Liu JY, Friedman M, Brody AR: Upregulation of the PDGF-alpha receptor precedes asbestos-induced lung fibrosis in rats. *Am J Respir Crit Care Med* 157:1652–1657, 1998.

180. Mossman BT, Faux S, Janssen Y, Jimenez LA, Timblin C, Zanella C, Goldberg J, Walsh E, Barchowsky A, Driscoll K: Cell signaling pathways elicited by asbestos. *Environ Health Perspect* 105[Suppl 5]:1121–1125, 1997.

181. Ding M, Dong Z, Chen F, Pack D, Ma WY, Ye J, Shi X, Castranova V, Vallyathan V: Asbestos induces activator protein-1 transactivation in transgenic mice. *Cancer Res* 59:1884–1889, 1999.

182. Robledo RF, Buder-Hoffmann SA, Cummins AB, Walsh ES, Taatjes DJ, Mossman BT: Increased phosphorylated extracellular signal-regulated kinase immunoreactivity associated with proliferative and morphologic lung alterations after chrysotile asbestos inhalation in mice. *Am J Pathol* 156:1307–1316, 2000.

183. Schoenberger CI, Hunninghake GW, Kawanami O, Ferrans VJ, Crystal RG: Role of alveolar macrophages in asbestosis: modulation of neutrophil migration to the lung after acute asbestos exposure. *Thorax* 37:803–809, 1982.

184. Doll NJ, Stankus RP, Goldbach S, Salvaggio JE: In vitro effect of asbestos fibers on polymorphonuclear leukocyte function. *Int Arch Allergy Appl Immunol* 68:17–21, 1982.

185. Elferink JG, Deierkauf M, Kramps JA, Koerten HK: An activating and cytotoxic effect of asbestos on polymorphonuclear leukocytes. *Agents Actions* 26:213–215, 1989.

186. Kamp DW, Dunne M, Weitzman SA, Dunn MM: The interaction of asbestos and neutrophils injures cultured human pulmonary epithelial cells: role of hydrogen peroxide. *J Lab Clin Med* 114:604–612, 1989.

187. Donaldson K, Brown GM, Brown DM, Bolton RE, Davis JM: Inflammation generating potential of long and short fibre amosite asbestos samples. *Br J Ind Med* 46:271–276, 1989.

188. Arden MG, Adamson IY: Collagen synthesis and degradation during the development of asbestos-induced pulmonary fibrosis. *Exp Lung Res* 18:9–20, 1992.

189. Kagan E: Current perspectives in asbestosis. *Ann Allergy* 54:464–473, 1985.

190. deShazo RD, Daul CB, Morgan JE, Diem JE, Hendrick DJ, Bozelka BE, Stankus RP, Jones R, Salvaggio JE, Weill H: Immunologic investigations in asbestos-exposed workers. *Chest* 89:162S–165S, 1986.

191. Barbers RG, Shih WW, Saxon A: In vitro depression of human lymphocyte mitogen response (phytohaemagglutinin) by asbestos fibres. *Clin Exp Immunol* 48:602–610, 1982.

192. Miller K, Weintraub Z, Kagan E: Manifestations of cellular immunity in the rat after prolonged asbestos inhalation. I. Physical interactions between alveolar macrophages and splenic lymphocytes. *J Immunol* 123:1029–1038, 1979.

193. Miller K, Kagan E: Manifestations of cellular immunity in the rat after prolonged asbestos inhalation. II. Alveolar macrophage-induced splenic lymphocyte proliferation. *Environ Res* 26:182–194, 1981.

194. Scheule RK, Holian A: IgG specifically enhances chrysotile asbestos-stimulated superoxide anion production by the alveolar macrophage. *Am J Respir Cell Mol Biol* 1:313–318, 1989.

195. Begin R, Cantin A, Masse S, Cote Y, Fabi D: Effects of cyclophosphamide treatment in experimental asbestosis. *Exp Lung Res* 14:823–836, 1988.

196. Brody AR, Hill LH: Initial epithelial and interstitial events following asbestos inhalation, In: *Health Issues Related to Metal and Nonmetallic Mining*, (Wagner WL, Rom WN, Merchant JA, eds.) Boston: Butterworth, 1983, pp. 161–172.

197. Brody AR: Pulmonary cell interactions with asbestos fibers in vivo and in vitro. *Chest* 89:155S-159S, 1986.

198. Brody AR, Hill LH, Warheit DB: Induction of early alveolar injury by inhaled asbestos and silica. *Fed Proc* 44:2596–2601, 1985.

199. Webster I, Goldstein B, Coetzee FS, van Sittert GC: Malignant mesothelioma induced in baboons by inhalation of amosite asbestos. *Am J Ind Med* 24:659–666, 1993.

200. Kannerstein M, Churg J: Mesothelioma in man and experimental animals. *Environ Health Perspect* 34:31–36, 1980.

201. Davis JM: Histogenesis and fine structure of peritoneal tumors produced in animals by injections of asbestos. *J Natl Cancer Inst* 52:1823–1837, 1974.

202. Muhle H, Pott F: Asbestos as reference material for fibre-induced cancer. *Int Arch Occup Environ Health* 73[Suppl]:S53–59, 2000.

203. Rodelsperger K, Woitowitz HJ: Airborne fibre concentrations and lung burden compared to the tumour response in rats and humans exposed to asbestos. *Ann Occup Hyg* 39:715–725, 1995.

204. Davis JM, Cowie HA: The relationship between fibrosis and cancer in experimental animals exposed to asbestos and other fibers. *Environ Health Perspect* 88:305–309, 1990.

205. McConnell EE, Wagner JC, Skidmore JW, Moore JA: A comparative study of the fibrogenic and carcinogenic effects of UICC Canadian chrysotile B asbestos and glass microfibre (JM100), In: *Biological Effects of Man-Made Mineral Fibers*, (Wagner JC, ed.) Copenhagen: World Health Oraganization, 1985, pp. 234–252.

206. Wagner JC, Berry GB, Hill RJ, Munday DE, Skidmore JW: Animal experiments with man-made mineral (vitreous) fibers: Effects of inhalation and intrapleural inoculation in rats, In: *Biological Effects of Man-Made Mineral Fibers*, (Wagner JC, ed.) Copenhagen: World Health Organization, 1985, pp. 209–233.

207. Jones RN, Hughes JM, Weill H: Asbestos exposure, asbestosis, and asbestos-attributable lung cancer. *Thorax* 51[Suppl 2]:S9–15, 1996.

208. Billings CG, Howard P: Asbestos exposure, lung cancer and asbestosis. *Monaldi Arch Chest Dis* 55:151–156, 2000.

209. Maltoni C, Minardi F, Morisi L: Pleural mesotheliomas in Sprague-Dawley rats by erionite: first experimental evidence. *Environ Res* 29:238–244, 1982.

210. Ozesmi M, Patiroglu TE, Hillerdal G, Ozesmi C: Peritoneal mesothelioma and malignant lymphoma in mice caused by fibrous zeolite. *Br J Ind Med* 42:746–749, 1985.

211. Suzuki Y: Carcinogenic and fibrogenic effects of zeolites: preliminary observations. *Environ Res* 27:433–445, 1982.

212. Fasske E: Experimental lung tumors following specific intrabronchial application of chrysotile asbestos. Longitudinal light and electron microscopic investigations in rats. *Respiration* 53:111–127, 1988.

213. Stanton MF, Layard M, Tegeris A, Miller E, May M, Kent E: Carcinogenicity of fibrous glass: pleural response in the rat in relation to fiber dimension. *J Natl Cancer Inst* 58:587–603, 1977.

214. Stanton MF, Layard M, Tegeris A, Miller E, May M, Morgan E, Smith A: Relation of particle dimension to carcinogenicity in amphibole asbestoses and other fibrous minerals. *J Natl Cancer Inst* 67:965–975, 1981.
215. Hesterberg TW, Barrett JC: Dependence of asbestos- and mineral dust-induced transformation of mammalian cells in culture on fiber dimension. *Cancer Res* 44:2170–2180, 1984.
216. Kogan FM, Nikitina OV: Solubility of chrysotile asbestos and basalt fibers in relation to their fibrogenic and carcinogenic action. *Environ Health Perspect* 102 [Suppl 5]:205–206, 1994.
217. Bonneau L, Malard C, Pezerat H: Studies on surface properties of asbestos. II. Role of dimensional characteristics and surface properties of mineral fibers in the induction of pleural tumors. *Environ Res* 41:268–275, 1986.
218. Coffin DL, Peters SE, Palekar LD, Stahel EP: A study of the biological activity of erionite in relation to its chemical and structural characteristics, In: *Biological interactions of inhaled mineral fibers and cigarette smoke*, (Wehner AP, ed.) Columbus: Battelle Memorial Institution, 1989, pp. 313–323.
219. Vasilewa LA, Pylev LN, Wozniak H, Wiecek E: Biological activity of synthetic amphibole asbestos. *Pol J Occup Med* 4:33–41, 1991.
220. Adachi S, Kawamura K, Kimura K, Takemoto K: Tumor incidence was not related to the thickness of visceral pleura in female Syrian hamsters intratracheally administered amphibole asbestos or manmade fibers. *Environ Res* 58:55–65, 1992.
221. Rossiter CE, Chase JR: Statistical analysis of results of carcinogenicity studies of synthetic vitreous fibres at Research and Consulting Company, Geneva. *Ann Occup Hyg* 39:759–769, 1995.
222. Barrett JC, Lamb PW, Wiseman RW: Multiple mechanisms for the carcinogenic effects of asbestos and other mineral fibers. *Environ Health Perspect* 81:81–89, 1989.
223. Chamberlain M, Tarmy EM: Asbestos and glass fibres in bacterial mutation tests. *Mutat Res* 43:159–164, 1977.
224. Light WG, Wei ET: Surface charge and a molecular basis for asbestos toxicity, In: *In Vitro Effects Of Mineral Dusts*, (Brown RC, Gormley JP, Chamberlain M, Davies R, eds.) Berlin: Springer-Verlag, 1980, pp. 139–146.
225. Reiss B, Solomon S, Tong C, Levenstein M, Rosenberg SH, Williams GM: Absence of mutagenic activity of three forms of asbestos in liver epithelial cells. *Environ Res* 27:389–397, 1982.
226. Oshimura M, Hesterberg TW, Tsutsui T, Barrett JC: Correlation of asbestos-induced cytogenetic effects with cell transformation of Syrian hamster embryo cells in culture. *Cancer Res* 44:5017–5022, 1984.
227. Brown DG, Johnson NF, Wagner MM: Multipotential behaviour of cloned rat mesothelioma cells with epithelial phenotype. *Br J Cancer* 51:245–252, 1985.
228. Jaurand MC, Bernaudin JF, Renier A, Kaplan H, Bignon J: Rat pleural mesothelial cells in culture. *In Vitro* 17:98–106, 1981.
229. Rennard SI, Jaurand MC, Bignon J, Kawanami O, Ferrans VJ, Davidson J, Crystal RG: Role of pleural mesothelial cells in the production of the submesothelial connective tissue matrix of lung. *Am Rev Respir Dis* 130:267–274, 1984.
230. Thiollet J, Jaurand MC, Kaplan H, Bignon J, Hollande E: Culture procedure of mesothelial cells from the rat parietal pleura. *Biomedicine* 29:69–73, 1978.
231. Jaurand MC, Kaplan H, Thiollet J, Pinchon MC, Bernaudin JF, Bignon J: Phagocytosis of chrysotile fibers by pleural mesothelial cells in culture. *Am J Pathol* 94:529–538, 1979.

232. Jaurand MC, Bastie-Sigeac I, Bignon J, Stoebner P: Effect of chrysotile and crocidolite on the morphology and growth of rat pleural mesothelial cells. *Environ Res* 30:255–269, 1983.

233. Paterour MJ, Bignon J, Jaurand MC: In vitro transformation of rat pleural mesothelial cells by chrysotile fibres and/or benzo[a]pyrene. *Carcinogenesis* 6:523–529, 1985.

234. Wang NS, Jaurand MC, Magne L, Kheuang L, Pinchon MC, Bignon J: The interactions between asbestos fibers and metaphase chromosomes of rat pleural mesothelial cells in culture. A scanning and transmission electron microscopic study. *Am J Pathol* 126:343–349, 1987.

235. Pass HI, Mew DJ: In vitro and in vivo studies of mesothelioma. *J Cell Biochem Suppl* 24:142–151, 1996.

236. Libbus BL, Craighead JE: Chromosomal translocations with specific breakpoints in asbestos-induced rat mesotheliomas. *Cancer Res* 48:6455–6461, 1988.

237. Fatma N, Khan SG, Aslam M, Rahman Q: Induction of chromosomal aberrations in bone marrow cells of asbestotic rats. *Environ Res* 57:175–180, 1992.

238. Tiainen M, Tammilehto L, Rautonen J, Tuomi T, Mattson K, Knuutila S: Chromosomal abnormalities and their correlations with asbestos exposure and survival in patients with mesothelioma. *Br J Cancer* 60:618–626, 1989.

239. Tiainen M, Tammilehto L, Mattson K, Knuutila S: Nonrandom chromosomal abnormalities in malignant pleural mesothelioma. *Cancer Genet Cytogenet* 33:251–274, 1988.

240. Popescu NC, Chahinian AP, DiPaolo JA: Nonrandom chromosome alterations in human malignant mesothelioma. *Cancer Res* 48:142–147, 1988.

241. Lechner JF, Tokiwa T, LaVeck M, Benedict WF, Banks-Schlegel S, Yeager H, Banerjee A, Harris CC: Asbestos-associated chromosomal changes in human mesothelial cells. *Proc Natl Acad Sci U S A* 82:3884–3888, 1985.

242. Olofsson K, Mark J: Specificity of asbestos-induced chromosomal aberrations in short-term cultured human mesothelial cells. *Cancer Genet Cytogenet* 41:33–39, 1989.

243. Achard S, Perderiset M, Jaurand MC: Sister chromatid exchanges in rat pleural mesothelial cells treated with crocidolite, attapulgite, or benzo 3–4 pyrene. *Br J Ind Med* 44:281–283, 1987.

244. Rihn B, Coulais C, Kauffer E, Bottin MC, Martin P, Yvon F, Vigneron JC, Binet S, Monhoven N, Steiblen G, Keith G: Inhaled crocidolite mutagenicity in lung DNA. *Environ Health Perspect* 108:341–346, 2000.

245. Yamaguchi R, Hirano T, Ootsuyama Y, Asami S, Tsurudome Y, Fukada S, Yamato H, Tsuda T, Tanaka I, Kasai H: Increased 8-hydroxyguanine in DNA and its repair activity in hamster and rat lung after intratracheal instillation of crocidolite asbestos. *Jpn J Cancer Res* 90:505–509, 1999.

246. Appel JD, Fasy TM, Kohtz DS, Kohtz JD, Johnson EM: Asbestos fibers mediate transformation of monkey cells by exogenous plasmid DNA. *Proc Natl Acad Sci U S A* 85:7670–7674, 1988.

247. Dubes GR, Mack LR: Asbestos-mediated transfection of mammalian cell cultures. *In Vitro Cell Dev Biol* 24:175–182, 1988.

248. Kenne K, Ljungquist S, Ringertz NR: Effects of asbestos fibers on cell division, cell survival, and formation of thioguanine-resistant mutants in Chinese hamster ovary cells. *Environ Res* 39:448–464, 1986.

249. Lipkin LE: Cellular effects of asbestos and other fibers: correlations with in vivo induction of pleural sarcoma. *Environ Health Perspect* 34:91–102, 1980.

250. Jaurand MC, Fleury J, Monchaux G, Nebut M, Bignon J: Pleural carcinogenic potency of mineral fibers (asbestos, attapulgite) and their cytotoxicity on cultured cells. *J Natl Cancer Inst* 79:797–804, 1987.

251. Versnel MA, Hagemeijer A, Bouts MJ, van der Kwast TH, Hoogsteden HC: Expression of c-sis (PDGF B-chain) and PDGF A-chain genes in ten human malignant mesothelioma cell lines derived from primary and metastatic tumors. *Oncogene* 2:601–605, 1988.

252. Marsella JM, Liu BL, Vaslet CA, Kane AB: Susceptibility of p53-deficient mice to induction of mesothelioma by crocidolite asbestos fibers. *Environ Health Perspect* 105 [Suppl 5]:1069–1072, 1997.

253. Lechner JF, LaVeck MA, Gerwin BI, Matis EA: Differential responses to growth factors by normal human mesothelial cultures from individual donors. *J Cell Physiol* 139:295–300, 1989.

254. Bielefeldt-Ohmann H, Fitzpatrick DR, Marzo AL, Jarnicki AG, Himbeck RP, Davis MR, Manning LS, Robinson BW: Patho- and immunobiology of malignant mesothelioma: characterisation of tumour infiltrating leucocytes and cytokine production in a murine model. *Cancer Immunol Immunother* 39:347–359, 1994.

255. Bielefeldt-Ohmann H, Fitzpatrick DR, Marzo AL, Jarnicki AG, Musk AW, Robinson BW: Potential for interferon-alpha-based therapy in mesothelioma: assessment in a murine model. *J Interferon Cytokine Res* 15:213–223, 1995.

256. Schwarzenberger P, Byrne P, Kolls JK: Immunotherapy-based treatment strategies for malignant mesothelioma. *Curr Opin Mol Ther* 1:104–111, 1999.

257. Moalli PA, MacDonald JL, Goodglick LA, Kane AB: Acute injury and regeneration of the mesothelium in response to asbestos fibers. *Am J Pathol* 128:426–445, 1987.

258. Branchaud RM, MacDonald JL, Kane AB: Induction of angiogenesis by intraperitoneal injection of asbestos fibers. *FASEB J* 3:1747–1752, 1989.

259. Suzuki Y, Chahinian AP, Ohnuma T: Comparative studies of human malignant mesothelioma in vivo, in xenografts in nude mice, and in vitro. Cell origin of malignant mesothelioma. *Cancer* 60:334–344, 1987.

260. Linden CJ, Johansson L: Progressive growth of a human pleural mesothelioma xenografted to athymic rats and mice. *Br J Cancer* 58:614–618, 1988.

261. Linden CJ, Johansson L: Xenografting of human pleural mesotheliomas to athymic rats and mice. *In Vivo* 2:345–348, 1988.

262. Mossman BT, Craighead JE: Use of hamster tracheal organ cultures for assessing the cocarcinogenic effects of inorganic particulates on the respiratory epithelium. *Prog Exp Tumor Res* 24:37–47, 1979.

263. Mossman BT, Craighead JE, MacPherson BV: Asbestos-induced epithelial changes in organ cultures of hamster trachea: inhibition by retinyl methyl ether. *Science* 207:311–313, 1980.

264. Holtz G, Bresnick E: Ascorbic acid inhibits the squamous metaplasia that results from treatment of tracheal explants with asbestos or benzo[a]pyrene-coated asbestos. *Cancer Lett* 42:23–28, 1988.

265. Wehner AP: *Biological Interactions of Inhaled Mineral Fibers and Cigarette Smoke*, Columbus: Battelle Memorial Institution, 1989.

266. Harvey G, Page M, Dumas L: Binding of environmental carcinogens to asbestos and mineral fibres. *Br J Ind Med* 41:396–400, 1984.

267. Kimizuka G, Azuma M, Ishibashi M, Shinozaki K, Hayashi Y: Cocarcinogenic effect of chrysotile and amosite asbestos with benzo(a)pyrene in the lung of hamsters. *Acta Pathol Jpn* 43:149–153, 1993.

268. Gerde P, Scholander P: Adsorption of benzo(a)pyrene on to asbestos and manmade mineral fibres in an aqueous solution and in a biological model solution. *Br J Ind Med* 45:682–688, 1988.

269. Mossman BT, Craighead JE: Mechanisms of asbestos carcinogenesis. *Environ Res* 25:269–280, 1981.

270. Lu YP, Lasne C, Lowy R, Chouroulinkov I: Use of the orthogonal design method to study the synergistic effects of asbestos fibres and 12-O-tetradecanoylphorbol-13-acetate (TPA) in the BALB/3T3 cell transformation system. *Mutagenesis* 3:355–362, 1988.

271. Mossman BT, Craighead JE: Comparative cocarcinogenic effects of crocidolite asbestos, hematite, kaolin and carbon in implanted tracheal organ cultures. *Ann Occup Hyg* 26:553–567, 1982.

272. Harrison PT, Heath JC: Apparent synergy between chrysotile asbestos and N-nitrosoheptamethyleneimine in the induction of pulmonary tumours in rats. *Carcinogenesis* 9:2165–2171, 1988.

273. Warren S, Brown CE, Chute RN, Federman M: Mesothelioma relative to asbestos, radiation, and methylcholanthrene. *Arch Pathol Lab Med* 105:305–312, 1981.

274. Gerde P, Scholander P: A hypothesis concerning asbestos carcinogenicity: the migration of lipophilic carcinogens in adsorbed lipid bilayers. *Ann Occup Hyg* 31:395–400, 1987.

275. Jung M, Davis WP, Taatjes DJ, Churg A, Mossman BT: Asbestos and cigarette smoke cause increased DNA strand breaks and necrosis in bronchiolar epithelial cells in vivo. *Free Radic Biol Med* 28:1295–1299, 2000.

276. Sekhon H, Wright J, Churg A: Effects of cigarette smoke and asbestos on airway, vascular and mesothelial cell proliferation. *Int J Exp Pathol* 76:411–418, 1995.

277. Churg A, Hobson J, Berean K, Wright J: Scavengers of active oxygen species prevent cigarette smoke-induced asbestos fiber penetration in rat tracheal explants. *Am J Pathol* 135:599–603, 1989.

278. Hei TK, Hall EJ, Osmak RS: Asbestos, radiation and oncogenic transformation. *Br J Cancer* 50:717–720, 1984.

279. Bernstein DM, Mast R, Anderson R, Hesterberg TW, Musselman R, Kamstrup O, Hadley J: An experimental approach to the evaluation of the biopersistence of respirable synthetic fibers and minerals. *Environ Health Perspect* 102 [Suppl 5]:15–18, 1994.

280. Bellmann B, Muhle H, Kamstrup O, Draeger UF: Investigation on the durability of man-made vitreous fibers in rat lungs. *Environ Health Perspect* 102 [Suppl 5]:185–189, 1994.

281. Brown RC, Hoskins JA, Glass LR: The in vivo biological activity of ceramic fibres. *Ann Occup Hyg* 39:705–713, 1995.

282. Dufresne A, Perrault G, Yamato H, Masse S, Begin R: Clearance of man-made mineral fibres from the lungs of sheep. *Occup Environ Med* 56:684–690, 1999.

283. Searl A, Buchanan D, Cullen RT, Jones AD, Miller BG, Soutar CA: Biopersistence and durability of nine mineral fibre types in rat lungs over 12 months. *Ann Occup Hyg* 43:143–153, 1999.

284. Donaldson K, Brown DM, Miller BG, Brody AR: Bromo-deoxyuridine (BRDU) uptake in the lungs of rats inhaling amosite asbestos or vitreous fibres at equal airborne fibre concentrations. *Exp Toxicol Pathol* 47:207–211, 1995.

285. Rogers RA, Antonini JM, Brismar H, Lai J, Hesterberg TW, Oldmixon EH, Thevenaz P, Brain JD: In situ microscopic analysis of asbestos and synthetic vitreous fibers retained in hamster lungs following inhalation. *Environ Health Perspect* 107:367–375, 1999.

286. McConnell EE: Synthetic vitreous fibers—inhalation studies. *Regul Toxicol Pharmacol* 20:S22–34, 1994.
287. Adamson IY, Prieditis H, Hedgecock C: Pulmonary response of mice to fiberglass: cytokinetic and biochemical studies. *J Toxicol Environ Health* 46:411–424, 1995.
288. Ellouk SA, Jaurand MC: Review of animal/in vitro data on biological effects of man-made fibers. *Environ Health Perspect* 102 [Suppl 2]:47–61, 1994.
289. Wheeler CS: Exposure to man-made mineral fibers: a summary of current animal data. *Toxicol Ind Health* 6:293–307, 1990.
290. Everitt JI: Mechanisms of fiber-induced diseases: implications for the safety evaluation of synthetic vitreous fibers. *Regul Toxicol Pharmacol* 20:S68–75, 1994.
291. Guthrie GD, Jr.: Mineral properties and their contributions to particle toxicity. *Environ Health Perspect* 105 [Suppl 5]:1003–1011, 1997.
292. Musselman RP, Miller WC, Eastes W, Hadley JG, Kamstrup O, Thevenaz P, Hesterberg TW: Biopersistences of man-made vitreous fibers and crocidolite fibers in rat lungs following short-term exposures. *Environ Health Perspect* 102 [Suppl 5]:139–143, 1994.
293. Searl A: A comparative study of the clearance of respirable para-aramid, chrysotile and glass fibres from rat lungs. *Ann Occup Hyg* 41:217–233, 1997.
294. Warheit DB: A review of inhalation toxicology studies with para-aramid fibrils. *Ann Occup Hyg* 39:691–697, 1995.
295. Warheit DB, Hartsky MA, Frame SR: Pulmonary effects in rats inhaling size-separated chrysotile asbestos fibres or p-aramid fibrils: differences in cellular proliferative responses. *Toxicol Lett* 88:287–292, 1996.
296. Warheit DB, Snajdr SI, Hartsky MA, Frame SR: Lung proliferative and clearance responses to inhaled para-aramid RFP in exposed hamsters and rats: comparisons with chrysotile asbestos fibers. *Environ Health Perspect* 105 [Suppl 5]:1219–1222, 1997.
297. Hesterberg TW, Miller WC, Mast R, McConnell EE, Bernstein DM, Anderson R: Relationship between lung biopersistence and biological effects of man-made vitreous fibers after chronic inhalation in rats. *Environ Health Perspect* 102 [Suppl 5]:133–137, 1994.
298. Hesterberg TW, Miller WC, Thevenaz P, Anderson R: Chronic inhalation studies of man-made vitreous fibres: characterization of fibres in the exposure aerosol and lungs. *Ann Occup Hyg* 39:637–653, 1995.
299. Hesterberg TW, Miller WC, Musselman RP, Kamstrup O, Hamilton RD, Thevenaz P: Biopersistence of man-made vitreous fibers and crocidolite asbestos in the rat lung following inhalation. *Fundam Appl Toxicol* 29:269–279, 1996.
300. Mossman BT, Gee JB: Asbestos-related diseases. *N Engl J Med* 320: 1721–1730, 1989.
301. Mossman B, Light W, Wei E: Asbestos: mechanisms of toxicity and carcinogenicity in the respiratory tract. *Annu Rev Pharmacol Toxicol* 23:595–615, 1983.
302. Fraire AE, Greenberg SD, Spjut HJ, Roggli VL, Dodson RF, Cartwright J, Williams G, Baker S: Effect of fibrous glass on rat pleural mesothelium. *Am J Respir Crit Care Med* 150:521–527, 1994.
303. Fraire AE, Greenberg SD, Spjut HJ, Dodson RF, Williams G, Lach-Pasko E, Roggli VL: Effect of erionite on pleural mesothelium of the Fischer 344 rat. *Chest* 111:1375–1380, 1997.
304. Oury TD, Day BJ, Crapo JD: Extracellular superoxide dismutase: a regulator of nitric oxide bioavailability. *Lab Invest* 75:617–636, 1996.

305. Craighead JE, Kane AB: The pathogenesis of malignant and nonmalignant serosal lesions in body cavities consequent to asbestos exposure. In: *The mesothelial cell and mesothelioma*, (Jaurand MC, Bignon J, eds.), New York: Marcel Dekker, 1994.

306. Gerwin BI: Mesothelial carcinogenesis. In: *The mesothelial cell and mesothelioma*, (Jaurand MC, Bignon J, eds.), New York: Marcel Dekker, 1994.

307. Mast RW, McConnell EE, Anderson R, Chevalier J, Kotin P, Bernstein DM, Thevenaz P, Glass LR, Miller WC, Hesterberg TW: Studies on the chronic toxicity (inhalation) of four types of refractory ceramic fiber in male Fischer 344 rats. *Inhal Toxicol* 7:425–467, 1995.

308. Mast RW, McConnell EE, Hesterberg TW, Chevalier J, Kotin P, Thevenaz P, Bernstein DM, Glass LR, Miller W, Anderson R: Multiple-dose chronic inhalation toxicity study of size-separated kaolin refractory ceramic fiber in male Fischer 344 rats. *Inhal Toxicol* 7:469–502, 1995.

309. McConnell EE, Mast RW, Hesterberg TW, Chevalier J, Kotin P, Bernstein DM, Thevenaz P, Glass LR, Anderson R: Chronic inhalation toxicity of a kaolin-based refractory ceramic fiber in Syrian golden hamsters. *Inhal Toxicol* 7:503–532, 1995.

11

Analysis of Tissue Mineral Fiber Content

Victor L. Roggli and Anupama Sharma

Introduction

The development of techniques for assaying the mineral fiber content of tissues has provided the opportunity to correlate the occurrence of various fiber-related diseases with the cumulative fiber burdens in the target organ. Exposure to mineral fibers generally occurs through the inhalation of airborne fibers, and thus the respiratory tract is the site of most asbestos-related diseases. Consequently, most studies of tissue fiber burdens have concentrated on the analysis of lung parenchyma.[1] It is the purpose of this chapter to review the various techniques which have been developed for the analysis of tissue fiber burdens, noting the advantages and limitations of each. The morphologic, crystallographic, and chemical features of the various types of asbestos are reviewed in Chapter 1, and the structure and nature of asbestos bodies in Chapter 3. In addition, the relationship between tissue asbestos burden and the various asbestos-associated diseases (see Chapters 4–7) and the various categories of occupational and environmental exposures (see Chapter 2) will also be explored in the present chapter. Finally, the overall contribution of the various types of asbestos and nonasbestos mineral fibers to the total mineral fiber burden will be discussed in relationship to the biological activity and pathogenicity of the various fiber types.

Historical Background

Throughout the twentieth century, there was considerable interest in the correlation of dusts in the workplace environment with lung diseases resulting from the inhalation of these dusts (i.e., the pneumoconioses). Analysis of lung dust burdens required considerable cooperation between the basic physical sciences and the biological and medical sciences. The distinctive behavior of fibrous materials as compared to other particulates has required many pointed studies as to inhalability, deposition, and subsequent disposal or accumulation of airborne fibers (see Chapter 10). The techniques employed were generally bulk analytical techniques such as x-ray diffraction, chemical analysis or polarizing microscopy, which were adequate in most circumstances because of the well-defined source of the dust in the workplace and the relatively large amounts of dust recoverable from the lungs of patients dying with pneumoconiosis. However, analysis of dust content from individuals exposed to asbestos posed a number of difficulties for the traditional bulk analytical approaches. First, the quantities of dust present within the lung samples were often relatively small. Second, the size of the particles posed some difficulty, since most of the asbestos fibers were less than a micron in diameter. Third, other dusts were often present in similar or even greater amounts than the asbestos component. Fourth, alteration of the chemical or crystalline properties of some types of fibers during prolonged residence in tissues complicated the precise identification of such agents. Furthermore, many of the techniques used for microfiber extraction from tissues tended to alter or destroy some of the mineral phases that were present.[2]

Clearly, the development of unique approaches for the identification of asbestos fibers in tissues was necessary before progress in this area could become possible. In the 1970s, the use of analytical electron microscopy for the identification and characterization of individual asbestos fibers isolated from human tissues was pioneered in large part by the innovative studies of investigators such as Arthur Langer in the United States and Fred Pooley in Great Britain.[3–8] The usefulness of these techniques has since been confirmed by other investigators,[9–14] and from the 1980s to the present time, these techniques have been employed to correlate the tissue asbestos burden with various asbestos-related diseases.[11,15–19]

Methods for Analysis of Tissue Mineral Fiber Content

Tissue Selection

As noted in the introduction, most studies of tissue mineral fiber content have examined lung parenchyma. There is no inherent reason why the techniques developed for this purpose cannot be applied to other tissues. However, little information has been published on the expected values of mineral fiber content of tissues other than the lung. Therefore, any investigator wishing to study such tissues must establish normal ranges for his or her laboratory and the analytical technique employed. In this regard, it should be noted that the expected levels of fibers in extrapulmonary tissues would be at or below the limits of detection for current techniques, and background contamination can be a considerable problem. In this section, comments regarding selection of tissue for mineral fiber analysis will be confined to lung parenchyma.

In most circumstances, formalin-fixed lung tissue is utilized, although fresh specimens work just as well. In some instances, paraffin-embedded tissue is all that is available. Such samples can be deparaffinized in xylene and rehydrated to 95% ethanol. The dehydration process removes some components of tissue, mainly lipids, so that a correction factor must be applied to equate the values obtained from paraffin blocks to those obtained from formalin-fixed tissue. In the authors' laboratory, the correction factor has been determined to be approximately 0.7 (i.e., the asbestos fiber concentration determined from a paraffin block should be multiplied by 0.7).[17]

In selecting tissue for digestion, areas of consolidation, congestion, or tumor should be avoided as much as possible. Such pathologic alterations would affect the denominator in calculations of the tissue concentration of fibers or asbestos bodies. Because there is some site-to-site variation of mineral fiber content within the lung, the more tissue that is available for analysis the better. Ideal specimens include autopsy, pneumonectomy, or lobectomy specimens, with analysis of multiple sites. In the authors' laboratory, two or three samples are typically analyzed for a lobectomy or pneumonectomy specimen, whereas four sites (upper and lower lobes of each lung) are sampled when both lungs are available at autopsy. Samples usually include lung parenchyma abutting against the visceral pleura, with each sample typically weighing 0.25 to 0.35 gm (wet weight). However, analyses may be performed on as little as 0.1 gm or less of wet tissue. Although some studies have reported analyses of transbronchial biopsy specimens,[20–22] the small size of such samples (usually 2–5 mg of tissue at best) makes them unlikely to be representative.[23,24]

Digestion Technique

Techniques for mineral fiber analysis generally involve three basic steps. First, there is dissolution and removal of the organic matrix material of the lung in which the fibers are embedded. Second, the mineral fibers are recovered and concentrated. Third, the fiber content is analyzed by some form of microscopy.[1] Dissolution steps involve either wet chemical digestion or ashing. Wet chemical digestion can be accomplished with sodium or potassium hydroxide, hydrogen peroxide, 5.25% sodium hypochlorite solution (commercial bleach), formamide, or proteolytic enzymes.[12] Most investigators prefer an alkali wet chemical digestion using either sodium hypochlorite or sodium or potassium hydroxide. Tissue ashing is an alternative approach. Ashing in a muffle furnace at 400°C to 500°C is unsuitable, because the drying and shrinkage of the tissue causes fragmentation of the fibers, artefactually increasing fiber numbers and decreasing mean fiber lengths. This problem is largely avoided by ashing the sample in a low temperature plasma asher.[25]

Once the digestion of the tissue is complete, the inorganic residue may then be collected on an acetate or polycarbonate filter, or an aliquot can be transferred into a Fuchs–Rosenthal counting chamber for direct counting of fibers by phase contrast light microscopy.[15] However, a permanent sample cannot be prepared with this latter technique, so most investigators prefer filtration, with a pore size of 0.2 to 0.45 μm. Use of a pore size which is too large in relation to the size of the fibers to be analyzed can result in significant loss of fibers and underestimation of the mineral fiber content of the sample.[26] Details of the digestion procedure employed by the authors are provided in the Appendix.

Fiber Identification and Quantification

A number of analytical techniques have been used for the identification of asbestos fibers in bulk samples, including x-ray diffractometry, infrared spectroscopy, differential thermal analysis, and polarization microscopy with dispersion staining.[2,6,11] For a variety of reasons as noted above in the section on "Historical Background," these techniques have severe limitations in regard to the identification of fibers from human lung tissue samples, and in practice bulk analytical techniques have been ineffective for this purpose.[2,6,11] As a result, investigators have turned to the use of various forms of microscopy for the analysis of pulmonary mineral fiber content. These include conventional bright field light microscopy, phase contrast light microscopy, scanning electron microscopy, and transmission electron microscopy.

Conventional bright field light microscopy is a simple, inexpensive technique that requires no special instrumentation. This technique, detailed in Chapter 3, is ideal for the quantification of asbestos bodies.[1–14,17] A few uncoated asbestos fibers can also be observed, but the vast majority of fibers are beyond the resolution of this technique. Furthermore, conventional light microscopy cannot distinguish among the various fiber types. Asbestos bodies can be counted at a magnification of 200 to 400×, and the results reported as numbers per gram of wet lung tissue.[12,17] Alternatively, a piece of lung tissue adjacent to the one actually analyzed can be dried to constant weight to obtain a wet-to-dry weight ratio, and the results reported as asbestos bodies per gram of dry weight.[11,14]

Phase contrast light microscopy (PCLM) has also been used by investigators to quantify the tissue mineral fiber burden.[15,18,19] This technique can resolve fibers with a diameter of 0.2 μm or greater, and it reveals that uncoated fibers greatly outnumber the coated ones (i.e., asbestos bodies).[27] However, a substantial proportion of asbestos fibers have diameters less than 0.2 μm, and thus are not detectable by PCLM. As is the case for conventional light microscopy, one cannot distinguish among the various types of asbestos fibers or differentiate asbestos from nonasbestos fibers by PCLM. Investigators using this technique have generally reported results as total fibers/gm dry lung tissue or separately as asbestos bodies and uncoated fibers/gm dry lung tissue.[15,28] Some investigators have also reported results as fibers per cm^3 of lung tissue.[29] As a rule of thumb, one fiber/gm wet lung (approximately equals to) ≅ one fiber/cm^3 ≅ ten fibers/gm dry lung.[23]

Scanning electron microscopy (SEM) has been used by some investigators for the quantification of tissue mineral fiber content.[17,24,30] This technique offers several advantages over PCLM and conventional bright field light microscopy. At low magnifications (1000×), asbestos bodies and uncoated fibers can be counted yielding quantitative results similar to those obtained with PCLM (Figure 11-1).[17] At higher magni-

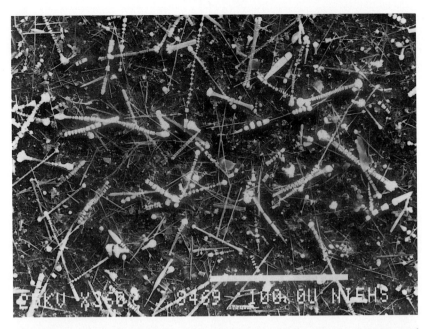

Figure 11-1. Scanning electron micrograph of Nuclepore filter preparation of lung tissue from an asbestos insulator with malignant pleural mesothelioma and asbestosis. Numerous asbestos bodies and uncoated asbestos fibers are visible. This patient's lung tissue contained nearly 3 million asbestos bodies and more than 9 million uncoated fibers 5 μm or greater in length per gram of wet lung. Magnified ×360.

fications (10,000–20,000×), the superior resolution of SEM permits the detection of fibers not visible by PCLM, with fibers as small as 0.3 μm long and 0.05 μm in diameter detected by this technique.[30] Furthermore, SEM can be coupled with energy dispersive x-ray analysis (EDXA) to determine the chemical composition of individual fibers (Figure 11-2). This information can in turn be used to classify a fiber as asbestos or nonasbestos and to determine the specific asbestos fiber type.[17,30–32] Sample preparation for SEM is relatively simple, requiring only that the filter be mounted on a suitable substrate (such as a carbon disc) with carbon paste, and then coated with a suitable conducting material (such as carbon, platinum or gold). Also, SEM analysis of mineral fibers has the potential for automation using commercially available automated image x-ray analyzers[33] and software programs which discriminate between fibers and other particles.[34,35] Disadvantages of SEM include the high cost of the instrumentation and the considerable time required for analysis (an hour or more per sample).

Transmission electron microscopy (TEM) is the analytical technique that has been preferred by most investigators for the determination of mineral fiber content in tissue digest preparations.[7,8,11,16,18,21,28] This technique provides the highest resolution for the identification of the smallest fibrils and can be coupled with EDXA for determination of the chemical composition of individual fibers. TEM has the further advantage that selected area electron diffraction (SAED) can also be performed, providing information regarding the crystalline structure of an

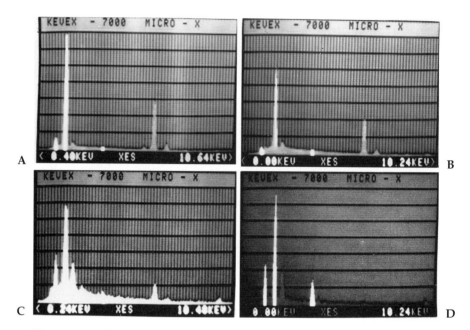

Figure 11-2. Energy dispersive x-ray spectra of four different amphibole asbestos fibers. **(A)** Amosite has peaks for Si, Fe, Mg, and sometimes Mn. **(B)** Crocidolite has peaks for Si, Fe, Na, and Mg. **(C)** Anthophyllite has peaks for Si, Mg, and Fe. **(D)** Tremolite has peaks for Si, Mg, and Ca. Peak in each spectrum immediately to right of Si is due to Au used to coat specimen. (Reprinted from Ref. 17, with permission.)

individual particle. The diffraction pattern of a fiber (Figure 11-3) can provide information useful for identification purposes, especially when the chemical compositions of two fibers are similar.[36,37] For example, SAED can readily distinguish chrysotile from anthophyllite asbestos, or anthophyllite from talc.[37] Methods for preparation of tissue samples for TEM analysis have been described;[37,38] however, these techniques are more complex than preparative steps for light microscopy or SEM. Therefore, there is increased opportunity for loss of fibers or contamination of the sample. Also, only a small proportion of a filter can be mounted on a TEM grid, so that one must be concerned with whether the portion of the filter sampled is truly representative.[23] As is the case for SEM, analysis of mineral fiber content of tissue by TEM is both time-consuming and expensive. Results are generally reported in terms of fibers per gram of wet or dry lung tissue. The magnifications used are generally too high to accurately assess the tissue asbestos body content by TEM.

Two other techniques deserve brief mention as potentially useful for tissue mineral fiber analysis. The confocal scanning optical microscope uses a focused light beam to scan across the sample and the image is detected and processed electronically.[39,40] This light microscopic technique has a resolution of 0.1 μm or better, which is superior to that of PCLM and thus would permit detection of considerably more fibers. The image is focused in a discrete plane with a thickness of less than

1 μm. Because asbestos fibers may be present at different depths in a filter preparation, quantitative examination of a filter with this imaging technique could be time-consuming. Another technique with potential value is scanning transmission electron microscopy (STEM). This technique has the high resolution and the capacity for electron diffraction that are characteristic of TEM.[41,42] Furthermore, the scanning mode of operation produces an image that is amenable to automated analysis. Hence STEM has many characteristics that would be ideal for a standardized and automated approach to mineral fiber analysis.

Variability of Results

The wide variety of preparative techniques and analytical methodologies that have been employed by various investigators make it difficult to extrapolate results from one laboratory to another. The actual analytical result obtained on any one sample can be profoundly influenced by the steps employed in the analytical procedure (Table 11-1).[1] Interlaboratory comparison trials demonstrate that striking differences can

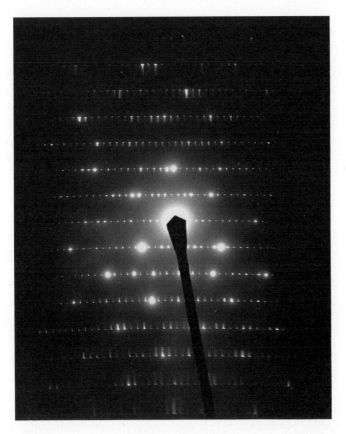

Figure 11-3. Selected area electron diffraction pattern obtained from an asbestos body core of an insulation worker. The pattern shows discrete dots along each layer line, with a calculated 5.3Å interlayer-line spacing typical for amphibole asbestos. (Reprinted from Roggli VL et al.: New techniques for imaging and analyzing lung tissue. Environ Hlth Persp. 56:163–183, 1984; Figure 4.)

Table 11-1. Factors affecting fiber burden data*

I. Digestion Procedure
   A. Wet chemical digestion (alkali, enzymes)
   B. Low temperature plasma ashing
   C. Number of sites sampled
II. Recovery Procedure
   A. Use of centrifugation step
   B. Use of a sonication step
   C. Filtration step (type of filter, pore size)
III. Analytical Procedure
   A. Microscopic technique (LM, PCLM, SEM, TEM)
   B. Magnification used
   C. Sizes of fibers counted and other "counting rules"
   D. Numbers of fibers or fields actually counted
IV. Reporting of Results
   A. Asbestos bodies or fibers (or both)
   B. Sizes of fibers counted
   C. Concentration of fibers (per gm wet or dry lung or per em³)

LM = light microscopy; PCLM = phase contrast light microscopy
SEM = scanning electron microscopy; TEM = transmission electron microscopy
*Reprinted from Ref. 1

occur among laboratories even when the same sample is analyzed.[43] Some asbestos bodies and fibers may be lost during the preparation process,[44,45] and some of the smallest fibers are difficult to recognize and count in a reproducible fashion.[46] On the other hand, use of a sonication step or ashing of the specimen can enhance the fragmentation of chrysotile fibers, artefactually increasing fiber numbers.[22,44] Nonetheless, there is evidence for internal consistency within individual laboratories, with similar ranking of samples among different laboratories from the lowest to the highest tissue fiber concentration. Still, one must use caution in comparing results between laboratories, bearing in mind any differences in the analytical procedures employed.[1]

In addition to interlaboratory variation, intralaboratory variation can occur, which may be due either to changes in a laboratory's procedures over time[47] or to variation in fiber content from one site to another within the lung.[27,48] Morgan and Holmes[27,48] have reported a five- to tenfold site-to-site variation based on analyses of multiple samples from a single lung using phase contrast light microscopy. In the authors' experience using light microscopy for asbestos body quantification (Figure 11-4) or SEM for asbestos body and uncoated fiber quantification (Figure 11-5), paired samples have asbestos body and fiber concentration values ranging from identical to within a factor of two or three. Rarely, two samples from the same patient may differ by as much as a factor of 10. The coefficient of variation for counting the same sample on multiple occasions is on the order of 10%.[49] When interpreting fiber burden data, one must keep in mind that the analysis is occurring at a single point in time, usually when advanced disease is present. The fiber burden at that time may or may not relate to the tissue fiber content at the time when disease was actively evolving.[1] Nonetheless, there is a growing consensus that the fiber burdens that persist in the lung are the primary determinant of subsequent disease.[50,51]

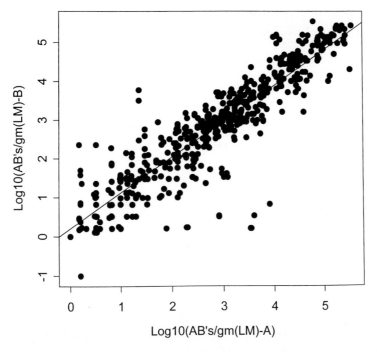

Figure 11-4. Correlation of asbestos body counts by light microscopy in 420 cases where multiple sites were sampled. Graph shows all pairwise comparisons, with the linear regression equation given by $\log y = 0.92 \log x + 0.20$ (correlation coefficient $r = 0.91$, $p = 0.0000$). Statistical analysis per Dr. Robin Vollmer, Durham VA Medical Center, Durham, NC.

Asbestos Content of Lung Tissue in Asbestos-Associated Diseases

Asbestosis

Relatively few studies have been published in which the asbestos content of lung tissue was examined in a series of patients with asbestosis.[15,16,18,28,52] The data from these studies are summarized in Table 11-2. Except for the unusually high median count for asbestos bodies in the study by Ashcroft and Heppleston,[28] and the high mean count for uncoated fibers by electron microscopy in the study by Wagner et al.,[18] the values are roughly similar among the reported series. This is rather remarkable when one considers the wide range of values obtained when different laboratories examine the same sample[43] and the different techniques employed in the various studies referred to in Table 11-2. For example, Whitwell et al.[15] used PCLM and counted all fibers greater than or equal to 6μm in length, counting asbestos bodies and uncoated fibers together. Ashcroft and Heppleston[28] used PCLM at a magnification of 400× and counted all visible fibers, reporting coated and uncoated fibers separately. Warnock et al.[16] used TEM and counted all fibers exceeding 0.25μm in length and with an aspect ratio (length to width) of three or greater. The study by Warnock et al.[16] also counted asbestos bodies by conventional light microscopy. Wagner et al.[18] used

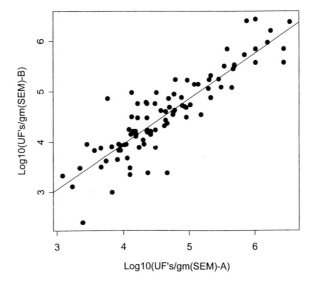

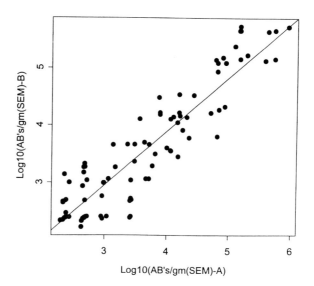

Figure 11-5. (Top) Correlation of uncoated fiber concentrations for fibers 5 μm or greater in length by SEM in 67 cases where multiple sites were sampled. Graph shows all pairwise comparisons, with the linear regression equation given by $\log y = 0.91 \log x + 0.33$ (r = 0.88, p = 0.0000). **(Bottom)** Correlation of asbestos body counts by scanning electron microscopy (SEM) in 66 cases where multiple sites were sampled. Graph shows all pairwise comparisons, with the linear regression equation given by $\log y = 0.94 \log x + 0.12$ (correlation coefficient r = 0.92, p = 0.0000). Statistical analysis per Dr. Robin Vollmer, Durham VA Medical Center, Durham, NC.

Table 11-2. Asbestos content of lung tissue in reported series of patients with asbestosis*

Source	No. of cases	Method[t]	Asbestos bodies/gm	Uncoated fibers/gm
Whitwell et al.[15]	23	PCLM	—	8 (1.0–70)
Ashcroft and Heppleston[28]	22	PCLM	12.2 (0.49–192)	32 (1.3–493)
Warnock et al.[16]	22	TEM[t]	0.123 (0.001–7.38)	5.68 (1.6–121)
Wagner et al.[18]	100	PCLM	—	1.5 (0.001–31.6)
	170	TEM	—	372 (<1.0–10,000)
Churg and Vedal[53]	23	TEM	—	10 (±6.6)

*Values reported as the median counts for millions (10[6]) of asbestos bodies or uncoated fibers per gram of dried lung tissue, with ranges indicated in parentheses, except for the study of Wagner et al.[18] where only the mean value could be determined from the data presented, and the study by Churg and Vedal,[53] where results are reported as geometric mean and standard deviation.
[t]In this study, asbestos bodies were counted by conventional light microscopy.
PCLM = phase contrast light microscopy; TEM = transmission electron microscopy.

the PCLM method of Ashcroft and Heppleston[28] as well as TEM. Churg and Vedal[53] used TEM and counted all fibers exceeding 0.5 µm in length. The median uncoated fiber count exceeds one million fibers per gram of dried lung tissue in all five studies.

The asbestos content of the lung in 170 patients with histologically confirmed asbestosis from the authors' laboratory is summarized in Table 11-3. Our laboratory employs SEM at a magnification of 1000×, counting all fibers with a length greater than or equal to 5 µm. Asbestos bodies are counted also by light microscopy. The median asbestos body count for patients with asbestosis is 22,000 asbestos bodies per gram of wet lung tissue. The median uncoated fiber count in 142 asbestosis cases examined by SEM is 179,000 fibers per gram of wet lung. The results can be approximately converted to bodies or fibers per gram of dry lung tissue by multiplying by a factor of 10.[11] For comparison, the median asbestos body count from individuals with normal lungs and no known occupational asbestos exposure is 0.4 AB/gm. The median count by SEM for uncoated fibers 5 µm or greater in length for our control cases is approximately 3100 fibers/gm. In 95% of the cases of asbestosis, the asbestos body content is 1200 AB/gm or greater. At this tissue asbestos body concentration, several asbestos bodies should be observed on most 2 × 2 cm histologic sections stained for iron and examined systematically (Chapter 3).[52] Thus the finding of asbestos

Table 11-3. Asbestos content of lung tissue in 170 cases of asbestosis[a]

	N	AB/gm (LM)	N	UF/gm (SEM)
Asbestosis[b]	52	17,100 (250–1,400,000)	48	152,000 (5,960–12,500,000)
Asbestosis plus lung cancer	74	28,600 (150–343,000)	71	180,000 (18,500–7,810,000)
Asbestosis plus peritoneal mesothelioma	9	140,000 (340–684,000)	9	380,000 (38,100–788,000)
Asbestosis plus pleural mesothelioma	35	14,900 (1,570–1,600,000)	36	77,800 (12,800–9,310,000)

[a]Asbestos bodies per gram of wet lung tissue as determined by light microscopy (LM) and uncoated fibers 5 µm or greater in length per gram of wet lung tissue as determined by scanning electron microscopy (SEM). Values reported as median with range in parentheses.
[b]Cases of asbestosis with neither lung cancer nor mesothelioma.

bodies in histologic sections is a reasonable histopathologic criterion for the diagnosis of asbestosis (Chapter 4).[54]

A few studies have investigated the relationship between tissue asbestos burden and the fibrotic response in human lungs (Table 11-4). Whitwell et al.[15] found a progressive increase in median total coated and uncoated fiber count from patients with mild (1+) to severe (3+) fibrosis. Ashcroft and Heppleston[28] also reported a progression in the severity of fibrosis with increasing uncoated fiber count from no fibrosis to moderate (2+) fibrosis, but no further increase in fiber count from moderate to severe disease. These authors concluded that additional factors other than tissue fiber burden must be involved in progression from moderate to severe fibrosis.[28] Warnock et al.[16] graded the severity of fibrosis on a scale of 0 to 3+ based on visual inspection of the cut surface of inflation fixed specimens, with 1/2+ defined as microscopic fibrosis only. These authors found no apparent correlation between the severity of fibrosis and total fiber content for all fibers $0.25\,\mu m$ or greater in length as assessed by TEM.[16] Wagner et al.[18] graded the severity of fibrosis microscopically on a scale of 0 to 4. Their data are summarized in Table 11-4, and for the sake of convenience have been tabulated as 0 to 3 with their grade 1 fibrosis listed under 1/2+. These authors found a progressive increase in optically visible and electron microscopically enumerated fibers with increasing severity of asbestosis.[18]

The relationship between the tissue content of uncoated fibers $5\,\mu m$ or greater in length as assessed by SEM in the authors' laboratory and the histologic asbestosis score as determined by the method proposed by the Pneumoconiosis Committee of the College of American Pathologists[55] is shown in Figure 11-6. These data are based on 36 cases of asbestosis for which tissue was available for analysis of asbestos content.[56] There is a statistically significant relationship ($p < 0.01$) between fiber content and histologic score, although there is a wide range of scatter of the data points. It is likely that the degree of correlation would improve with more extensive histologic and mineralogical sampling of the lungs and expression of the data as total lung burden rather than fiber concentration.[17] This is because of the fact that accumulation of collagen and other cellular components as a result of

Table 11-4. Severity of asbestosis vs. tissue asbestos content as total fibers/gm dried lung*

Study	Asbestosis grade				
	0	1/2+	1+	2+	3+
Whitwell et al.[15]			8×10^6	14×10^6	37×10^6
Ashcroft and Heppleston[28]	2.4×10^6		20×10^6	200×10^6	144×10^6
Warnock et al.[16]	4.8×10^6	5.7×10^6	48×10^6	11×10^6	3.6×10^6
Wagner et al.[18]	0.005×10^6	0.009×10^6	0.015×10^6	0.12×10^6	1.2×10^6
	1.3×10^6	31.6×10^6	44×10^6	68×10^6	464×10^6

*Values indicated represent the median counts derived from the data presented in the reference that is cited. Asbestosis grade is as defined in each original source. First two studies employed phase contrast light microscopy whereas the study by Warnock et al.[16] used transmission electron microscopy and the study of Wagner et al.[18] used both (phase contrast results from Figure 11-2 of the latter study listed first, and EM results from Figure 11-1 listed below). Wagner et al.[18] grading scheme of 0 to 4 has been modified to 0 to 3 simply for purposes of tabulation.
Source: Reprinted from Ref. 54, with permission.

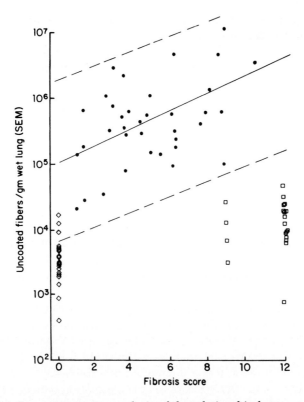

Figure 11-6. Linear regression analysis of the relationship between the severity of fibrosis and the pulmonary concentration of uncoated fibers 5 µm or greater in length as determined in 36 autopsied cases of asbestosis by SEM. The regression equation is given by $\log y = 0.117x + 5.05$ and is indicated by the solid black line. Dashed lines mark the 95% confidence limits. Asbestosis (•), diffuse pulmonary fibrosis of unknown cause (□), and normal autopsied lung (◇). (Reprinted from Ref. 56, with permission.)

the scarring process increases the weight of the lungs and hence dilutes the concentration of fibers in the parenchyma, a point often overlooked in dust analysis studies.[57] There is a statistically significant association between histologic score and total (coated plus uncoated) fiber content as assessed by SEM, but not between histologic score and asbestos body content as measured by light microscopy (Table 11-5). Furthermore, there was no significant association between histologic score and patient age, duration of occupational exposure, or pack-years of smoking.[54]

Figure 11-6 also shows the fiber content of the lung in 24 cases with diffuse pulmonary fibrosis and some history of asbestos exposure, but lacking histologic criteria for the diagnosis of asbestosis (Chapter 4). In every case, the fiber count is below the 95% confidence interval for bona fide cases of asbestosis. Very few patients with grade 4 or higher asbestosis have uncoated fiber counts below 100,000 per gram, although some patients with fibrosis confined to the walls of small airways (grade 3 or less) have values well below this level.[54] This observation is in agreement with the findings of Churg[58] that relatively low tissue asbestos burdens occur in chrysotile miners and millers with

Table 11-5. Correlation of histologic grade of asbestosis with tissue asbestos content and other parameters

	Correlation coefficient (r)	P
Uncoated fibers/gm (>5μm), SEM	0.46	<0.01
Total fibers/gm (coated and uncoated), SEM	0.44	<0.01
Asbestos bodies/gm, LM	0.26	NS
Smoking history, pk-yrs.	0.22	NS
Age	0.12	NS
Duration of exposure, yr.	0.06	NS

SEM = scanning electron microscopy; LM = light microscopy; pk-yr = packs smoked daily × no. years smoked; NS = not significant (p > 0.05). Reprinted from Ref. 54, with permission.

fibrosis confined to the walls of small airways. It should be noted that the intercept of the regression line in Figure 11-6 is approximately 100,000 fibers per gram of wet lung (or one million fibers per gram of dried lung), which coincides with the lower limit of the range of values shown in Table 11-2. Figure 11-6 also shows the fiber burden level for 20 cases with normal lungs and no history of asbestos exposure. The median fiber count for these cases is one and a half orders of magnitude less than the intercept at zero fibrosis for asbestosis cases. This observation indicates that there is a threshold for asbestos exposure and the development of any degree of lung fibrosis.

Thus, there generally appears to be a correlation between the severity of fibrosis in patients with asbestosis and the tissue mineral fiber burden, although there is a wide scatter in the data.[28,54] In this regard, studies by Timbrell et al.[59] (reviewed by Lippmann[60]) have shown that among individuals exposed to the various types of amphibole asbestos, the severity of pulmonary fibrosis correlates better with the relative fiber surface area per unit weight of tissue than with the relative fiber number or mass, as determined by magnetic alignment and light scattering. On the other hand, Churg et al.,[61] in a study of asbestosis among chrysotile miners and millers, found no correlation between fibrosis and fiber size, surface area, or mass for chrysotile, and an inverse correlation with fiber length, aspect ratio, and surface area for contaminating tremolite asbestos. These authors did show a direct correlation between fiber concentration and severity of fibrosis for both chrysotile and tremolite fibers.[61] Further studies of the mineralogical correlates of fiber-induced pulmonary fibrosis are needed in order to resolve these discrepancies.[1]

In summary, analysis of tissue mineral fiber burdens in patients with asbestosis indicates a heavy lung asbestos burden in the vast majority of cases. This observation is consistent with epidemiologic evidence that asbestosis occurs primarily in individuals with direct and prolonged occupational exposure to asbestos.[1] Since no uniform method for the analysis of tissue mineral fiber content has been established, it is not presently possible to recommend a specific tissue asbestos fiber content to be used as a criterion for the pathologic diagnosis of asbestosis. Nonetheless, based on the data summarized in Table 11-2 and Figure 11-6, it seems unlikely that a patient with clinically significant pulmonary interstitial fibrosis (i.e., symptomatic with substantial phys-iologic impairment) who has fewer than 10^6 fibers 5 μm or greater in length per gram of dried lung (10^5 fibers/gm wet lung) tissue is suf-fering from asbestosis.[54] Whereas the fibrogenicity of asbestos fibers 5 μm or greater in length is well established,[62–66] the fibrogenicity of fibers less than 5 μm in length remains unproven[67] (see Chapter 10). Therefore, no tissue level of fibers in the latter size range should be pro-posed as a criterion for the diagnosis of asbestosis.[54]

Malignant Mesothelioma

Several studies have examined the asbestos content of lung tissue in series of patients with mesothelioma.[15,22,53,68–72] The data from these studies are summarized in Table 11-6. Whitwell et al.[15] studied 100 patients with malignant mesothelioma by means of PCLM. The median count was 750,000 combined fibers and bodies per gram of dried lung, with a range of 0 to 70 million fibers per gram. In only seven cases was the combined count less than 20,000 per gram, and in six of these, there was no identifiable occupational exposure to asbestos. In contrast, the count was less than 20,000 per gram in 71% of the normal control series in the same study.[15] Gylseth et al.[68] examined 15 cases of malignant mesothelioma counting fibers by means of SEM at a magnification of 4500×, and compared the results with those of 14 cases of parietal pleural plaques and 12 control cases without cancer or chronic respi-ratory disease. The median fiber count in the patients with mesothe-lioma was 11 million per gram of dried lung as compared to 2.2 million per gram in the pleural plaque cases and 0.6 million per gram among the control cases. Mowe et al.[69] used SEM at a magnification of 4500× to analyze the asbestos fiber content of lung tissue from 14 cases of mesothelioma and 28 controls matched for age, sex, year of death, and county of residence. These investigators reported a median fiber count of 2.4 million fibers per gram of dried lung among the mesothelioma

Table 11-6. Asbestos content of lung tissue in reported series of patients with mesothelioma*

Source	No. of cases	Method†	Asbestos bodies/gm dried lung	Uncoated fibers/gm dried lung
Whitwell et al.[15]	100	PCLM	—	0.75 (0–70)
Gylseth et al.[68]	15	SEM	—	11 (2–490)
Mowe et al.[69]	14	SEM	—	2.4 (0.4–37)
Dodson et al.[70]	55	TEM‡	9.56 (0.06–1250)	0.70 (0.022–69.0)
Churg and Vedal[53]	83	TEM	—	0.92
Churg et al.[71]	15	TEM	—	214 (SD ± 9)
Gaudichet et al.[72]	20	TEM‡	3.2 (0.04–450)	18
Warnock[73]	27	TEM‡	18.5 (1.9–3800)	4.9 (0.57–137)

*Values reported are the median counts for thousands (10^3) of asbestos bodies or millions (10^6) of uncoated fibers per gram of dried lung tissue, with ranges indicated in parentheses. The studies by Churg and Vedal,[53] Churg et al.,[71] and Gaudichet et al.[72] provided the mean value for total fibers per gm dried lung. Geometric standard deviation is given in parentheses for the study by Churg et al.[71]
†PCLM = phase contrast light microscopy; SEM = scanning electron microscopy; TEM = transmission electron microscopy.
‡In these three studies, asbestos bodies were counted by conventional light microscopy.

patients as compared to 0.25 million fibers per gram among the controls. Dodson et al.[70] used TEM to study the asbestos content of 55 patients with mesothelioma, and reported a median value of 698,000 fibers per gram. Churg and Vedal[53] examined the mineral fiber content of lung tissue by TEM from 83 patients with malignant mesothelioma and heavy mixed amosite and chrysotile exposure. The geometric mean asbestos fiber count was 920,000 fibers per gram of dried lung. Churg et al.[71] also studied 15 cases of mesothelioma in chrysotile miners and millers. The geometric mean asbestos fiber count in this group was 214 million fibers per gram of dried lung. These authors concluded that patients with mesothelioma due to exposure to chrysotile from mining and milling have large pulmonary fiber burdens relative to patients with mesothelioma secondary to exposure to amosite or crocidolite asbestos.

Gaudichet et al.[72] examined lung tissue in 20 patients with mesothelioma and compared the results with those from 40 lung cancer cases and 20 patients who died from nonmalignant, nonasbestos-related processes. The mean total fiber burden for the patients with mesothelioma was 18 million fibers per gram of dried lung, as compared to 16 million fibers per gram for the lung cancer cases and 11.2 million fibers per gram for the nonmalignant control group. The main difference between the mesothelioma cases and the other comparison groups was in regard to the greater numbers of commercial amphibole fibers (amosite and crocidolite) in the former as compared to the latter. Warnock[73] studied the mineral fiber content of lung tissue in 27 shipyard and construction workers with mesothelioma. The median total fiber count by TEM was 4.9 million fibers per gram of dried lung. In contrast, the median count in 19 unexposed controls was 0.85 million fibers per gram.

Although valuable information can also be obtained from an analysis of the tissue asbestos body content in mesothelioma cases, only a few studies have reported such data in a series of patients with malignant mesothelioma. Dodson et al.[70] reported a median asbestos body count of 9560 asbestos bodies per gram dried lung in 55 patients with mesothelioma. Gaudichet et al.[72] reported a median asbestos body concentration of 3200 asbestos bodies per gram of dried lung tissue in 20 patients with mesothelioma. The concentration exceeded 1000 asbestos bodies/gm in 70% of mesothelioma patients, but in only 10% of 80 age- and sex-matched control cases. Warnock[73] found a median asbestos body count of 18,500 bodies per gram of dried lung in 27 patients with mesothelioma, as compared to 300 bodies/gm in 19 nonexposed controls. Kishimoto et al.[74] reported a median asbestos body concentration of 1360 asbestos bodies per gram of wet lung (approximately 13,600 bodies/gm dried lung) in eight Japanese workers with mesothelioma.

The asbestos content of the lung in 281 patients with malignant mesothelioma from the authors' laboratory is summarized in Table 11-7. The median asbestos body count for mesothelioma cases that also had asbestosis is much higher than cases that had parietal pleural plaques without asbestosis, which in turn is much higher than cases that had neither plaques nor asbestosis. In addition, the median

Table 11-7. Asbestos content of lung tissue in 281 cases of mesothelioma[a]

	N	AB/gm (LM)	N	UF/gm (SEM)
Pleural Mesothelioma				
Asbestosis	35	14,900 (1,570–1,600,000)	36	77,800 (12,800–9,310,000)
PPP	85	900 (2.2–74,500)	79	24,900 (950–781,000)
Other	143	97 (0.8–84,100)	137	18,900 (670–1,040,000)
Peritoneal Mesothelioma				
Asbestosis	9	140,000 (340–684,000)	9	380,000 (38,100–788,000)
PPP	3	1,450 (14.4–23,100)	2	122,000 (39,800–205,000)
Other	6	10 (1.0–590)	6	6,520 (2,430–23,900)

[a] Asbestos bodies per gram of wet lung tissue as determined by light microscopy (LM) and uncoated fibers 5 μm or greater in length per gram of wet lung tissue as determined by scanning electron microscopy (SEM). Values reported as median with range in parentheses.
PPP = parietal pleural plaques; Other = cases with neither asbestosis nor plaques (or uninformative cases with regard to plaques or asbestosis)

asbestos body count for each of these categories is higher for patients with peritoneal as compared to pleural mesotheliomas. A similar trend is observed for uncoated fibers as measured by SEM (Table 11-7). These findings are consistent with the observation that, on average, greater exposure to asbestos is necessary for the development of peritoneal mesothelioma than is needed to develop pleural mesothelioma.[75] The asbestos body counts and fiber levels in the authors' laboratory are reported per gram of wet lung, and can be compared with those of other investigators by multiplying by a factor of 10 to convert to counts per gram of dried lung.

The asbestos body content was within our normal range of 0–20 AB/gm in 48 cases, or 17% of the total. In 18 of these 48 cases, the fiber content was found to be elevated by SEM.[76] Hence, the asbestos content was indistinguishable from that of a background population in 11% of cases (Figure 11-7). The median asbestos body count for 33 women with mesothelioma was 31 AB/gm (range: 1.6–14,100 AB/gm). The median uncoated fiber count by SEM for 31 women was 13,000 fibers/gm (range: 1570–162,000 fibers/gm). Fifteen cases had asbestos body counts within background range, and six of these had an elevated fiber count by SEM. Hence, approximately 27% of mesotheliomas in women had an asbestos content indistinguishable from background. Most of the cases with a normal-range asbestos body count and an elevated fiber content by SEM had predominantly noncommercial amphiboles (mostly tremolite). These fibers typically were in the size range between 5 and 20 μm. Asbestos bodies usually form on fibers that are greater than 20 μm in length (see Chapter 3).

The predominant fiber type identified in patients with mesothelioma is commercial amphibole (amosite or crocidolite).[53,70,72,73,77–79] In a study of 94 cases from the United States, Roggli et al. found that 58% of more than 1500 fibers analyzed were amosite, whereas only 3% were crocidolite.[77] In a separate study, the concentration of commercial amphibole fibers showed a significant correlation with the duration of asbestos exposure.[80] Patients with direct exposures to asbestos had on average higher lung fiber burdens than patients with indirect (i.e.,

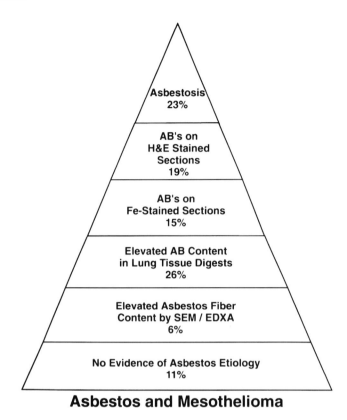

Asbestos and Mesothelioma

Figure 11-7. Pyramid showing the relationship between asbestos exposure and mesothelioma. At the upper range of exposures, 23% of patients have histologically confirmed asbestosis. An additional 34% have asbestos bodies on hematoxylin and eosin (H & E) or iron-stained sections. At the next level, 26% of patients will have an elevated pulmonary asbestos body content even though asbestos bodies are not observed in histologic sections. A further 6% will have an elevated lung fiber burden as determined by scanning electron microscopy even though asbestos body counts are within the background range of 0 to 20 AB/gm. Finally, in 11% of cases, there is no pathologic evidence for an asbestos etiology. (Reprinted from Ref. 19, with permission.)

bystander) exposures, and shipyard exposures had on average higher burdens than non-shipyard exposures. When cases were grouped by exposure category, more than 94% of 1445 cases fit into one or more of 12 different industrial, six different occupational, or one non-occupational categories (Table 11-8).[81] The one nonoccupational category, that of a household contact of an asbestos worker, accounted for 6% of all cases and more than half of mesotheliomas among women.[82]

In view of the experimental observations that fibers 8.0 μm or greater in length and 0.25 μm or less in diameter are the most efficient at producing mesotheliomas,[83] it is of interest to examine fiber dimension data in studies of human cases of malignant mesothelioma. In a study of amphibole asbestos-induced mesotheliomas, Churg and Wiggs[84] reported that 39% of amosite fibers and 23% of crocidolite fibers exceeded 5 μm in length. In contrast, a study of chrysotile-related mesotheliomas showed that only 11% of chrysotile fibers and 13% of tremolite fibers were 5 μm or greater in length.[85] The vast majority of fibers in both studies were less than 0.25 μm in diameter.[84,85] The biopersistence of relatively long amphibole fibers in lung tissues is the likely reason for the greater potency of amosite and crocidolite fibers in the production of mesothelioma as compared to chrysotile. The latter tends to fragment into shorter fibers and has a much shorter half-life within the lung.[53,71]

It should be noted that most of the studies of fiber burdens in mesothelioma patients have examined lung parenchyma. It is reasonable to assume that fibers actually reaching the pleura are the ones responsible for pleural disease, and the dimensions and types of fibers accumulating in the pleura are of interest in this regard. Sebastien et al.[29] reported that in individuals exposed to mixtures of fibers, short chrysotile fibers (<5 μm) tended to accumulate in the pleura whereas longer amphibole fibers accumulated in the lung parenchyma. Suzuki and Yuen[86] also reported primarily short chrysotile fibers in the pleura and in mesothelial tissues. Churg et al.,[85] on the other hand, found no difference in the length, diameter, or type of fibers isolated from peripheral versus central lung parenchyma in Canadian chrysotile workers. Dodson et al.[87] found long commercial amphibole fibers in samples of pleural plaque from asbestos workers, and Gibbs et al.[88] also identified similar fibers in pleural samples of patients with diffuse visceral pleural thickening. Boutin et al.[89] found a preferential concentration of long commercial amphibole fibers in black spots on the parietal pleura. Dodson et al.[90] recovered long commercial amphibole fibers from samples of peritoneum and mesentery. Clearly, fibers of the type and size known to be associated with the greatest risk of mesothelioma do in fact migrate to pleural tissues. The identification of short chrysotile fibers in these tissues is of questionable relevance, since there is no convincing data that these fibers are pathogenic (see Chapter 10). Before analysis of pleural tissues can be substituted for lung tissue analyses, proper controls will have to be established, including values expected

Table 11-8. Exposure categories in 94% of 1445 cases with malignant mesothelioma

Industry	Occupation	Nonoccupational exposure
Shipbuilding	Pipefitter/welder	Household contact
U.S. Navy/merchant marine	Boiler worker	
Construction	Maintenance	
Insulation	Machinist	
Oil and chemical	Electrician	
Power plant	Sheet metal worker	
Railroad		
Automotive		
Steel/metal		
Asbestos manufacture		
Paper mill		
Ceramics/glass		

Source: Modified from Ref. 81.

for normal pleura from nonexposed individuals and for metastatic tumor to the pleura in patients with malignancies not known to be asbestos related.

In summary, patients with mesothelioma who do not also have asbestosis have on average smaller pulmonary asbestos burdens than do patients with asbestosis. This observation is consistent with epidemiologic evidence that mesothelioma can occur in individuals with brief, low level, or indirect exposures to asbestos.[1] In over half of the patients with mesothelioma in the authors' series, asbestos bodies can be detected in histologic sections with careful scrutiny, and in more than 80%, tissue digestion studies show an elevated tissue asbestos body content (Figure 11-7). The distribution of asbestos body counts in patients with mesothelioma appears to be bimodal, suggesting that there are two distinct populations.[19,24,76] One group has elevated tissue asbestos content and is asbestos related, while the other has a tissue asbestos content indistinguishable from a reference population and may be considered to be "spontaneous" or idiopathic.[15,24] Analysis of tissue asbestos content in an individual case can thus provide useful information with regard to an etiologic role for asbestos in the production of a mesothelioma.

Benign Asbestos-Related Pleural Diseases

Several studies have examined the asbestos content of lung tissue in series of patients with benign asbestos-related pleural disease.[68,91–94] Most of these have dealt with parietal pleural plaques, and the studies are summarized in Table 11-9. Gylseth et al.[68] studied 14 cases of parietal pleural plaques by means of SEM and found a median of 2.2 million fibers per gram of dried lung as compared to 0.6 million fibers per gram in 12 control cases. Warnock et al.[91] reported a median of 0.54 million fibers per gram dried lung in 20 cases of parietal pleural plaques studied by TEM, whereas Churg[92] found 1.14 million fibers per gram in 29 cases of pleural plaques. Both studies showed a significant

Table 11-9. Asbestos content of lung tissue in reported series of patients with benign asbestos-related pleural disease*

Source	No. of cases	Method[t]	Asbestos bodies/gm dried lung	Uncoated fibers/gm dried lung
Gylseth et al.[68]	14	SEM	—	2.2 (0.1–13)
Warnock et al.[91]	20	TEM	7.8[§] (0.3–9,600)	0.54[§] (0.018–71)
Churg[92]	29	TEM	17.3[§] (0–194)	1.14[§] (ND)
Stephens et al.[93]	7**	PCLM	—	0.131 (0.029–0.378)
		TEM	—	28.9 (9.2–83.5)
Voisin et al.[94]	6**	LM	3[§] (0.1–40)	—

*Values reported are the median counts for thousands (10^3) of asbestos bodies or millions (10^6) of uncoated fibers per gram of dried lung tissue, with ranges indicated in parentheses, except for the study of Churg,[92] where only the mean value for total fibers per gm was given and a range could not be determined (ND).
[t]PCLM = phase contrast light microscopy; SEM = scanning electron microscopy; TEM = transmission electron microscopy; LM = light microscopy.
[§]In these three studies, asbestos bodies were counted by conventional light microscopy.
**Cases in series of Stephens et al.[93] are diffuse pleural fibrosis, and those of Voisin et al.[94] are rounded atelectasis. All others are parietal pleural plaques.

Table 11-10. Asbestos content of lung tissue in 197 cases of benign asbestos-related pleural disease[a]

	N	AB/gm (LM)	N	UF/gm (SEM)
PPP + Mesothelioma	88	970 (2.2–74,500)	81	25,100 (950–781,000)
PPP + Lung Cancer	54	710 (1.5–18,900)	54	19,200 (280–399,000)
PPP (Other)	43	330 (3.5–91,500)	40	14,800 (400–980,000)
Rounded Atelectasis	8	680 (5.5–1980)	9	22,100 (400–189,000)

[a] Asbestos bodies per gram of wet lung tissue as determined by light microscopy (LM) and uncoated fibers 5 µm or greater in length per gram of wet lung tissue as determined by scanning electron microscopy (SEM). Values reported as median with range in parentheses.
PPP = parietal pleural plaques; Other = cases with neither mesothelioma nor lung cancer. Cases with asbestosis excluded.

increase in the concentrations of commercial amphiboles (amosite or crocidolite) in the lungs of patients with plaques as compared to a reference population, but no significant differences for chrysotile or noncommercial amphiboles. Whitwell et al.[15] included 21 patients with pleural plaques in their normal control series of 100 cases, and found that 55% of the cases with more than 20,000 fibers/gm as determined by PCLM but only 5.5% of cases with fewer than 20,000 fibers/gm had plaques. All of these observations support a role for asbestos fibers in the production of pleural plaques.[1]

The authors have had the opportunity to examine the asbestos content of the lung in 189 patients with parietal pleural plaques but with no evidence of parenchymal asbestosis (Table 11-10). The median asbestos body concentration by light microscopy in 184 patients was 680 AB/gm (range: 1.5–91,500). This is similar to the median value of 780 bodies per gram in the study by Warnock et al.[91] and the value of 1730 per gram wet lung in the series reported by Churg.[92] The median fiber count by SEM for uncoated fibers 5 µm or greater in length in 175 patients from the authors' series was 19,600 fibers per gram wet lung, which is about 10% of the median level in patients with asbestosis[54] (Table 11-3). Among the 184 patients with plaques alone, 18 (10%) had asbestos body counts within our normal range of 0–20 AB/gm, as compared to 0% of patients with asbestosis (Table 11-2). Among these 18, an additional 8 had elevated fiber levels by SEM. Thus in our series, 95% of patients with pleural plaques (174/184) had an elevated tissue asbestos content. Andrion et al.[95] reported a highly significant association between pleural plaques and the finding of asbestos bodies in 30 µm thick histologic sections by light microscopy in a study of 191 cases of pleural plaques from a series of 996 consecutive autopsies in Torino, Italy. The median asbestos body count tends to be higher in patients with bilateral plaques when compared to those with unilateral plaques.[17] In addition, the asbestos body count in histologic sections seems to correlate positively with the severity and extent of plaque formation.[95]

Benign asbestos-related pleural diseases that occur less frequently than pleural plaques include diffuse pleural fibrosis, rounded atelectasis, and benign asbestos effusions (see Chapter 6). Stephens et al.[93] examined the pulmonary mineral fiber content in seven patients with diffuse pleural fibrosis (Table 11-9). The median uncoated fiber count in these seven cases by PCLM was 0.131 million fibers per gram dried lung, and by TEM was 28.9 million fibers/gm. These patients on the average have a greater fiber burden than patients with pleural plaques alone, but less than patients with asbestosis (Tables 11-2 and 11-9). The asbestos body content of lung parenchyma was examined in six patients with rounded atelectasis by Voisin et al.[94] These authors found a median value of 3000 AB/gm dry lung, with a range of 100–40,000 AB/gm (Table 11-9). Eight cases of rounded atelectasis have been studied in the authors' laboratory (Table 11-10). All were men, and their age ranged from 42 to 72 years. Five patients also had parietal pleural plaques and one had bilateral areas of rounded atelectasis. The median asbestos body count by light microscopy was 680 AB/gm wet lung tissue (range: 5.5–1980 AB/gm). The median uncoated fiber concentration (fibers 5 μm or greater in length) as assessed by SEM in 7 cases was 22,100 fibers per gram of wet lung tissue (range: 400–189,000 fibers per gram). These levels are essentially identical to the values we have observed for patients with pleural plaques. We are not aware of any reports in the literature of pulmonary mineral fiber content in series of patients with benign asbestos effusion.

In summary, patients with parietal pleural plaques who do not also have asbestosis have considerably smaller pulmonary asbestos burdens than patients with asbestosis, and levels that are somewhat lower than but of about the same order of magnitude as patients with malignant mesothelioma. This observation is consistent with epidemiologic evidence that pleural plaques can occur in individuals with brief, low level, or indirect exposures to asbestos.[1] Limited information is available regarding the pulmonary mineral fiber content of patients with other benign asbestos-related pleural diseases. Published findings in this regard seem to indicate that patients with rounded atelectasis have tissue asbestos levels similar to those of patients with plaques, whereas patients with diffuse pleural fibrosis have levels intermediate between those of patients with plaques and patients with asbestosis.

Carcinoma of the Lung

The association between asbestos exposure and an increased risk for lung cancer has been well-established in epidemiological studies, and cigarette smoking and asbestos appear to act in a synergistic fashion to increase this risk.[1] The data supporting these observations and the pathologic features of lung cancers occurring among asbestos-exposed individuals are described in Chapter 7. Although the association between asbestos exposure and lung cancer among individuals with asbestosis is universally accepted, the causative role for asbestos among asbestos workers with lung cancer but without asbestosis is controversial. It is therefore of interest to review what has been learned from fiber burden analysis in this regard.

Table 11-11. Asbestos content of lung tissue in reported series of patients with carcinoma of the lung*

Source	No. of cases	Selection criteria	Method	Asbestos bodies/gm dried lung	Uncoated fibers/gm dried lung
Whitwell et al.[15]	100	General population	PCLM	—	0.009 (0–0.115)
Gaudichet et al.[72]	40	General population	TEM+	0.16 (0–290)	16
Warnock et al.[16]	9	Asbestos workers	TEM+	35.6 (0.41–840)	5.83 (3.10–73.3)
Warnock and Isenberg[96]	75	Asbestos workers	TEM+	3.75 (0–1000)	2.18 (0.077–97)
Anttila et al.[97]	22	Construction workers	TEM	—	2.1 (0.3–49.9)

*Values reported are the median counts for thousands (10^3) of asbestos bodies or millions (10^6) of uncoated fibers per gram of dried lung tissue, with ranges indicated in parentheses, except for the study of Gaudichet et al.,[72] where only the mean value for total fibers per gm dried lung could be obtained from the data presented.
+In these three studies, asbestos bodies were counted by conventional light microscopy.
PCLM = phase contrast light microscopy; TEM = transmission electron microscopy

Studies which have examined the asbestos content of lung tissue in series of patients with lung cancer are summarized in Table 11-11.[15,16,72,96,97] The values reported are influenced not only by the investigative and analytical techniques employed, but also by the way the cases were selected. Whitwell et al.[15] examined 100 consecutive cases of lung cancer by PCLM and found a similar distribution of fiber content between cancer cases and controls. Gaudichet et al.[72] included 20 patients with squamous carcinoma and 20 with adenocarcinoma of the lung, and found similar asbestos body counts by light microscopy and fiber counts by TEM in these two groups as compared to 20 patients with pulmonary metastases and 20 with cardiovascular disease. The series of Warnock et al.[16] included 7 of 9 cases with histologically confirmed asbestosis, and the series of Warnock and Isenberg[96] included 12 of 62 cases with asbestosis. The authors of the latter study concluded that an asbestos body concentration of 1000 or more per gram of dried lung tissue or a combined amosite and crocidolite fiber concentration of 100,000 or more per gram of dried lung should be used as an indication that a lung cancer may be asbestos related.[96] Anttila et al.[97] studied 22 cases of lung cancer among construction workers, and concluded that fiber number and size correlated with location of tumors in the lower lobes.

We have had the opportunity to study the asbestos content of lung tissue in 273 cases of lung cancer, and the results of our analyses are summarized in Table 11-12. Seventy-four patients also had asbestosis, 54 had parietal pleural plaques without asbestosis, and 145 had neither plaques nor asbestosis. All had some alleged degree of asbestos exposure. Smoking histories were available in 180 cases. All but 16 were cigarette smokers or ex-smokers; 267 of the cases occurred in men. The six women included one with asbestosis, one with pleural plaques, and four "other" lung cancer cases. The data from Table 11-12 show that patients with asbestosis had a median asbestos body count that was

Table 11-12. Asbestos content of lung tissue in 273 cases of lung cancer[a]

	N	AB/gm (LM)	N	UF/gm (SEM)
Lung cancer plus asbestosis	74	28,600 (150–343,000)	71	180,000 (18,500–7,810,000)
Lung cancer plus PPP	54	710 (1.5–18,900)	54	19,200 (280–399,000)
Lung cancer (Other)[b]	145	68 (1.5–45,800)	137	12,400 (210–262,000)

[a] Asbestos bodies per gram of wet lung tissue as determined by light microscopy (LM) and uncoated fibers 5 μm or greater in length per gram of wet lung tissue as determined by scanning electron microscopy (SEM). Values reported as median with range in parentheses.
[b] Cases of lung cancer with neither asbestosis nor PPP, or uninformative cases with respect to asbestosis or plaques.
PPP = parietal pleural plaques.

about 40 times that of pleural plaque cases, and an uncoated fiber count that was almost 10 times greater. Similarly, patients with pleural plaques alone had an asbestos body count that was ten times as great and an uncoated fiber content about 1.5 times as great as lung cancer patients with neither plaques nor asbestosis. Although all cases had some history of asbestos exposure, 48 of the 145 patients (33%) with neither plaques nor asbestosis had asbestos body counts within our normal range of 0 to 20 AB/gm.

Epidemiologic studies have generally failed to present convincing evidence that patients with pleural plaques alone have a significantly increased risk for developing lung cancer (see Chapter 6). Our 145 lung cancer patients with neither plaques nor asbestosis are a very heterogeneous group with regard to type, duration, and intensity of exposure to asbestos. Nonetheless, comparison of their pulmonary fiber burdens with that of the 54 patients with plaques alone would suggest that as a *group*, they would be unlikely to have a significantly increased risk for lung cancer as a result of exposure to asbestos. Others have argued that in an *individual* case, it is the fiber burden rather than the fibrogenic response that is likely the important determinant of carcinogenic risk. Therefore, according to this line of argument, patients with a fiber burden within the range of values observed for patients with asbestosis would have a similar lung cancer risk as patients with asbestosis[96] (see also Chapter 7).

Karjalainen et al.[98] in 1994 published the results of a study of the pulmonary asbestos concentration in 113 surgically resected specimens and compared them with 297 autopsy cases serving as referents. These authors were able to demonstrate that a fiber burden exceeding one million amphibole fibers per gram of dry lung as measured by SEM was associated with an overall lung cancer odds ratio of 1.7. When the value exceeded five million fibers per gram, the odds ratio increased to 5.3. The elevated risk persisted after controlling for smoking and asbestosis. The odds ratio was greatest for adenocarcinoma and lower lobe cancers. Roggli and Sanders[99] studied 234 cases of lung cancer by

SEM, dividing them into patients with asbestosis, with plaques alone, or with neither asbestosis nor plaques. The fiber burden exceeded 50 thousand amphibole fibers 5 μm or greater in length per gram of wet lung tissue in 82% of cases with asbestosis, which is roughly equivalent to one million amphibole fibers per gram of dry lung as determined by Karjalainen et al.[98] However, only 10% of patients with plaques alone and 5% of patients with neither plaques nor asbestosis had fiber burdens exceeding this level. The odds were approximately 100 to 1 against finding 50,000 or more amphibole fibers per gram of wet lung when asbestos bodies were not detected in H&E or iron-stained histologic sections. Fiber burden studies are most useful in lung cancer patients that do not meet histologic criteria for a diagnosis of asbestosis but for whom asbestos bodies are identified in histologic sections of lung.

In summary, tissue asbestos analysis has shown that in populations with no appreciable occupational exposure to asbestos and with substantial exposure to cigarette smoke, there is no evidence for a contributing role for asbestos in any lung cancers which occur.[15,72] This observation is not surprising when one considers that 90% or more of lung cancers occurring annually in the United States are attributable to cigarette smoking, whereas as few as 2% of cases may be related to asbestos exposure.[100] In populations with some occupational exposure to asbestos, the presence of either histologically or clinically confirmed asbestosis or a tissue asbestos burden equivalent to that seen in asbestotic subjects is the most useful marker for an asbestos-related lung cancer. It should be noted that fiber dimensions are probably important with regard to the carcinogenic potential of asbestos. Lippmann[60] concluded in his review of the human and animal data that it is primarily fibers greater than 10 μm in length and greater than 0.15 μm in diameter that are responsible for the development of lung cancer.[1]

Normal Lungs (Nonexposed Individuals)

Determination of background levels of fibers to be expected in the general population is an extraordinarily difficult task, since it is no simple matter to define what is normal or to exclude unknown exposures. Several investigators have established ranges of fiber burdens identified in control or reference populations,[15,30,69,72,101,102] and these are summarized in Table 11-13. Methodological differences and patient selection criteria largely account for the variations in reported values. Our own control cases were selected on the basis of having macroscopically normal lungs at autopsy and an asbestos body count within our previously determined normal range.[17,76] Two cases with grossly normal lungs but with asbestos body counts of 620 and 300 per gram of wet lung were excluded. Although there is substantial difference in fiber counts between laboratories, there is a remarkable similarity for asbestos body counts. Three separate laboratories have identified 0 to 20 AB/gm as the background or reference value. These include the laboratories of Ron Dodson in Tyler, Texas, Sam Hammar in Bremerton,

Table 11-13. Asbestos content of lung tissue in reference or control populations*

Source	No. of cases	Method	Asbestos bodies/gm dried lung	Uncoated fibers/gm dried lung
Whitwell et al.[15]	100	PCLM		0.007 (0–0.521)
Mowe et al.[69]	28	SEM		0.25 (0–4.8)
Gaudichet et al.[72]	20	TEM[t]	0.18 (0–3.2)	11.2
Churg and Warnock[101]	20	TEM[t]	0.28[§] (0.02–0.84)	1.29[§] (0.260–7.55)
Case et al.[102]	23	TEM		0.62
Roggli et al. (present study)	20	SEM[t]	0.029[§] (0–0.22)	0.031[§] (0.004–0.169)

*Values reported are the median counts for thousands (10^3) of asbestos bodies or millions (10^6) of uncoated fibers per gram of dried lung tissue, with ranges indicated in parentheses, except for the study of Gaudichet et al.,[72] where only the mean value for total fibers per gm dried lung could be obtained from the data presented.
[t] In these three studies, asbestos bodies were counted by conventional light microscopy.
[§] Values multiplied by a factor of 10 (approximate ratio of wet to dry lung weight) for purposes of comparison.
PCLM = phase contrast light microscopy; SEM = scanning electron microscopy; TEM = transmission electron microscopy.

Washington, and Victor Roggli in Houston, Texas and Durham, North Carolina.[103] In any analysis of fiber burden data in a population with a given disease, it is of paramount importance to compare the findings with those of an appropriate reference or control population for which the same analytical technique was employed.[1]

Asbestos Content of Lung Tissue by Exposure Category

There have been relatively few studies that attempted to correlate tissue asbestos burdens with occupational exposures. Whitwell et al.[15] reported that the number of asbestos fibers found in the lungs correlated closely with patient occupations but not with their home environment. Patients living near likely sources of atmospheric asbestos pollution had asbestos fiber counts that were similar to the remainder of the patients. Sebastien et al.[29] described the tissue asbestos content in six asbestos workers with heavy exposure, six subjects who handled small amounts of asbestos during their professional life, and six randomly selected cases with no known asbestos exposure history. The mean fiber count by PCLM (400× magnification) for these three groups was 2,000,000, 2000, and 200 fibers per cubic centimeter of lung parenchyma, respectively. However, the difference between the first two groups was much less striking in terms of fiber counts by TEM: ten million for the six heavily exposed as compared to one million fibers/cm^3 for the casually exposed subjects.

Churg and Warnock[104] reported pulmonary asbestos body counts in 252 urban patients over 40 years of age, and found that 32% of blue-collar men but less than 12% of white-collar men and blue- or white-collar women had more than 100 asbestos bodies per gram of wet lung tissue. In addition, 45% of steelworkers and 65% of construction workers had more than 100 asbestos bodies per gram. Tuomi et al.[105] correlated occupational exposure to asbestos and lung fiber burdens in 23 Finnish mesothelioma cases. Two patients had definite and seven probable occupational exposure to asbestos. Six patients had possible and eight unlikely or unknown exposures. All nine patients with definite or probable asbestos exposure had one million or more fibers per gram of dry lung as determined by SEM, whereas only three of eight with unlikely or unknown exposure had more than a million fibers per gram.

The authors have had the opportunity to examine the pulmonary asbestos content by LM and SEM in 405 patients with diseases known to be associated with asbestos exposure whose occupational category was also known. The occupational categories for these patients are summarized by disease classification in Table 11-14. The results of tissue asbestos analysis by occupational category are summarized in Table 11-15 and compared with 19 patients with normal lungs at autopsy. The various categories are discussed in more detail in the following sections.

Insulators

The highest levels of pulmonary asbestos content were found in patients who were categorized as asbestos insulators. These included individuals whose job descriptions involved work as an insulator, pipe coverer, asbestos sawyer, and asbestos sprayer (Table 11-14). The median asbestos body content among 68 insulators was 55,600 AB/gm, with a range of 32 to 1,600,000 ABs/gm, as determined by LM. The uncoated fiber content was 342,000 uncoated fibers $5\,\mu m$ or greater in length per gram of wet lung, with a range of 3480 to 12,500,000 fibers/gm, as determined by SEM. Forty-six of 67 insulators had histologically confirmed asbestosis (Table 11-14). Insulators have higher asbestos body and uncoated fiber content of the lung than other

Table 11-14. Occupational category for 405 patients with asbestos-associated diseases

Exposure category	Asbestosis	Mesothelioma	PPP	Lung cancer
Asbestos insulator	46	27	40	29
Asbestos manufacturing	5	3	5	6
Shipyard worker	40	35	57	51
Power plant worker	4	9	7	5
Household contact	3	22	8	4
Molten metal worker	0	6	5	5
U.S. Navy/merchant marine	2	19	9	10
Construction worker	10	26	14	11
Oil/chemical refinery	3	9	12	8
Railroad worker	2	7	4	8
Brake repair worker	0	11	5	5
Bldg. occupant	0	8	1	1

Asbestos insulator: Insulator, pipe coverer, asbestos sawyer, asbestos sprayer
Shipyard worker: Joiner, welder, rigger, sandblaster, fitter, shipwright, electrician, draftsman, handyman, engineer and estimator (excluding asbestos insulator)
Molten metal worker: steel mill, iron foundry, aluminum plant worker
Construction worker: Brickmason, carpenter, construction worker, drywall finisher, electrician, laborer, machinist, painter, plasterer, project engineer, and roofer
Bldg. occupant: Worked in building containing asbestos materials as only known exposure.

Table 11-15. Asbestos content of lung tissue by exposure category*

	N	AB/gm (LM)	UF/gm (SEM)
Asbestos insulator	68	55,600 (32–1,600,000)	342,000 (3,480–12,500,000)
Asbestos manufacturing	13	3,090 (2–79,000)	104,000 (1,410–1,220,000)
Shipyard worker (other than insulator)	114	2,560 (3.3–1,400,000)	38,600 (280–4,790,000)
Power plant worker	16	860 (12.6–58,800)	34,000 (2,430–195,000)
Household contact	28	260 (2.0–14,100)	24,300 (17,000–120,000)
Molten metal worker	13	260 (3.3–4,070)	21,800 (4,380–132,000)
U.S. Navy/merchant marine	34	220 (1.5–8,020)	17,400 (1,470–399,000)
Construction worker	44	220 (1.5–83,500)	14,000 (195–2,360,000)
Oil/chemical refinery	22	180 (1.5–2,750)	17,100 (275–158,000)
Railroad worker	20	55 (1.7–10,000)	15,900 (950–111,000)
Brake repair worker	23	19 (1.5–7,740)	9,710 (670–54,100)
Bldg. occupant	10	1.7 (<0.2–14)	13,000 (3,750–25,100)
Reference population	19	2.9 (0–22)	3,100 (870–12,700)

Data are presented as median values, with range indicated in parentheses, of asbestos bodies per gram of wet lung as determined by light microscopy or uncoated fibers 5 μm or greater in length per gram of wet lung as determined by SEM. Exposure categories as defined in Table 11-14, with N representing the number of cases in each category.

categories of asbestos-exposed individuals, even when the duration of exposure is similar.[24] These observations correlate well with the reported high prevalence of asbestos-associated diseases among asbestos insulators.[106]

Asbestos Manufacturing Plant Workers

Exposure to asbestos in plants that manufactured asbestos products in the past was quite heavy, resulting in many cases of asbestos-related diseases.[49,107–109] The authors have studied lung tissue from 13 workers at asbestos manufacturing plants with various diseases that have been associated with exposure to asbestos (Table 11-14). The median asbestos body content among these workers was 3090 AB/gm, with a range of 2 to 79,000 AB/gm, as determined by LM. The uncoated fiber content was 104,000 uncoated fibers 5 μm or greater in length per gram of wet lung, with a range of 1410 to 1,220,000 fibers/gm, as determined by SEM. Five of 13 cases had histologically confirmed asbestosis. One reason for the somewhat lower asbestos content for asbestos plant workers as compared to insulators is the shorter duration of exposure for the former (13 years for 11 cases with information, range: 4 mos. to 42 years) as compared to the latter (27 years for 60 cases, range: 1 to 49 years).

Shipyard Workers (Other Than Insulators)

This category includes individuals whose job descriptions listed their primary occupation as a joiner, welder, rigger, sandblaster, fitter, shipwright, electrician, draftsman, handyman, engineer, painter and estimator. Shipyard workers whose primary occupation was as an insulator are included in the previous category of asbestos insulators. There were 114 individuals in this group of shipyard workers (Table 11-15), and most of these individuals did not work directly with asbestos products but were rather exposed as bystanders. The median asbestos body content among these shipyard workers was 2560 AB/gm, with a range of 3.3 to 1,400,000 AB/gm, as determined by LM. The uncoated fiber content was 38,600 uncoated fibers 5 μm or greater in length per gram of wet lung, with a range of 280 to 4,790,000 fibers/gm, as determined by SEM. Forty of 111 shipyard workers had histologically confirmed asbestosis (Table 11-14). The relatively high pulmonary asbestos burden among individuals with a bystander type of exposure can be related to the fact that these individuals worked side by side with others who directly handled asbestos within the tight confines of the holds of ships. Shipyard workers represented the largest single exposure category in a study of 1445 mesothelioma cases by Roggli et al.,[81] accounting for 289 (20%) of the cases studied. The wide range of values observed in this and other categories of occupational asbestos exposure may be explained by variation in duration and intensity of exposure, cofactors such as cigarette smoking, and individual variability in clearance efficiency.

Power Plant Workers

Cross-sectional studies have demonstrated the presence of asbestos-related diseases among workers in power plants.[110] Exposures to these individuals derive from insulation used on turbines, generators, boilers, and pipes carrying steam. The authors have studied 16 power plant workers with various diseases associated with asbestos exposure (Table 11-14). The results of tissue asbestos analysis in these cases are summarized in Table 11-15. The median asbestos body content in this category was 860 AB/gm, with a range of 12.6 to 58,800 AB/gm. The median uncoated fiber content was 34,000 fibers 5 μm or greater in length per gram of wet lung, with a range of 2430 to 195,000 fibers/gm. The asbestos body count in power plant workers is intermediate between that of shipyard workers versus U.S. Navy/merchant marine or oil and chemical refinery workers, but the uncoated fiber content is more similar to that of shipyard workers. Asbestosis was present in 4 of 15 cases. Amosite was the main fiber type identified. Exposure to asbestos in power plants was a common cause of mesothelioma in both the study of Roggli et al.[81] and the Australian Mesothelioma Surveillance study.[111]

Molten Metal Workers

Industries such as steel manufacture, iron foundries, and aluminum smelting and manufacture involve intense heat, so it is not surprising that such industries might afford the opportunity for exposure to asbestos that had been used for insulating purposes. The authors have studied 13 workers from the molten metal industry (nine steel workers, three iron workers, and one aluminum potroom worker) with various diseases associated with asbestos exposure (Table 11-14). The results of tissue asbestos analysis in these cases are summarized in Table 11-15. The median asbestos body content in this category was 260 AB/gm, with a range of 3.3 to 4070 AB/gm. The median uncoated fiber content was 21,800 fibers 5 μm or greater in length per gram of wet lung, with a range of 4380 to 132,000 fibers/gm. Asbestosis was not present in any of these cases. Amosite was the main fiber type identified.

U.S. Navy/Merchant Marine

As a result of the large amount of asbestos aboard ships, servicemen in the U.S. Navy and seamen in the merchant marine had the opportunity for significant asbestos exposure. This is especially true for those who worked around boilers in the engine room. The authors have studied 34 such patients with various diseases associated with asbestos exposure (Table 11-14). The results of tissue asbestos analysis in these cases are displayed in Table 11-15. The median asbestos body content in this category was 220 AB/gm, with a range of 1.5 to 8020 AB/gm. The median uncoated fiber content was 17,400 fibers 5 μm or greater in length per gram of wet lung, with a range of 1470 to 399,000 fibers/gm. Asbestosis was confirmed histologically in 2 of 33 cases. In the study of 1445 mesothelioma cases by Roggli et al.,[81] U.S. Navy/merchant marine seamen were second only to shipyard workers as the major source of mesothelioma cases in the United States. In comparison, the median asbestos body count in shipyard workers is about 10 times as high and the uncoated fiber content about twice as high (vide supra). As in the case of shipyard workers, amosite was the predominant fiber type identified.

Construction Workers

This group encompasses a variety of occupations in the construction industry not covered in any of the prior categories. Job titles include brickmason, carpenter, construction worker, drywall finisher, electrician, laborer, machinist, painter, plasterer, project engineer, and roofer. The authors have studied 44 construction workers with various diseases associated with asbestos exposure (Table 11-14). The results of tissue asbestos analysis in these cases are summarized in Table 11-15. The median asbestos body content in this category was 220 AB/gm, with a range of 1.5 to 83,500 AB/gm. The median uncoated fiber content was 14,000 fibers 5 μm or greater in length per gram of wet lung, with a range of 195 to 2,360,000 fibers/gm. Asbestosis was present in 10 of 42 cases. Amosite was the main fiber type identified. Twenty-six of our construction workers had mesothelioma. In the Australian Mesothelioma Surveillance Program, construction trades were the most common cause of mesothelioma.[111]

Oil and Chemical Refinery Workers

Studies have shown that oil and chemical refinery workers are at risk for asbestos-related diseases.[112,113] This is primarily the result of the presence of boilers and miles of pipeline in these facilities and the consequent requirement for pipe and boiler insulation. The authors have studied 22 refinery workers with various diseases associated with asbestos exposure (Table 11-14). The results of tissue asbestos analysis in these cases are summarized in Table 11-15. The median asbestos body content in this category was 180 AB/gm, with a range of 1.5 to 2750 AB/gm. The median uncoated fiber content was 17,100 fibers 5 μm or greater in length per gram of wet lung, with a range of 275 to 158,000 fibers/gm. Asbestosis was confirmed histologically in 3 of 20 cases. The tissue asbestos content in these workers is quite similar to that of U.S. Navy/merchant marine seamen. Amosite was the predominant fiber type identified.

Railroad Workers

Railroad workers during the steam engine era often had the opportunity for occupational exposure to asbestos, especially workers in the machine shops or those involved with ripping out old insulation from the steam boilers and replacing it with new insulation. Such exposures virtually disappeared with the replacement of steam locomotives with diesel engines. The authors have had the opportunity to examine the tissue asbestos content of the lungs in 20 individuals whose primary exposure to asbestos was as a railroad worker during the steam engine era (Table 11-15). The median asbestos body content among these workers was 55 AB/gm, with a range of 1.7 to 10,000 AB/gm. The median uncoated fiber content was 15,900 fibers 5 μm or greater in length per gram of wet lung, with a range of 950 to 111,000 fibers/gm. Only two of the 20 workers had histologically confirmed asbestosis (Table 11-14). The median uncoated fiber content for the railroad workers was less than half that for the shipyard workers (15,900 vs. 38,600 fibers/gm), but the asbestos body counts are strikingly less (55 vs. 2560 AB/gm). This may be due to the fact that chrysotile was the primary type of fiber to which the railroad workers were exposed,[114] and chrysotile is less efficient at forming asbestos bodies than are the amphiboles (see Chapter 3). Nonetheless, railroad workers were also exposed to amosite asbestos,[115] and amosite fibers have been identified by the authors in many of these workers' lungs by means of EDXA.[81,99]

Brake Repair Workers

Large numbers of workers are involved with the repair and replacement of brake linings and clutch facings in the course of their daily work. Since these friction products contain asbestos, there has been some concern that these workers are at risk for the development of asbestos-associated diseases. The results of tissue asbestos analysis of 23 brake repair workers are summarized in Table 11-15. The median asbestos body count among these workers was 19 AB/gm, with a range of 1.5 to 7740 AB/gm. The median uncoated fiber content was 9710 fibers 5 μm or greater in length per gram of wet lung, with a range of 670 to 54,100 fibers/gm. The patient with the highest asbestos body count was a brake line grinder in a manufacturing plant for many years, who died at age 85 with advanced pulmonary fibrosis. At autopsy, the uncoated fiber content was only 13,000 fibers/gm, and most of these were amosite. None of the 23 patients had histologically confirmed asbestosis, although five patients (including the 85-year-old man noted above) had idiopathic pulmonary fibrosis and one had desquamative interstitial pneumonia.[56] A few cases of mesothelioma among auto mechanics have been described in the literature.[116–119] Eleven cases of pleural mesothelioma are also included among the 23 brake repair workers we have studied.[81] Fiber analyses in these cases have shown either normal range asbestos content or elevated commercial amphibole fibers.

Our fiber burden studies are in accord with epidemiologic studies, which have failed to demonstrate an association between exposure to asbestos as an automotive mechanic and the development of mesothelioma.[120] The lack of significant risk of asbestos-related diseases among brake repair workers and their low pulmonary asbestos content are apparently related to the nature of brake dust. It contains a low level of asbestos (about 1%), most of which is short chrysotile fibers (less than 1.0 μm in length). The crystalline structure of much of the chrysotile in the dust has been altered due to the heat generated during the braking process.[121] Experimental animal studies have confirmed the lack of fibrogenic and carcinogenic potential of short asbestos fibers (see Chapter 10).

Household Exposures

An increased risk of developing an asbestos-associated disease has been reported among household contacts of asbestos workers,[122,123] apparently secondary to asbestos fibers brought home on the worker's clothing. Whitwell et al.[15] reported a case of mesothelioma in the son of a worker from a gas-mask factory where the workers took crocidolite home to pack into canisters. The worker's son was found to have between 50,000 and 100,000 fibers per gram of dry lung tissue as determined by PCLM. Huncharek et al.[124] reported another case of mesothelioma in the 76-year-old wife of a shipyard machinist who dismantled boilers and other shipyard machinery for 34 years. She was found to have 6.5 million fibers per gram of dry lung as determined by TEM. Gibbs et al.[125] reported 10 cases of malignant pleural mesothelioma among household contacts of asbestos workers. The total fiber count in these individuals ranged from 5.3 to 320 million per gram of dry lung tissue. Amosite and/or crocidolite were found at elevated levels in eight of the ten cases, whereas two cases had fiber counts within the range of a reference population. The occupations of the asbestos workers included shipyard working, lagging, building and ordnance, and the household contacts were presumably exposed through fibers brought home on the workers' clothing. In general, the fiber burdens in the lungs of the household contacts were similar to other groups of workers with light or moderate direct industrial exposure to asbestos.

The authors have had the opportunity to examine the pulmonary asbestos content in 28 household contacts of asbestos workers, including 22 with mesothelioma and 4 with lung cancer (Table 11-14). Twenty-six of these cases were women,[82] including 16 wives, 9 daughters, and one mother of an asbestos worker. The other two cases were sons of asbestos workers. The occupation of the worker was known in 24 cases, and included 11 insulators, 5 shipyard workers, three power plant workers, two pipefitters, one chemical plant worker, one vinyl floor installer, and one tool grinder/glass plant worker. The median asbestos body count for these cases was 260 AB/gm, with a range of 2.0 to 14,100 AB/gm. The median uncoated fiber content was 22,400 fibers 5μ or greater in length per gram of wet lung, with a range of 2920 to 162,000 fibers/gm (Table 11-15). It should be noted that the tissue asbestos content in household contacts is of the same order of magnitude as that of molten metal workers, U.S. Navy/merchant marine seamen, construction workers, and oil and chemical refinery workers (Table 11-15). Our findings are thus similar to those reported by Gibbs et al.[125] Asbestosis was confirmed histologically in 3 of 27 cases. Amosite was the major fiber type identified.

Building Occupants

There has been considerable scientific and public debate concerning possible risks of asbestos-induced disease derived from living and working (or attending school) in buildings containing asbestos. Certainly the measured fiber levels in buildings are extremely low,[126] and no adverse health effects have been observed in at least one study of workers in buildings with and without asbestos insulation.[127] There are two case reports in the literature of patients with pleural mesothelioma whose only known asbestos exposure was that of an occupant of a building with asbestos-containing materials. One is that of a 54-year-old woman with pleural mesothelioma whose only known exposure to asbestos was as an office worker in a building with ceiling material composed of 70% amosite asbestos.[128] Analysis of lung tissue demonstrated 31 million fibers per gram of dry lung by TEM, the vast majority of which were found to be amosite asbestos by EDXA. The other is that of a teacher's aide with pleural mesothelioma and parietal pleural plaques.[129] Analysis of lung tissue demonstrated elevated concentrations of tremolite asbestos and a particle content consistent with exposure to dust from acoustical ceiling tiles.

The authors have examined the pulmonary asbestos content in 10 patients whose alleged exposure was in buildings containing asbestos. The median age was 50 years with a range of 28 to 64. Five had been exposed within school buildings. Eight patients had mesothelioma (7 pleural, one peritoneal), one was a nonsmoking man with pulmonary adenocarcinoma who had worked for 20 years in a building containing asbestos, and one was a patient with idiopathic pulmonary fibrosis (Table 11-14). The median asbestos body count in these cases was 1.7 AB/gm, with a range of less than 0.2 to 14 AB/gm. The median uncoated fiber content was 13,000 fibers 5μ or greater in length per gram of wet lung, with a range of 3750 to 25,100 fibers/gm (Table 11-15). The asbestos body counts are indistinguishable from those of 20 individuals with no known occupational exposure to asbestos. Of course, the possibility of living or working in a building containing asbestos cannot be excluded in these latter 20 cases. The tissue asbestos content was elevated in three cases. All were pleural mesotheliomas.

Two were exposed in schools, and one was exposed while supervising construction of a medical center. These three cases had elevated lung content of noncommercial amphibole fibers (e.g., tremolite).

The available information indicates that the asbestos content of the lungs in patients with building exposures is often within the background range (Table 11-15). In a series of 1445 mesotheliomas, only three cases were identified that may be related to exposure as a building occupant.[81] No cases of asbestosis or asbestos-related lung cancer were identified among the patients we studied. The authors' view is that at these levels of exposure, asbestos-related diseases are extremely unlikely to occur.[130]

Identification of Fiber Types

As noted in the previous section on fiber quantification, analytical electron microscopy can be used to also identify the types of mineral fibers present in a tissue sample. A number of studies have reported the results of EDXA of mineral fibers from human lung samples.[3–5,16–19,24,30,44,49,51,54,58,73,77,78,81,84,91,92,96,99,101,102,131–135] These studies have confirmed the observations from animal experimentation (i.e., that amphibole fibers accumulate within the lung parenchyma to a much greater degree than chrysotile fibers, which over long periods of time are more readily cleared from the lungs). The observations regarding types of mineral fibers present in human lung tissue samples from our laboratory as well as results reported in the literature are summarized in the following sections.

Asbestos Fibers

McDonald et al.[136] examined the mineral fiber content of lung tissue in 99 mesothelioma cases and an equal number of age- and sex-matched controls. These investigators noted an excess of amphibole fibers (amosite and crocidolite) in cases as compared to controls, but equal quantities of chrysotile fibers in cases and controls. In a study of 78 additional cases of mesothelioma and matched referents in Canada, McDonald et al.[78] reported that relative risk was related to the concentration of long ($\geq 8\,\mu m$) amphibole (amosite, crocidolite, or tremolite) fibers with no additional information provided by shorter fibers. The distribution of chrysotile, anthophyllite, and talc fibers and all other inorganic fibers in the two groups were quite similar. The relationship between commercial amphibole fibers and mesothelioma has been confirmed by other investigators, with amosite as the major fiber type identified in cases from North America.[53,77,81] Furthermore, studies from Finland have indicated that anthophyllite is also associated with the development of mesothelioma.[137]

Similar observations have been reported with regard to asbestos fiber types in the lungs of individuals with asbestosis. Warnock et al.[16] found large numbers of commercial amphiboles, noncommercial amphiboles, and chrysotile fibers in patients with asbestosis. Churg[58] reported the presence of both chrysotile and tremolite fibers in the lungs of chrysotile miners and millers with asbestosis, although tremolite fibers were more abundant in the lungs of these miners when compared to the mine dust. Wagner et al.,[18] in a study of naval dockyard workers, found significantly elevated levels of commercial amphiboles in the lungs of workers with asbestosis, whereas chrysotile fibers did not show the same degree of elevation. An elevated pulmonary content of commercial amphibole fibers but not of chrysotile has also been reported for individuals with parietal pleural plaques.[91,92]

The situation with respect to chrysotile and mesothelioma is somewhat more complex. There is a consensus among investigators that a fiber gradient exists with respect to fiber type and mesothelioma, with crocidolite more potent than amosite and amosite more potent than chrysotile on a fiber per fiber basis. However, the steepness of this gradient is a matter of controversy. Some investigators have suggested that the ratio of crocidolite versus chrysotile potency is as low as twofold.[138] More recently, Hodgson and Darnton have suggested that the ratio is as high as 500 to 1 for crocidolite versus chrysotile and 100 to 1 for amosite versus chrysotile.[139] In this regard, it is of interest that McDonald et al. have reported that chrysotile miners and millers with a cumulative exposure of 1000 to 1500 fiber/cc-years have a 300-fold increased risk of mesothelioma.[140] Investigators from Australia have estimated that exposure to Wittenoom crocidolite at levels as low as 0.53 fiber/cc-year is associated with an increased risk of mesothelioma.[141] These observations add further support to the existence of a fiber gradient between commercial amphibole fibers such as crocidolite and chrysotile.

Investigators have debated as to whether chrysotile or its non-commercial amphibole contaminants are responsible for mesothelioma development. Despite the epidemiologic evidence to the contrary,[142] some have gone so far as to claim that chrysotile is the primary cause of pleural mesothelioma.[143] Begin et al.[144] noted that the rates of mesothelioma were similar among miners in Thetford as compared to the township of Asbestos, although tremolite contamination was much less in chrysotile from the latter mines. However, subsequent studies showed that some of the mesothelioma cases from miners in Asbestos contained commercial amphibole fibers in their lung tissue samples.[145] In contrast, Thetford miners and millers with mesothelioma contained only chrysotile and tremolite in their lung samples. Tremolite levels usually exceeded chrysotile, even though tremolite accounted for only a small fraction of the mine dust. In addition, the five central mines around Thetford with the highest levels of tremolite contamination had the highest mesothelioma rates.[140] Although Yano et al.[146] reported that workers exposed to Chinese chrysotile that was tremolite-free had an elevated mesothelioma risk, subsequent studies showed that Chinese chrysotile is in fact contaminated with tremolite.[147] Furthermore, the ratio of tremolite to chrysotile among the Chinese workers was similar to that of Canadian chrysotile miners and millers. Taken together, these data strongly suggest that tremolite contamination is the major factor in the mesotheliogenic properties of chrysotile dust. There is no convincing evidence for a causative relationship between peritoneal mesothelioma and exposure to chrysotile dust.[139]

Some investigators have claimed that tremolite is removed from chrysotile during processing, implying that exposure to chrysotile-containing products is unlikely to cause mesothelioma.[148] Churg studied the tremolite-to-chrysotile ratio in chrysotile miners and millers with mesothelioma as well as in mesothelioma patients with heavy mixed exposure to amosite and chrysotile as insulators or shipyard workers.[53,85] The ratio of tremolite to chrysotile was indistinguishable in these two groups, and there was a strong correlation between tremolite and chrysotile concentrations. These findings suggest that there is little if any removal of tremolite from chrysotile during processing. Roggli et al.[149] performed lung fiber burden analyses in more than 300 mesothelioma patients exposed to asbestos as users of end-products. Tremolite was detected in more than 50% of the cases and was elevated above background levels in at least 25%. Cases with elevated tremolite levels represented a wide range of occupational exposures. In about 3% of cases, tremolite was the only fiber type found in excess concentrations. Tremolite correlated with both talc and chrysotile levels within the lung. The weight of the evidence does not support the claim that chrysotile from end-products is free of contamination by tremolite.

The results of analysis of more than 11,000 fibers from more than 500 patients in our laboratory are summarized in Table 11-16. The data reported are for fibers 5µm or greater in length per gram of wet lung tissue. Values below the detection limits for any fiber type were recorded as half the detection limit for that case. Analysis of the types of fibers identified according to disease category indicates that as the pulmonary fiber burden increases, the proportion of commercial amphiboles (amosite or crocidolite) also increases. These fiber types are generally below detection limits from individuals with background exposure (i.e., controls), but as much as 100% of the fiber burden among individuals with asbestosis. The highest levels occurred among patients with asbestosis, and the lowest levels among patients with neither plaques nor asbestosis. Patients with parietal pleural plaques tended to have intermediate values of commercial amphibole fibers. Patients with peritoneal mesothelioma had on average higher values than patients with pleural mesothelioma. Noncommercial amphiboles were present at higher levels than chrysotile, and both were present at much lower levels than commercial amphiboles for most categories. In general, the percentage of noncommercial amphiboles and chrysotile fibers correlated inversely with the total pulmonary fiber burden.

Nonasbestos Mineral Fibers

If one defines a fiber as an inorganic particle with an aspect (length-to-diameter) ratio of three or more and with roughly parallel sides, then studies have shown that a number of nonasbestos mineral fibers (NAMF) can be recovered from human lung tissue samples.[150] Among members of the general population, NAMF actually outnumber asbestos fibers by a ratio of about four to one. In a study employing transmission electron microscopy with EDXA and electron diffraction, Churg reported that calcium phosphate (apatite), talc, silica,

Table 11-16. Energy dispersive x-ray analysis of 11,052 fibers from 576 cases[a]

	N	AC	TAA	Chrys	NAMF
Asbestosis[b]	48	157,000	11,000	8,820	18,700
		(2,060–7,530,000)	(920–499,000)	(970–376,000)	(2,370–376,000)
Pleural Mesothelioma					
Asbestosis	35	94,500	6,700	6,060	13,400
		(3,060–11,900,000)	(1,770–211,000)	(560–211,000)	(1,840–541,000)
PPP	79	14,500	2540	1,100	7,000
		(120–933,000)	(240–79,800)	(60–124,000)	(240–454,000)
Other[c]	135	3,300	2000	700	7,220
		(120–142,000)	(90–454,000)	(90–80,000)	(240–146,000)
Peritoneal Mesothelioma					
Asbestosis	9	533,000	25,200	25,200	31,500
		(36,700–1,970,000)	(1,900–49,200)	(950–49,200)	(3810–59,200)
PPP	2	121,000	5,300	16,000	21,400
		(29,700–213,000)	(1,990–8,610)	(1270–30,800)	(11,900–30,800)
Other[c]	6	300	1190	300	5,340
		(240–2.920)	(340–7,170)	(240–840)	(1,940–16,700)
Lung Cancer					
Asbestosis	70	252,000	15,700	11,400	22,800
		(5.600–8,540,000)	(970–427,000)	(240–427,000)	(490–427,000)
PPP	52	9,410	1,590	1,030	5,870
		(150–118,000)	(220–48,400)	(150–9980)	(380–380,000)
Other[c]	121	2,640	1,580	850	6,000
		(190–113,000)	(160–144,000)	(80–11,600)	(200–105,000)
Reference Population	19	300	300	300	2,830
		(50–1,270)	(85–2,540)	(50–1,270)	(210–10,200)

[a] Values reported are the median of fibers 5 μm or greater in length per gram of wet lung tissue, with range in parentheses, as determined by SEM.
[b] Asbestosis cases without mesothelioma or lung cancer.
[c] Other represents cases with neither asbestosis nor plaques (or uninformative cases).
AC = amosite and crocidolite; Chrys = chrysotile; NAMF = nonasbestos mineral fibers; PPP = parietal pleural plaques without asbestosis; TAA = tremolite, anthophyllite, and actinolite.

rutile, kaolinite, micas, feldspar, and other silicates (in decreasing order of frequency) accounted for most NAMF recovered from the human lung.[150] These minerals also account for the majority of nonfibrous particulates which can be recovered from human lung samples.[151]

The authors have analyzed more than 3100 NAMF from more than 500 patients (Table 11-16). NAMF account for about 80% of the fiber burden from individuals with background exposure, but for fewer than 5% of the fiber burden among individuals with asbestosis. In general, the percentage of NAMF correlated inversely with the total pulmonary fiber burden. The most commonly encountered fibers in decreasing order were talc, silica, rutile (titanium dioxide), aluminum silicate, potassium aluminum silicates, and iron oxides.[152] The remainder were mostly silicates, with various combinations of Si with Na, Mg, Al, K, Ca, and Fe. Metal oxides other than titanium or iron were uncommon and included aluminum, iron-chromium, iron-aluminum, copper-zinc, and tin fibers. Endogenous calcium fibers (mostly calcium phosphate or apatite) represented less than 1% of the total. Fibrous erionite, a hydrated aluminum silicate belonging to the zeolite family of minerals and known to be associated with malignant mesothelioma and pleural calcification (see Chapters 3, 5, and 6), has also been identified in human lung tissue samples. Nonetheless, it has thus far not been reported in lung specimens from North America.

Manmade mineral fibers (MMMF) represent another class of non-asbestos mineral fibers that occasionally are identified in human lung samples. Fibers with a morphology and composition consistent with fibrous glass represented less than 3% of the NAMF that we have analyzed. These fibers are soluble in lung tissue and thus lack the biopersistence of amphibole asbestos fibers. However, some less common MMMF, namely, refractory ceramic fibers (RCF), are considerably more bio-persistent and thus are of some concern. We have detected RCF in lung tissue from 17 cases, including 7 RCF manufacturing plant workers. Six patients had lung cancer, and four had pleural plaques. Among the 10 cases who were not RCF workers were six patients with mesothelioma.[81] In two of these cases, RCF were the most frequent fibers identified. In both cases, however, elevated levels of commercial amphibole fibers were also detected. There is currently insufficient information to implicate MMMF (including RCF) as a cause of mesothelioma in humans.[153]

Although the biologic significance of nonasbestos mineral fibers is largely unknown, there is no evidence to date (with the exception of erionite) that they are of any significance in the causation of mesothelioma. One study has demonstrated a statistically significant increase in the pulmonary content of fibrous and nonfibrous particulates among patients with lung cancer as compared to noncancer controls matched for age, smoking history, and general occupational category.[154] Although it has been suggested that these mineral fibers and particles may play a pathogenetic role in the development of lung cancer, these observations may merely imply that smokers who develop lung cancer have less efficient clearance mechanisms for fibers, particles, tars, and associated carcinogens that may find their way into the respiratory tract.[1]

References

1. Roggli VL: Human disease consequences of fiber exposures—A review of human lung pathology and fiber burden data. *Environ Health Perspect* 88:295–303, 1990.
2. Berkley C, Langer AM, Baden V: Instrumental analysis of inspired fibrous pulmonary particulates. *NY Acad Sci Trans* 30:331–350, 1967.
3. Langer AM, Selikoff IJ, Sastre A: Chrysotile asbestos in the lungs of persons in New York City. *Arch Environ Health* 22:348–361, 1971.
4. Langer AM, Rubin IB, Selikoff IJ: Chemical characterization of asbestos body cores by electron microprobe analysis. *J Histochem Cytochem* 20:723–734, 1972.
5. Langer AM, Rubin IB, Selikoff IJ, Pooley FD: Chemical characterization of uncoated asbestos fibers from the lungs of asbestos workers by electron microprobe analysis. *J Histochem Cytochem* 20:735–740, 1972.

6. Langer AM, Ashley R, Baden V, Berkley C, Hammond EC, Mackler AD, Maggiore CJ, Nicholson WJ, Rohl AN, Rubin IB, Sastre A, Selikoff IJ: Identification of asbestos in human tissues. *J Occup Med* 15:287–295, 1973.

7. Langer AM, Mackler AD, Pooley FD: Electron microscopical investigation of asbestos fibers. *Environ Health Perspect* 9:63–80, 1974.

8. Pooley FD: The identification of asbestos dust with an electron microscope analyser. *Ann Occup Hyg* 18:181–186, 1975.

9. Hayashi H: Energy dispersive x-ray analysis of asbestos fibers. *Clay Sci* 5:145–154, 1978.

10. Abraham JL: Recent advances in pneumoconiosis: The pathologists' role in etiologic diagnosis, In: *The Lung*, IAP Monograph 19. Baltimore: Williams & Wilkins, 1978, pp. 96–137.

11. Churg A: Fiber counting and analysis in the diagnosis of asbestos-related disease. *Hum Pathol* 13:381–392, 1982.

12. Roggli VL, Shelburne JD: New concepts in the diagnosis of mineral pneumoconioses. *Sem Respir Med* 4:128–138, 1982.

13. Vallyathan V, Green FHY: The role of analytical techniques in the diagnosis of asbestos-associated disease. *CRC Crit Rev Clin Lab Sci* 22:1–42, 1984.

14. Churg A: Analysis of asbestos fibers from lung tissue: Research and diagnostic uses. *Sem Respir Med* 7:281–288, 1986.

15. Whitwell F, Scott J, Grimshaw M: Relationship between occupations and asbestos fibre content of the lungs in patients with pleural mesothelioma, lung cancer, and other diseases. *Thorax* 32:377–386, 1977.

16. Warnock ML, Kuwahara TJ, Wolery G: The relation of asbestos burden to asbestosis and lung cancer. *Pathol Annu* 18(2):109–145, 1983.

17. Roggli VL, Pratt PC, Brody AR: Asbestos content of lung tissue in asbestos associated diseases: A study of 110 cases. *Br J Ind Med* 43:18–28, 1986.

18. Wagner JC, Moncrief CB, Coles R, Griffiths DM, Munday DE: Correlation between fibre content of the lungs and disease in naval dockyard workers. *Br J Ind Med* 43:391–395, 1986.

19. Roggli VL: Fiber analysis. In: *Environmental and Occupational Medicine*, 3rd ed. (Rom WN, ed.), New York: Lippincott-Raven, 1998, pp. 335–347.

20. Kane PB, Goldman SL, Pillai BH, Bergofsky EH: Diagnosis of asbestosis by transbronchial biopsy: A method to facilitate demonstration of ferruginous bodies. *Am Rev Respir Dis* 115:689–694, 1977.

21. Dodson RF, Hurst GA, Williams MG, Corn C, Greenberg SD: Comparison of light and electron microscopy for defining occupational asbestos exposure in transbronchial lung biopsies. *Chest* 94:366–370, 1988.

22. Kohyama N, Hiroko K, Kunihiko Y, Yoshizumi S: Evaluation of low level asbestos exposure by transbronchial lung biopsy with analytical electron microscopy. *J Electron Microsc* 42:315–327, 1992.

23. Roggli VL: Preparatory techniques for the quantitative analysis of asbestos in tissues. *Proceedings of the 46th Annual Meeting of the Electron Microscopy Society of America* (Bailey GW, ed.), San Francisco: San Francisco Press, Inc, 1988, pp. 84–85.

24. Roggli VL: Mineral fiber content of lung tissue in patients with malignant mesothelioma. Ch. 6 In: *Malignant Mesothelioma* (Henderson DW, Shilkin KB, Langlois SLP, Whitaker D, eds.), Washington, DC: Hemisphere Pub. Corp., 1991, pp. 201–222.

25. Gylseth B, Baunan RH, Bruun R: Analysis of inorganic fiber concentrations in biological samples by scanning electron microscopy. *Scand J Work Environ Health* 7:101–108, 1981.

26. O'Sullivan MF, Corn CJ, Dodson RF: Comparative efficiency of Nuclepore filters of various pore sizes as used in digestion studies of tissue. *Environ Res* 43:97–103, 1987.

27. Morgan A, Holmes A: The distribution and characteristics of asbestos fibers in the lungs of Finnish anthophyllite mineworkers. *Environ Res* 33:62–75, 1984.

28. Ashcroft T, Heppleston AG: The optical and electron microscopic determination of pulmonary asbestos fiber concentration and its relation to the human pathological reaction. *J Clin Pathol* 26:224–234, 1973.

29. Sebastien P, Fondimare A, Bignon J, Monchaux G, Desbordes J, Bonnaud G: Topographic distribution of asbestos fibers in human lung in relation to occupational and nonoccupational exposure. In: *Inhaled Particles IV* (Walton WH, McGovern B, eds.), Oxford: Pergamon Press, 1977, pp. 435–444.

30. Roggli VL: Scanning electron microscopic analysis of mineral fibers in human lungs. Ch. 5 In: *Microprobe Analysis in Medicine* (Ingram P, Shelburne JD, Roggli VL, eds.), New York: Hemisphere Pub. Corp., 1989, pp. 97–110.

31. Ferrell RE, Jr., Paulson GG, Walker CW: Evaluation of an SEM-EDS method for identification of chrysotile. *Scanning Electron Microscopy* 11:537–546, 1975.

32. Millette JR, McFarren EF: EDS of waterborne asbestos fibers in TEM, SEM and STEM. *Scan Electron Microsc* 111:451–460, 1976.

33. Johnson GG, White EW, Strickler D, Hoover R: Image analysis techniques, In: *Symposium on Electron Microscopy of Microfibers: Proceedings of the First FDA Office of Science Summer Symposium* (Asher IM, McGrath PP, eds.), Washington, DC: Government Printing Office, 1976, pp. 76–82.

34. Kenny LC: Asbestos fibre counting by image analysis—The performance of the Manchester Asbestos Program on Magiscan. *Ann Occup Hyg* 28:401–415, 1984.

35. Kenny LC: Automated analysis of asbestos clearance samples. *Ann Occup Hyg* 32:115–128, 1988.

36. Ruud CO, Barrett CS, Russell PA, Clark RL: Selected area electron diffraction and energy dispersive x-ray analysis for the identification of asbestos fibres, a comparison. *Micron* 7:115–132, 1976.

37. Churg A: Quantitative methods for analysis of disease induced by asbestos and other mineral particles using the transmission electron microscope. Ch. 4 In: *Microprobe Analysis in Medicine* (Ingram P, Shelburne JD, Roggli VL, eds.), New York: Hemisphere Pub. Corp., 1989, pp. 79–95.

38. Churg A, Sakoda N, Warnock ML: A simple method for preparing ferruginous bodies for electron microscopic examination. *Am J Clin Pathol* 68:513–517, 1977.

39. Schraufnagel D, Ingram P, Roggli VL, Shelburne JD: An introduction to analytical electron microscopy and microprobe analysis: Techniques and tools to study the lung. In: *Electron Microscopy of the Lung* (Schraufnagel D, ed.), New York: Marcel Dekker, 1990, pp. 1–46.

40. Yatchmenoff B: A new confocal. scanning optical microscope. *Amer Lab* 20:58, 60–62, 64, 66, 1988.

41. MacDonald JL, Kane AB: Identification of asbestos fibers within single cells. *Lab Invest* 55:177–185, 1986.

42. Geiss RH: Electron diffraction from submicron areas using STEM. *Scanning Electron Microscopy* 11:337–344, 1976.

43. Gylseth B, Churg A, Davis JMG, Johnson N, Morgan A, Mowe G, Rogers A, Roggli V: Analysis of asbestos fibers and asbestos bodies in tissue samples from human lung: An international interlaboratory trial. *Scand J Work Environ Health* 11:107–110, 1985.

44. Gylseth B, Baunan RH, Overaae L: Analysis of fibers in human lung tissue. *Br J Ind Med* 39:191–195, 1982.

45. Corn CJ, Williams MG, Jr., Dodson RF: Electron microscopic analysis of residual asbestos remaining in preparative vials following bleach digestion. *J Electron Microsc Tech* 6:1–6, 1987.

46. Steel EB, Small JA: Accuracy of transmission electron microscopy for the analysis of asbestos in ambient environments. *Anal Chem* 57:209–213, 1985.

47. Ogden TL, Shenton-Taylor T, Cherrie JW, Crawford NP, Moorcroft S, Duggan MJ, Jackson PA, Treble RD: Within-laboratory quality control of asbestos counting. *Ann Occup Hyg* 30:411–425, 1986.

48. Morgan A, Holmes A: Distribution and characteristics of amphibole asbestos fibres in the left lung of an insulation worker measured with the light microscope. *Br J Ind Med* 40:45–50, 1983.

49. Roggli VL, Greenberg SD, Seitzman LH, McGavran MH, Hurst GA, Spivey CG, Nelson KG, Hieger LR: Pulmonary fibrosis, carcinoma, and ferruginous body counts in amosite asbestos workers: A study of six cases. *Am J Clin Pathol* 73:496–503, 1980.

50. Wagner JC, Pooley FD: Mineral fibres and mesothelioma. *Thorax* 41:161–166, 1986.

51. Churg A: Chrysotile, tremolite, and malignant mesothelioma in man. *Chest* 93:621–628, 1988.

52. Roggli VL, Pratt PC: Numbers of asbestos bodies on iron-stained tissue sections in relation to asbestos body counts in lung tissue digests. *Hum Pathol* 14:355–361, 1983.

53. Churg A, Vedal S: Fiber burden and patterns of asbestos-related disease in workers with heavy mixed amosite and chrysotile exposure. *Am J Respir Crit Care Med* 150:663–669, 1994.

54. Roggli VL: Pathology of human asbestosis: A critical review, In: *Advances in Pathology*, (Vol. 2) (Fenoglio-Preiser CM, ed.), Chicago: Year Book Medical Publishers, Inc., 1989, pp. 31–60.

55. Craighead JE, Abraham JL, Churg A, Green FH, Kleinerman J, Pratt PC, Seemayer TA, Vallyathan V, Weill H: Pathology of asbestos associated diseases of the lungs and pleural cavities: Diagnostic criteria and proposed grading schema. *Arch Pathol Lab Med* 106:544–596, 1982.

56. Roggli VL: Scanning electron microscopic analysis of mineral fiber content of lung tissue in the evaluation of diffuse pulmonary fibrosis. *Scanning Microsc* 5:71–83, 1991.

57. Pratt PC: Role of silica in progressive massive fibrosis in coal workers' pneumoconiosis. *Arch Environ Health* 16:734–737, 1968.

58. Churg A: Asbestos fiber content of the lungs in patients with and without asbestos airways disease. *Am Rev Respir Dis* 127:470–473, 1983.

59. Timbrell V, Ashcroft T, Goldstein B, Heyworth F, Meurman LO, Rendall REG, Reynolds JA, Shilkin KB, Whitaker D: Relationships between retained amphibole fibers and fibrosis in human lung tissue specimens. *Ann Occup Hyg* 32:323–340, 1988.

60. Lippmann M: Asbestos exposure indices. *Environ Res* 46:86–106, 1988.

61. Churg A, Wright JL, De Paoli L, Wiggs B: Mineralogic correlates of fibrosis in chrysotile miners and millers. *Am Rev Respir Dis* 139:891–896, 1989.

62. Vorwald AJ, Durkan TM, Pratt PC: Experimental studies of asbestosis. *Arch Ind Hyg Occup Med* 3:1–43, 1951.

63. Wright GW, Kuschner M: The influence of varying lengths of glass and asbestos fibers on tissue response in guinea pigs, In: *Inhaled Particles IV* (Walton WH, ed.), Oxford: Pergamon Press, 1977, pp. 455–474.

64. Davis JMG, Beckett ST, Bolton RE, Collings P, Middleton AP: Mass and number of fibres in the pathogenesis of asbestos-related lung disease in rats. *Br J Cancer* 37:673–688, 1978.

65. Crapo JD, Barry BE, Brody AR, O'Neil JJ: Morphological, morphometric, and x-ray microanalytical studies on lung tissue of rats exposed to chrysotile asbestos in inhalation chambers, In: *Biological Effects of Mineral Fibres*, (Vol. 1) (Wagner JC, ed.), IARC Scientific Publications, Lyon, 1980, pp. 273–283.

66. Lee KP, Barras CE, Griffith FD, Waritz RS, Lapin CA: Comparative pulmonary responses to inhaled inorganic fibers with asbestos and fiberglass. *Environ Res* 24:167–191, 1981.

67. Gross P: Is short-fibered asbestos dust a biological hazard? *Arch Environ Health* 29:115–117, 1974.

68. Gylseth B, Mowe G, Skaug V, Wannag A: Inorganic fibers in lung tissue from patients with pleural plaques or malignant mesothelioma. *Scand J Work Environ Health* 7:109–113, 1981.

69. Mowe G, Gylseth B, Hartveit F, Skaug V: Fiber concentration in lung tissue of patients with malignant mesothelioma: A case-control study. *Cancer* 56:1089–1093, 1985.

70. Dodson RF, O'Sullivan M, Corn CJ, McLarty JW, Hammar SP: Analysis of asbestos fiber burden in lung tissue from mesothelioma patients. *Ultrastruct Pathol* 21:321–336, 1997.

71. Churg A, Wright JL, Vedal S: Fiber burden and pattern of asbestos-related disease in chrysotile miners and millers. *Am Rev Respir Dis* 148:25–31, 1993.

72. Gaudichet A, Janson X, Monchaux G, Dufour G, Sebastien P, DeLajartre AY, Bignon J: Assessment by analytical microscopy of the total lung fibre burden in mesothelioma patients matched with four other pathological series. *Ann Occup Hyg* 32[Suppl 1]:213–223, 1988.

73. Warnock ML: Lung asbestos burden in shipyard and construction workers with mesothelioma: Comparison with burdens in subjects with asbestosis or lung cancer. *Environ Res* 50:68–85, 1989.

74. Kishimoto T, Okada K, Sato T, Ono T, Ito H: Evaluation of the pleural malignant mesothelioma patients with the relation of asbestos exposure. *Environ Res* 48:42–48, 1989.

75. Browne K, Smither WJ: Asbestos-related mesothelioma: factors discriminating between pleural and peritoneal sites. *Br J Ind Med* 40:145–152, 1983.

76. Srebro SH, Roggli VL, Samsa GP: Malignant mesothelioma associated with low pulmonary tissue asbestos burdens: A light and scanning electron microscopic analysis of 18 cases. *Mod Pathol* 8:614–621, 1995.

77. Roggli VL, Pratt PC, Brody AR: Asbestos fiber type in malignant mesothelioma: An analytical electron microscopic study of 94 cases. *Am J Ind Med* 23:605–614, 1993.

78. McDonald JC, Armstrong B, Case B, Doell B, McCaughey WTE, McDonald AD, Sebastien P: Mesothelioma and asbestos fiber type: Evidence from lung tissue analyses. *Cancer* 63:1544–1547, 1989.

79. Rogers AJ, Leigh J, Berry G, Ferguson DA, Mulder HB, Ackad M: Relationship between lung asbestos fiber type and concentration and relative risk of mesothelioma: A case-control study. *Cancer* 67:1912–1920, 1991.

80. Roggli VL: Malignant mesothelioma and duration of asbestos exposure: Correlation with tissue mineral fiber content. *Ann Occup Hyg* 39:363–374, 1995.

81. Roggli VL, Sharma A, Butnor KJ, Sporn T, Vollmer RT: Malignant mesothelioma and occupational exposure to asbestos: A clinicopathological correlation of 1445 cases. *Ultrastruct Pathol* 26:1–11, 2002.

82. Roggli VL, Oury TD, Moffatt EJ: Malignant mesothelioma in women. In: *Anatomic Pathology*, (Vol. 2) (Rosen PP, Fechner RE, eds.), Chicago: ASCP Press, 1998, pp. 147–163.
83. Stanton MF, Layard M, Tegeris A, Miller E, May M, Morgan E, Smith A: Relation of particle dimension to carcinogenicity in amphibole asbestoses and other fibrous minerals. *J Natl Cancer Inst* 67:965–975, 1981.
84. Churg A, Wiggs B: Fiber size and number in amphibole-asbestos-induced mesothelioma. *Am J Pathol* 115:437–442, 1984.
85. Churg A, Wiggs B, De Paoli L, Kampe B, Stevens B: Lung asbestos content in chrysotile workers with mesothelioma. *Am Rev Respir Dis* 130:1042–1045, 1984.
86. Suzuki Y, Yuen SR: Asbestos tissue burden study on human malignant mesothelioma. *Ind Health* 39:150–160, 2001.
87. Dodson RF, Williams MG, Corn CJ, Brollo A, Bianchi C: Asbestos content of lung tissue, lymph nodes, and pleural plaques from former shipyard workers. *Am Rev Respir Dis* 142:843–847, 1990.
88. Gibbs AR, Stephens M, Griffiths DM, Blight BJN, Pooley FD: Fibre distribution in the lungs and pleura of subjects with asbestos related diffuse pleural fibrosis. *Br J Ind Med* 48:762–770, 1991.
89. Boutin C, Dumortier P, Rey F, Viallat JR, De Vuyst P: Black spots concentrate oncogenic asbestos fibers in the parietal pleura. *Am J Respir Crit Care Med* 153:444–449, 1996.
90. Dodson RF, O'Sullivan MF, Huang J, Holiday DB, Hammar SP: Asbestos in extrapulmonary sites—omentum and mesentery. *Chest* 117:486–493, 2000.
91. Warnock ML, Prescott BT, Kuwahara TJ: Numbers and types of asbestos fibers in subjects with pleural plaques. *Am J Pathol* 109:37–46, 1982.
92. Churg A: Asbestos fibers and pleural plaques in a general autopsy population. *Am J Pathol* 109:88–96, 1982.
93. Stephens M, Gibbs AR, Pooley FD, Wagner JC: Asbestos induced diffuse pleural fibrosis: Pathology and mineralogy. *Thorax* 42:583–588, 1987.
94. Voisin C, Fisekci F, Voisin-Saltiel S, Ameille J, Brochard P, Pairon J-C: Asbestos-related rounded atelectasis: Radiologic and mineralogic data in 23 cases. *Chest* 107:477–481, 1995.
95. Andrion A, Colombo A, Mollo F: Lung asbestos bodies and pleural plaques at autopsy. *La Ricerca Clin Lab* 12:461–468, 1982.
96. Warnock ML, Isenberg W: Asbestos burden and the pathology of lung cancer. *Chest* 89:20–26, 1986.
97. Anttila S, Karjalainen A, Taikina-aho O, Kyyronen P, Vainio H: Lung cancer in the lower lobe is associated with pulmonary asbestos fiber count and fiber size. *Environ Health Perspect* 101:166–170, 1993.
98. Karjalainen A, Anttila S, Vanhala E, Vainio H: Asbestos exposure and the risk of lung cancer in a general urban population. *Scand J Work Environ Health* 20:243–250, 1994.
99. Roggli VL, Sanders LL: Asbestos content of lung tissue and carcinoma of the lung: A clinicopathologic correlation and mineral fiber analysis of 234 cases. *Ann Occup Hyg* 44:109–117, 2000.
100. Gaensler EA, McLoud TC, Carrington CB: Thoracic surgical problems in asbestos-related disorders. *Ann Thorac Surg* 40:82–96, 1985.
101. Churg A, Warnock ML: Asbestos fibers in the general population. *Am Rev Respir Dis* 122:669–678, 1980.
102. Case BW, Sebastien P: Environmental and occupational exposures to chrysotile asbestos: A comparative microanalytic study. *Arch Environ Health* 42:185–191, 1987.

103. Hammar SP, Dodson RF: Asbestos. Ch. 28 In: *Pulmonary Pathology*, 2nd ed. (Dail DH, Hammar SP, eds.), New York: Springer-Verlag, 1994, pp. 901–983.

104. Churg A, Warnock ML: Correlation of quantitative asbestos body counts and occupation in urban patients. *Arch Pathol Lab Med* 101:629–634, 1977.

105. Tuomi T, Huuskonen MS, Tammilehto L, Vanhala E, Virtamo M: Occupational exposure to asbestos as evaluated from work histories and analysis of lung tissues from patients with mesothelioma. *Br J Ind Med* 48:48–52, 1991.

106. Hammond EC, Selikoff IJ, Seidman H: Asbestos exposure, cigarette smoking, and death rates. In: Health Hazards of Asbestos Exposure (Selikoff IJ, Hammond EC, eds.), *Ann NY Acad Sci* 330:473–490, 1979.

107. Talcott JA, Thurber WA, Kantor AF, Gaensler EA, Danahy JF, Antman KH, Li FP: Asbestos-associated diseases in a cohort of cigarette-filter workers. *N Engl J Med* 321:1220–1223, 1989.

108. Newhouse ML, Berry G: Patterns of mortality in asbestos factory workers in London. *Ann NY Acad Sci* 330:53–60, 1979.

109. Hughes JM, Weill H: Asbestosis as a precursor of asbestos related lung cancer: Results of a prospective mortality study. *Br J Ind Med* 48:229–233, 1991.

110. Hirsch A, Di Menza L, Carre A, Harf A, Perdrizet F, Cooreman J, Bignon J: Asbestos risk among full-time workers in an electricity-generating power station. *Ann NY Acad Sci* 330:137–145, 1979.

111. Leigh J, Davidson P, Hendrie L, Berry D: Malignant mesothelioma in Australia, 1945–2000. *Am J Ind Med* 41:188–201, 2002.

112. Eisenstadt HB: Asbestos pleurisy. *Dis Chest* 46:78–81, 1964.

113. Lilis R, Daum S, Anderson H, Sirota M, Andrews G, Selikoff IJ: Asbestos disease in maintenance workers of the chemical industry. *Ann NY Acad Sci* 330:127–135, 1979.

114. Mancuso TF: Relative risk of mesothelioma among railroad machinists exposed to chrysotile. *Am J Ind Med* 13:639–657, 1988.

115. Mancuso TF: Mesothelioma among machinists in railroad and other industries. *Am J Ind Med* 4:501–513, 1983.

116. Langer AM, McCaughey WTE: Mesothelioma in a brake repair worker. *Lancet* 2:1101–1103, 1982.

117. Huncharek M, Muscat J, Capotorto JV: Pleural mesothelioma in a brake mechanic. *Br J Ind Med* 46:69–71, 1989.

118. Jarvholm B, Brisman J: Asbestos associated tumors in car mechanics. *Br J Ind Med* 45:645–646, 1988.

119. Woitowitz HJ, Rodelsperger K: Mesothelioma among car mechanics? *Ann Occup Hyg* 38:635–638, 1994.

120. Wong O: Malignant mesothelioma and asbestos exposure among auto mechanics: appraisal of scientific evidence. *Reg Tox Pharmacol* 34:170–177, 2001.

121. Williams RL, Muhlbaier JL: Asbestos brake emissions. *Environ Res* 29:70–82, 1982.

122. Anderson HA, Lilis R, Daum SM, Selikoff IJ: Asbestosis among household contacts of asbestos factory workers. *Ann NY Acad Sci* 330:387–399, 1979.

123. Newhouse ML, Thompson H: Mesothelioma of pleura and peritoneum following exposure to asbestos in the London area. *Br J Ind Med* 22:261–269, 1965.

124. Huncharek M, Capotorto JV, Muscat J: Domestic asbestos exposure, lung fibre burden, and pleural mesothelioma in a housewife. *Br J Ind Med* 46:354–355, 1989.

125. Gibbs AR, Griffiths DM, Pooley FD, Jones JSP: Comparison of fibre types and size distributions in lung tissues of paraoccupational and occupational cases of malignant mesothelioma. *Br J Ind Med* 47:621–626, 1990.

126. Crump KS, Farrar DB: Statistical analysis of data on airborne asbestos levels collected in an EPA survey of public buildings. *Reg Toxicol Pharmacol* 10:51–62, 1989.

127. Cordier S, Lazar P, Brochard P, Bignon J, Ameille J, Proteau J: Epidemiologic investigation of respiratory effects related to environmental exposure to asbestos inside insulated buildings. *Arch Environ Health* 42:303–309, 1987.

128. Stein RC, Kitajewska JY, Kirkham JB, Tait N, Sinha G, Rudd RM: Pleural mesothelioma resulting from exposure to amosite asbestos in a building. *Respir Med* 83:237–239, 1989.

129. Roggli VL, Longo WE: Mineral fiber content of lung tissue in patients with environmental exposures: Household contacts vs. building occupants. *Ann NY Acad Sci* 643:511–519, 1992.

130. Mossman BT, Bignon J, Corn M, Seaton A, Gee JBL: Asbestos: scientific developments and implications for public policy. *Science* 247:294–301, 1990.

131. Pooley FD: An examination of the fibrous mineral content of asbestos lung tissue from the Canadian chrysotile mining industry. *Environ Res* 12:281–298, 1976.

132. Churg A, Warnock ML: Analysis of the cores of asbestos bodies from members of the general population: Patients with probable low-degree exposure to asbestos. *Am Rev Respir Dis* 120:781–786, 1979.

133. Gylseth B, Norseth T, Skaug V: Amphibole fibers in a taconite mine and in the lungs of the miners. *Am J Ind Med* 2:175–184, 1981.

134. Rowlands N, Gibbs GW, McDonald AD: Asbestos fibres in the lungs of chrysotile miners and millers—A preliminary report. *Ann Occup Hyg* 26:411–415, 1982.

135. Roggli VL: Analytical electron microscopy of mineral fibers from human lungs. *Proceedings of the 45th Annual Meeting of the Electron Microscopy Society of America* (Bailey GW, ed.), San Francisco: San Francisco Press, Inc, 1987, pp. 666–669.

136. McDonald AD, McDonald JC, Pooley FD: Mineral fibre content of lung in mesothelial tumours in North America. *Ann Occup Hyg* 26:417–422, 1982.

137. Karjalainen A, Meurman LO, Pukkala E: Four cases of mesothelioma among Finnish anthophyllite miners. *Occup Environ Med* 51:212–215, 1994.

138. Nicholson WJ: Comparative dose-response relationships of asbestos fiber types: Magnitudes and uncertainties. *Ann NY Acad Sci* 643:74–84, 1991.

139. Hodgson JT, Darnton A: The quantitative risk of mesothelioma and lung cancer in relation to asbestos exposure. *Ann Occup Hyg* 44:565–601, 2000.

140. McDonald AD, Case BW, Churg A, Dufresne A, Gibbs GW, Sebastien P, McDonald JC: Mesothelioma in Quebec chrysotile miners and millers: Epidemiology and aetiology. *Ann Occup Hyg* 41:707–719, 1997.

141. Hansen J, de Klerk NH, Musk AW, Hobbs MST: Environmental exposure to crocidolite and mesothelioma: Exposure-response relationships. *Am J Respir Crit Care Med* 157:69–75, 1998.

142. Churg A: Neoplastic Asbestos-Induced Diseases. Ch. 10 In: *Pathology of Occupational Lung Disease*, 2nd ed. (Churg A, Green FHY, eds.), Baltimore: Williams & Wilkins, 1998, pp. 339–391.

143. Smith AH, Wright CC: Chrysotile asbestos is the main cause of pleural mesothelioma. *Am J Ind Med* 30:252–266, 1996.

144. Begin R, Gauthier J-J, Desmeules M, Ostiguy G: Work-related mesothelioma in Quebec, 1967–1990. *Am J Ind Med* 22:531–542, 1992.

145. Dufresne A, Begin R, Churg A, Masse S: Mineral fiber content of lungs in patients with mesothelioma seeking compensation in Quebec. *Am J Respir Crit Care Med* 153:711–718, 1996.

146. Yano E, Wang Z-M, Wang X-R, Wang M-Z, Lan Y-J: Cancer mortality among workers exposed to amphibole-free chrysotile asbestos. *Am J Epidemiol* 154:538–543, 2001.

147. Tossavainen A, Kotilainen M, Takahashi K, Pan G, Vanhala E: Amphibole fibres in Chinese chrysotile asbestos. *Ann Occup Hyg* 45:145–152, 2001.

148. Craighead JE: Airways and Lung. Ch. 28 In: *Pathology of Environmental and Occupational Disease* (Craighead JE, ed.), St. Louis: Mosby, 1995, pp. 455–489.

149. Roggli VL, Vollmer RT, Butnor KJ, Sporn TA: Tremolite and mesothelioma. *Ann Occup Hyg* 46:447–453, 2002.

150. Churg A: Nonasbestos pulmonary mineral fibers in the general population. *Environ Res* 31:189–200, 1983.

151. Stettler LE, Groth DH, Platek SF, Burg JR: Particulate concentrations in urban lungs. Ch. 7 In: *Microprobe Analysis in Medicine* (Ingram P, Shelburne JD, Roggli VL, eds.), New York: Hemisphere Pub. Corp., 1989, pp. 133–146.

152. Roggli VL: *Nonasbestos mineral fibers in human lungs. Microbeam Analysis— 1989* (Russell PE, ed.), San Francisco: San Francisco Press, Inc., 1989, pp. 57–59.

153. Rodelsperger K, Jockel J-H, Pohlabeln H, Romer W, Woitowitz H-J: Asbestos and manmade vitreous fibers as risk factors for diffuse malignant mesothelioma: Results from a German hospital-based case-control study. *Am J Ind Med* 38:1–14, 2001.

154. Churg A, Wiggs B: Mineral particles, mineral fibers, and lung cancer. *Environ Res* 37:364–372, 1985.

12

Medicolegal Aspects of Asbestos-Related Diseases: A Plaintiff's Attorney's Perspective

Ronald L. Motley, Charles W. Patrick, Jr., and Anne McGinness Kearse

Background: History of Exposure and Disease

The widespread use of asbestos products, the ambient nature of asbestos fibers, and the debilitating effects of asbestos-related diseases have caused unprecedented human suffering and have resulted in an American tragedy. The association between exposure to asbestos fibers and disease is well documented. Asbestos has been used since prehistoric times, and its toxic effects on humans have been recognized for at least 2,000 years.[1] In the early 1900s, asbestos-related disease was associated with occupations that required working in mines, mills, and manufacturing plants, and it was during this time that reports of asbestosis began to appear in the published literature. In 1906, a London physician, H. Montague Murray, performed a postmortem examination on a thirty-three-year-old man who worked for fourteen years in an asbestos textile factory.[2] The patient was suffering from pulmonary fibrosis. At the autopsy, Dr. Murray found asbestos fibers in the lung tissue and linked the man's occupational exposure to asbestos to the disease that killed him. In 1924, the first death due to asbestosis appeared in the medical literature.[3] W.E. Cooke, an English physician, performed a postmortem autopsy on a thirty-three-year-old woman who had worked in an asbestos textile plant. The autopsy showed extensive pulmonary fibrosis and dense strands of abnormal fibrous tissue connecting the lungs and the pleural membranes surrounding them.

Conditions in the mills, mines, and manufacturing plants subjected workers to hazardous conditions on a daily basis. In 1930, Merewether and Price, Medical Inspectors with the Factory Department, reported on their research of the British asbestos textile industry. Merewether explained:

It is helpful to visualize fibrosis of the lungs as it occurs among asbestos workers as the slow growth of fibrous tissue (scar tissue) between the air cells of the lungs wherever the inhaled dust comes to rest. While new fibrous tissue is being laid down like a spider's web, that deposited earlier gradually contracts. This fibrous tissue is not only useless as a substitute for the air cells, but with continued inhalation of the causative dust, by its invasion of new territory and consolidation of that already occupied, it gradually, and literally strangles the essential tissues of the lungs.

In common with other essential organs of the body the lungs have a large reserve of tissue for use in emergencies and to permit of a diminution in functional capacity due to advancing age or disease. For this reason, and because fibrosis of the lungs is essentially a local disease, it is only when the fibrosis progresses to the extent of obliterating this reserve, that undue shortness of breath on any extra effort draws the worker's attention to the fact that his health is not what it should be. The other symptoms of the disease such as cough are equally unassuming, and are readily ascribed to some common and trivial cause.

From this point the progress of the disease is more rapid, since it is now encroaching on the remaining sound tissue of the lungs, already only just sufficient to maintain him in his ordinary daily activities. Ultimately, if no acute respiratory infection has precipitated a fatal termination, a stage is reached when the lungs can do little more than maintain life, and the shortness of breath becomes extreme.

This landmark study reported that of 363 asbestos textile workers examined, more than 25% showed evidence of pulmonary fibrosis.[4] The incidence of fibrosis increased with the number of years of exposure. As a result, legislation was passed in England that required improved methods of ventilation and dust suppression in asbestos textile factories, instituted periodical medical examinations for workers engaged in dusty processes in the asbestos textile industry, and made asbestosis a compensable disease. In the early 1930s, asbestos workers who had asbestosis began filing claims against Johns-Manville and Raybestos–Manhattan, the nation's largest asbestos manufacturers. In the United States, asbestosis would not become a compensable disease in most states until 10 or 15 years after the English regulations.

The manufacture of products containing asbestos as a key ingredient prevented this disease from being contained within these occupations. The application and use of asbestos products also subjected workers to breathing asbestos dust. The numbers of persons exposed from various trades and occupations using asbestos-containing products or working next to trades using asbestos-containing products was very large. Inadequate controls and warnings subjected hundreds of thousands of employees to breathing asbestos fibers. For many, their work cost them their lives. Exposure was not confined to the plants and worksites, and, in fact, dust-laden clothing brought home exposed whole households to asbestos. Dust emitted from the mines and plants exposed nearby neighborhoods to environmental pollution.

In 1964, Wilhelm Hueper, a pathologist with the National Cancer Institute, warned:

Cancers of all types and causes display, even under already existing conditions, all the characteristics of an epidemic in slow motion. Through a continued, unrestrained, needless, avoidable and in part reckless increasing contamination of the human environment with chemical and physical carcinogens, and with chemicals supporting and potentiating their action, the stage is being set indeed for a future occurrence of a catastrophic epidemic, which once present cannot be effectively checked for decades with the means available nor can its course appreciably be altered once it has been set in motion.[5]

Until around 1970, industry regulated itself as to permissible exposure levels. Occupational and environmental asbestos exposures today are regulated by the Occupational Safety and Health Administration (OSHA) under provisions of the Occupational Safety and Health Act and by the Environmental Protection Agency (EPA) under provisions of the Clean Air Act (CAA) and the Toxic Substances Control Act (TSCA). Consumer asbestos exposures are regulated by the Consumer Product Safety Commission. In March 1971, the EPA, under the Clean Air Act, listed asbestos as a hazardous air pollutant.[6] In April 1973, spray application of products containing more than 1 percent asbestos was banned except on equipment and machinery.[7] In 1975, demolition standards were revised and made more stringent concerning controls, use of asbestos in friable insulation, and waste disposal, and friable insulation products containing more than one percent asbestos were banned in the United States.[8] In addition, the EPA under the Toxic Substances Control Act has issued numerous regulations under its authority to regulate toxic substances if it finds that the manufacture, processing, distribution in commerce, use, or disposal of the chemical substance, or any combination of such activities, presents or will present an unreasonable risk of injury to human health or the environment.[9] In May 1971, OSHA issued initial regulations adopting the ACGIH Threshold Limit Value of 12f/cc.[10] OSHA has continually reduced by regulation permissible exposures to asbestos in the workplace.[11] In 1986, OSHA's overview of asbestos-related diseases described the magnitude of the problem, as it exists today:

OSHA is aware of no instance in which exposure to a toxic substance has more clearly demonstrated detrimental health effects on humans than has asbestos exposure. The diseases caused by asbestos exposure are life-threatening or disabling. Among these diseases are lung cancer, cancer of the mesothelial lining of the pleura and peritoneum, asbestosis, and gastrointestinal cancer.[12]

Still, even with government regulations reducing the possibility of exposures there is no known safe level of exposure to asbestos and government regulations do not differentiate between fiber types. OSHA has recognized that all types of asbestos fibers have fibrogenic and carcinogenic potential.[13]

Evolution of Legal Claims

Trial Courts

Just as Hueper predicted in 1964, the latent onset of disease from exposure has led to a catastrophic epidemic and a continuing onslaught of disease as a result of persons exposed in the 1940s, 1950s, and 1960s. Recently, the U.S. Supreme Court recognized the nightmare that asbestos exposure has inflicted on the American public and the American judicial system. In *Ortiz v. Fibreboard Corporation*, it commented that occupational asbestos exposure and its detrimental effects have created an "elephantine mass of asbestos cases."[14] The tide has yet to turn.

Although asbestos claims were filed before the 1960s, legal troubles began for the asbestos industry when Claude J. Tomplait, a forty-year-old Texas insulator sought legal representation from Ward Stephenson, an attorney in Orange, Texas, in 1969. For 20 years, Tomplait labored as an asbestos insulator. He insulated steam pipes, boilers, turbines, and other high-temperature equipment in the shipyards, power plants, oil refineries, and petrochemical factories. Recently diagnosed with pulmonary fibrosis as a result of inhaling asbestos fibers, Tomplait asked Stephenson if he would file a worker's compensation claim on his behalf. Stephenson filed not only a worker's compensation claim, but for the first time, brought suit against the asbestos manufacturers under the newly recognized doctrine of strict liability. Although unsuccessful in his suit against the manufacturers, this case served as a catalyst for future litigation. In 1969, Stephenson brought suit on behalf of a coworker of Tomplait, Clarence Borel, against eleven asbestos manufacturers.[15] *Borel v. Fibreboard Corporation* was filed in the District Court for the Eastern District of Texas and significantly changed the way the litigation would progress into the future. *Borel* was the first case in the country to recognize a manufacturer's duty to warn of asbestos product dangers. It became the seminal case standing for the manufacturer's responsibility to know and warn of the dangers of its products that may cause occupational disease.

When Judge John Minor Wisdom issued the opinion of the U.S. Court of Appeals for the Fifth Circuit in *Borel* on September 10, 1973, little did anyone expect that this decision—extending the doctrine of strict product liability to asbestos-related disease caused by the use of insulation materials—would engender a wave of personal injury litigation never before seen in American jurisprudence. Fewer than 10 years later, more than 16,000 asbestos-related personal injury cases had been filed in the United States, and, in the words of a subsequent opinion by the Fifth Circuit, asbestos litigation "had become the largest area of product liability litigation, far surpassing the number of cases generated by the controversies over Agent Orange, the drug DES, the Dalkon Shield intrauterine device, or even automobile defects."[16] In the year 2001, it is estimated that there are more than 200,000 asbestos cases pending nationwide.

Today there is no shortage of plaintiffs seeking compensation for asbestos-related disease. The courts, still backlogged from the impact of industrial exposures and disease-stricken plaintiffs, suffer from the filings of claims by persons exposed to asbestos fibers from a variety of sources. As buildings constructed with asbestos over the past six decades begin to age and deteriorate, asbestos disease among persons engaged in the repair, renovation, and demolition of these buildings is on the rise. Many still proceed by traditional jurisprudence of tort litigation—a single plaintiff suing for injury against a number of asbestos product manufacturers or suppliers. A traditional setting requires the plaintiff to prove his injuries, that the injuries are a result of exposure to asbestos-containing products, that the exposure from each defendant contributed to the disease, and that the asbestos defendant is legally liable for the asbestos-related injuries sustained by the plaintiff.

As the numbers of persons injured from exposure to asbestos grew, so did the flood of litigation in courts throughout the nation. It became obvious that to try each case one at a time would create a huge backlog of cases well past many of the lifetimes of the plaintiffs involved as well as the lawyers and judges.[17] To deal with the staggering numbers of cases, courts made efforts to streamline the cases by consolidating trials, conducting summary trials, and standardizing discovery and pleading forms. Still huge numbers of cases remained in the court system.

Asbestos cases such as those we are now considering present a complex pattern of legal, social, and political issues that threaten to cripple the common law system of adjudication, if for no other reason than by the sheer volume of cases.[18]

To date, Congress has not created any legislative solution to these problems nor, for that matter, has an effective or fair legislative scheme been proposed. In the absence of a workable statutory solution, Congress has effectively forced the courts to adopt diverse, innovative, and often nontraditional judicial management techniques to reduce the burden of asbestos litigation that seems to be paralyzing their active dockets.[19] In testimony offered to the Committee on the Judiciary of the U.S. House of Representatives on July 1, 1999, Professor William N. Eskridge of Yale Law School offered the following observations about the effects of asbestos litigation on the judiciary:

A big loser is the judiciary, which has a larger management problem than ever before. The courts continue to be deluged with asbestos lawsuits. There are now more than 200,000 of them in the system, and tens of thousands of new cases were added last year. . . . The asbestos litigation problem is one that has defeated the judiciary. An increasing number of judges are now admitting it.[20]

In an effort to deal with the growing number of claims, a national settlement class action was filed in 1993 in an attempt to resolve claims of present and future victims of asbestos disease.[21] Nevertheless, in 1997, the U.S. Supreme Court overturned the $1.3 billion class-action settlement that was forged between plaintiffs and the Center for Claims Resolution, a consortium of 20 former asbestos manufacturers.[22] Some view this decision as contributing to the resurgence of asbestos litigation, and in striking down this historic class-action settlement, plaintiffs and asbestos defendants were again forced to resolve these cases one at a time in what appears to be endless litigation.

Bankruptcy Court

Asbestos companies are increasingly seeking protection under the bankruptcy code. Since 1982, at least 42 firms with asbestos liabilities have sought chapter 11 bankruptcy protection with others inevitably to follow. Reorganization under chapter 11 of the bankruptcy code is one of the few methods by which a company can isolate its operations from its asbestos liabilities. Although bankruptcy may permit an asbestos defendant to put a permanent end to asbestos litigation against it and resolve liability issues in a coordinated and integrated fashion, it severely reduces compensation to diseased plaintiffs.[23] The first relief for a defendant in asbestos litigation after filing under chapter 11 is an immediate stay. Section 362 of the bankruptcy code, the "automatic stay" provision, enjoins virtually all litigation against the debtor immediately upon the filing of a bankruptcy case.[24] A claims process is established for which both present and future claims are eventually paid at a much reduced value than one would hope to receive in the civil court system. Depending on the bankruptcy, claimants submit information as part of a proof of claim that is then processed and paid if the claimant meets the criteria for payment.

In August 1982, Johns-Manville, the largest manufacturer of asbestos-containing products, filed for bankruptcy, and several years later, the Manville Asbestos Disease Compensation Fund (Manville Trust) was created to handle claims filed against Johns-Manville. At the end of 1999, the Manville Trust projected that it would receive almost 500,000 claims over the next four decades. In the year 2000, however, it received 58,600 new claims, an 81% rise over the prior year, and two years after its initial prediction, the Trust revised its projections and estimated that it will receive 1.5 million to 2.5 million future claims.[25]

As a result of the bankruptcies, the remaining defendants are increasingly pressed to help pay for the injuries suffered as a result of asbestos exposure. The dwindling number of manufacturing defendants left in civil litigation has caused plaintiffs' counsel to add as defendants those companies that, although not involved in the manufacture of asbestos products, were distributors of such products and have come to be known in asbestos litigation as "peripheral defendants."

Proving the Asbestos Disease Case

Knowledge of the Manufacturer

Under the product liability laws of most states, the plaintiff must prove that the manufacturers either knew or should have known that their asbestos-containing products were hazardous and that the manufacturers failed to give adequate warnings of those dangers. Establishing this burden can be accomplished in two ways. The plaintiff may prove through oral testimony or documentary evidence that a manufacturer was actually aware that its products containing asbestos could cause harm to the users of those products.[26] Alternatively, a plaintiff may prove that, if a manufacturer were to have reviewed the scientific and medical literature at the time its products were sold, such an analysis would have revealed that asbestos was known to be dangerous. Under the law of product liability, a manufacturer is presumed to know the hazards of its products, and *Borel* established that a manufacturer is considered to be an expert with regard to the dangers of its products.

At trial, a plaintiff may establish the manufacturers' actual knowledge and corporate misconduct by introducing as exhibits the internal correspondence and memoranda of the companies. Throughout the years internal documents located in corporate files reveal that many companies not only had actual knowledge of the hazards of asbestos, but also took active measures to thwart publication or mention of asbestos-related hazards. In 1935, Sumner Simpson, the president of the asbestos manufacturer Raybestos–Manhattan, wrote to Vandiver Brown, head of Johns-Manville's legal department, telling him, "I think the less said about asbestos the better off we are," Brown replied, "I quite agree with you that our interests are best served by having asbestosis receive the minimum of publicity."[27] In the following year, officials from asbestos manufacturing companies met in New York City to sign a secret agreement to finance animal experiments at the Trudeau Foundation's Saranac Laboratory at Saranac Lake, New York. The intent was to gather data that would support a defense to lawsuits beginning to be brought against asbestos manufacturers. Before final publication, the Saranac report originally made reference to the findings that animals exposed to asbestos developed cancer. The final report, however, published in 1951, deleted all reference to cancer. Furthermore, the revised report was absent in its criticism of the asbestos dust threshold limit value (TLV) and previously published studies linking asbestos with cancer. In 1952, a Saranac symposium that included discussions of asbestosis and cancer in product users was never published.[28]

The industry code of silence is also shown in a variety of ways, which includes the use of internal documents. In 1947, members of the Asbestos Textile Institute (ATI) sponsored a study of textile factories by the Industrial Hygiene Foundation. The study found asbestosis in workers, made recommendations about medical exams, and recommended re-evaluation of the industry's threshold limit value for asbestos. These findings were never circulated outside the ATI. In the mid-1950s, the Institute rejected funding for cancer studies because "such an investigation would stir up a hornet's nest and put the whole industry under suspicion."[29]

A number of internal documents reveal that the asbestos companies continued to be less than forthcoming with their increasing knowledge of asbestos and disease.[30] As information mounted, so did industry's fear that the dangers of asbestos would be publicized and adversely affect profits. For example, a once contemplated health and safety booklet was opposed by industry members because "the booklet creates fear in the minds of buyers, users, and workers without justification. These fears would be damaging to the entire industry."[31] The asbestos companies recognized this as an industrywide problem and, in fact, one such document revealed that the companies understood that "no one company acting independently could adequately or effectively represent an entire industry in dealing with the press and with government officials."[32]

Against this background of these and other documents that will be introduced at trial, evidence concerning the medical and scientific literature seems to pale in comparison. Yet, with the dwindling number of defendants who conspired to withhold knowledge of the dangers, the role of state-of-the art case, that is, what should have been known, is once again of central prominence because any manufacturer had the duty to keep abreast of the medical and scientific literature. The industrial physicians knew as much, if not more, about the hazards of asbestos-containing products than the rest of the scientific community. A plaintiff may present evidence through a medical historian or a scientist who lived and worked through that period of time that asbestos-related diseases have been recognized throughout the century. As stated by David Ozonoff, a professor of public health at Boston University and a medical historian:

> The knowledge that exposure to asbestos could cause a serious chronic pulmonary disease called asbestosis was irrefutable and generally accepted by 1930. The suspicion that asbestos could cause cancer of the lung was first voiced in the 1930s, was considered a probable relationship by 1942, and was generally accepted by 1949. Epidemiological studies in the mid-1950s left little room for doubt. The index of suspicion relating asbestos exposure to the rare tumors called mesothelioma was high by 1953, and by 1960, the full extent of the relationship was being revealed. Exposure to asbestos in the course of work with asbestos-containing products posed the same hazards as exposures in the factory setting. The simple fact that "asbestos was asbestos" was evident from the medical record and confirmed by numerous case reports and studies showing harm to those who worked with asbestos products.[33]

Asbestos companies usually present a medical historian to offer their defense that it was not until the publication of the Selikoff studies in 1964 that they either knew or should have known of the hazards of asbestos to insulation workers. The asbestos companies present evidence that the threshold limit value (TLV) for asbestos was established in 1946 as five million particles of asbestos per cubic foot of air and that this standard was not changed until 1969. Additionally, they contend that prior to 1964, it was thought that exposures to asbestos below this TLV were safe and that insulation work usually produced concentrations of atmospheric asbestos less than five million particles per cubic foot of air.

The weakness in this defense is that several of the companies had actual knowledge that the TLV was not reliable as noted above.[34] The medical director of Johns-Manville, Kenneth Smith, testified that he was aware in the late 1940s and early 1950s that insulation workers were developing asbestosis.[35] Indeed, insulation workers were filing workers' compensation claims against the companies throughout the 1950s and 1960s, and these companies included Fibreboard, Owens-Corning, and Armstrong Contracting and Supply.[36] One corporate executive, after reviewing the number of workers' compensation claims filed by insulators, wrote in 1962 that the list of claims was "rather imposing."[37] Although the state-of-the-art expert for the manufacturers may be able to construct a defense solely based on the medical literature, a review of the corporate documents reveals not only that the companies should have known of the hazards, but that they did know that asbestos was causing disease in the workers who were using their products.

Asbestos Fibers Are Released and Respirable

In addition to proving that the manufacturers knew or should have known about the hazards of asbestos, the plaintiff must demonstrate that he or she breathed asbestos fibers liberated from the use of one or more of the manufacturers' products. Since exposures to asbestos may have occurred decades earlier, recollection of the use of a specific product by name is extremely difficult. In some instances, a plaintiff or a coworker can establish the name and manufacturer of the asbestos-containing materials used by the plaintiff or in the vicinity of the plaintiff.[38] It is not unusual, however, that many persons who have developed asbestos-related disease cannot actually identify the specific product name because they were exposed from the work of nearby tradesmen and did not have the opportunity to observe product labels. The nature of asbestos and its ability to permeate a workplace exposed many persons working next to the asbestos trades. Evidence that a particular manufacturer sold its products to a specific shipyard or placed them on a specific job site is admissible in the form of sales records and may raise a presumption that a plaintiff was exposed to this product. A plaintiff may testify that he or she used a specific product over time, and this testimony may be buttressed by the testimony of coworkers that particular products were used. Court decisions concerning product identification evidence have usually required that, before a coworker may testify as to the use of specific products, the coworker must testify that the products were in the general vicinity of the plaintiffs.

Exposure Caused Injury: Asbestos-Related Disease

Finally, the plaintiff must prove that he or she developed an asbestos-related disease and has suffered damages. To prove medical causation, plaintiffs' counsel will usually retain an expert medical witness such as a pulmonary specialist, occupational physician, or lung pathologist. The role of the family physician should not be minimized, and even though the treating physician may not be an expert in the diagnosis of asbestosis, it is critical that the local doctor support the diagnosis.

Whether the diagnosis of an asbestos-related disease can be made is usually the most controversial issue in an asbestos trial. Unless there is no room for debate, the defendants will attempt to shift the focus of the trial from the evidence of corporate misconduct to creation of doubt in the jurors' minds about the propriety of the diagnosis. In essence, the victim is on trial as to whether or not he or she is suffering from an asbestos-related disease.

In an asbestosis case, where tissue is not available, the defendants argue that numerous criteria must be met before a diagnosis can be established. In 1986, the American Thoracic Society (ATS) issued a statement concerning the diagnosis of asbestosis, and the manufacturers have seized a misreading of that document in order to confuse juries about medical causation. The ATS statement reads as follows:

In the absence of pathologic examination of lung tissue, the diagnosis of asbestosis is a judgment based on a careful consideration of all relevant clinical findings. In our opinion, it is necessary that there be:

1. A reliable history of exposure.
2. An appropriate time interval between exposure and detection.

Furthermore, we regard the following clinical criteria to be of recognized value:

1. Chest roentgenographic evidence of type "s," "t," "u," small irregular opacifications of a profusion of 1/1 or greater.
2. A restrictive pattern of lung impairment with a forced vital capacity below the lower limit of normal.
3. A diffusing capacity below the lower limit of normal.
4. Bilateral late or pan inspiratory crackles at the posterior lung bases not cleared by cough.[39]

As can be seen from the statement itself, there are only two mandatory criteria that must be met before the diagnosis of asbestosis can be made. Obviously, there must be a history of exposure to asbestos, and a sufficient time must have passed between first exposure to asbestos and the development of the disease process. The defendants, however, argue that the other criteria that the ATS regards as "of recognized value" must all be met as well, and this reading, if accepted by the jury, would exclude many legitimate diagnoses.

One of the most controversial criteria in the ATS statement is the requirement for a chest x-ray reading of 1/1 according to the International Labor Organization's (ILO) profusion rating for interstitial fibrosis. From a pathologic standpoint, asbestosis can exist in the absence of the chest x-ray findings; and even from a clinical standpoint, other criteria can establish the diagnosis in the absence of a positive chest x-ray reading. Indeed, a 1/0 reading is considered by the ILO to be indicative of an abnormal chest x-ray.[40] Readings of 1/0 are often contested. Both plaintiff and defense counsel will usually hire qualified B-readers specifically trained in reviewing chest x-rays for pneumoconiosis-related diseases. Because B-reading is an interpretive science, plaintiffs will have to be prepared to defend their B-reader's findings.

Also hotly contested is the significance of pleural disease. In fact, pleural disease is notably absent from the ATS statement. Although there can be reasonable debate on the issue on the extent to which pleural disease can cause pulmonary dysfunction,[41] no one can argue that pleural plaques and thickening are almost always caused by asbestos in those persons who are occupationally exposed, and the existence of pleural disease in those people is strong evidence that fibrosis on the chest x-ray, however slight, is also due to asbestos exposure.

The remaining criteria, although "of recognized value" in establishing the diagnosis, are certainly not mandatory and are more helpful in assessing impairment. For instance, a reduction in the forced vital capacity (FVC) to below 80% of predicted certainly is indicative of an abnormal FVC, but the ATS document fails to take into consideration the extent to which the lung volumes may have declined over time. A worker with asbestosis, whose FVC has declined from 110% of predicted to 82% still has a "normal" FVC in the absolute sense, but the drop in values is anything but normal. Although more difficult to reproduce, the diffusing capacity shares the same problem.

The issue of restriction versus obstruction is also hotly debated in asbestos disease cases. The defendants argue that obstruction is not caused by asbestos exposure, but is most likely attributable to cigarette smoking if such history is present. Although cigarettes are a frequent cause of obstructive disease, recent data indicate that asbestos can also cause an obstructive disease process.[42]

The cigarette smoking defense is probably the most powerful argument offered by the asbestos manufacturers, and it is raised by them in cases ranging from pleural disease to mesothelioma. In asbestosis cases, the defendants argue that cigarette smoke may increase the presence of pleural plaques,[43] cause or contribute to interstitial fibrosis, reduce lung volumes,[44] and impair diffusing capacity.[45] In lung cancer cases, the defendants argue that cigarettes are a powerful carcinogen, and thus try to establish that smoking is the sole cause of the cancer.

Although the defendants cannot dispute that smoking is not a cause of mesothelioma, they argue that cigarette smoke paralyzes the defense mechanisms of the lungs and allows for increased penetration and retention of asbestos fibers that cause mesothelioma.[46] In 1986, OSHA concluded, "well-conducted studies demonstrate a substantially increased rate of lung cancer and mesothelioma mortality among workers having low cumulative exposures to asbestos."[47] In mesothelioma cases, the defendants argue to possible alternative causes even in the face of strong medical evidence that malignant mesotheliomas of the pleura and peritoneum are extremely rare in persons not exposed to asbestos.[48] Alternative causes of mesothelioma have recently been expanded to include evidence that some people who were inoculated with the polio vaccine contaminated with the SV40 virus are at greater risk of contracting this cancer. The defense of idiopathic or spontaneous mesothelioma is alleged in instances where exposure history is not sufficient to render an opinion based on asbestos exposure, or one's strict criteria will not allow a mesothelioma to be the result of asbestos exposure because underlying asbestos markers such as pleural plaques or asbestosis are not present.

In sum, establishing medical causation not only requires that the plaintiff present evidence of an asbestos-related disease, but forces the plaintiff to defuse defense arguments that the diagnosis is incorrect and should not be made on the evidence. Plaintiff's counsel must persuade the jury that the defendants have created unreasonable diagnostic criteria so that few, if any, claimants, will be able to prove the existence of the disease. The defendants' contentions require that the plaintiff offer a skilled pulmonary or occupational expert to testify and that plaintiff's counsel become well-versed in the medical criteria necessary to establish a diagnosis.

In Depth: The Pathologist's Role in Establishing Causation

With the increasing proliferation of mass trials in which liability issues are decided separately, and by different juries, from causation issues, and where once peripheral defendants are taking center stage, plaintiff's counsel must be prepared to present strong medical testimony[49] and cannot expect to rely on evidence of corporate misconduct to sway a jury in a difficult case. One of the best ways to demonstrate that a worker has developed an asbestos-related disease is to obtain a lung tissue specimen, have it analyzed, and demonstrate to the jury the presence of asbestos bodies or fibers. The results of chest x-rays, CT scans, and pulmonary function tests are all useful in demonstrating to the jury that an asbestos-related disease is present, but there is nothing more persuasive than evidence, preferably visual, that asbestos is in the plaintiff's lung tissue in elevated concentrations. Also considerably useful to the plaintiff is the detection of a particular type of asbestos fiber that may be in the defendants' products. As is often stated at trial, the pathologist has the "final word" on the diagnosis of asbestosis. And when there is enough lung tissue available for examination, this observation is certainly true. If a plaintiff's lawyer has tissue available, it is certainly advantageous to have the tissue examined by a pulmonary pathologist, and, if possible, to have it analyzed for the presence and type of asbestos fiber. If asbestosis is present, this establishes without question the existence of that disease process; and if lung cancer is coexistent, it is strong, if not conclusive, evidence that the lung cancer was caused by asbestos exposure.

In the absence of a fiber burden analysis, the diagnosis of asbestosis by light microscopy is usually debated only in borderline cases. If asbestosis is severe, multiple asbestos bodies can usually be found in the presence of diffuse interstitial fibrosis. In questionable cases, however, fibrosis may be present but asbestos bodies may be difficult to identify. In the asbestos trial setting, the debate usually centers on the number of asbestos bodies necessary to support the diagnosis. A publication by the College of American Pathologists suggests that a minimum of two asbestos bodies must be present in areas of fibrosis before the diagnosis can be established.[50] One of the members of the committee that issued this statement has remarked that "the requirement for two asbestos bodies is probably overcautious" and that "the chance of overdiagnosing asbestosis from the observation of only one asbestos body seems very small indeed."[51] Although he continues that "the problem is more theoretic than real,"[52] it unfortunately becomes a matter of frequent dispute in the courtroom. Sometimes only one asbestos body can be identified; in some cases, there are none. In the case of fibrosis alone, one may argue that it is *occult* asbestosis, but the frequency of such cases is probably rare.[53] In the courtroom, however, the frequency of the claim is not.

The type of fibrosis necessary to support the diagnosis of asbestosis is also a disputed subject. Although some lung pathologists require a pattern of peribronchiolar fibrosis,[54] it is not always present in cases that are taken to court. Once again, juries are asked to decide issues that are controversial even among the experts, and they are forced to decide whether peribronchiolar fibrosis is necessary to make the diagnosis or whether "its absence in no way militates against the diagnosis."[55] In cases that are not so clear-cut, the trial can indeed become a battle of the experts.

The pathologic diagnosis of asbestosis is not only central to the non-malignant case, but it is significant in relating a lung cancer to asbestos exposure. The problem lies not in those cases where asbestosis is readily diagnosed, because most commentators are willing to relate a bronchogenic carcinoma to asbestos if coexisting asbestosis can be found.[56] If asbestosis cannot be found but there are numerous asbestos bodies, a strong case can also be made that the underlying lung burden is sufficient to have triggered the cancerous process. Many defense experts, however, are unwilling to relate a cancer to asbestos exposure unless all of the diagnostic features of asbestosis are present. This idea has been criticized in a report to the British government, which argued that, because the mechanisms of fibrogenesis and carcinogenesis are separate, there is no good reason why asbestosis must necessarily be present.[57] A better indicator of whether lung cancer can be related to asbestos is an elevated fiber burden, and it has been suggested that a fiber burden in excess of 100,000 per gram of dry lung tissue should be used as a minimum for relating a lung cancer to asbestos.[58]

The use of electron microscopy to assess the lung burden of asbestos can be of enormous benefit to the plaintiff in relating a lung cancer or mesothelioma to asbestos exposure. Additionally, an energy-dispersive x-ray analysis that specifically identifies the asbestos fiber type can be used to determine which products may have caused the disease process. For instance, in a mesothelioma case where plaintiff's lung tissue reveals an elevated asbestos fiber count and the majority of asbestos fibers are amosite, the plaintiff can point as the cause to a defendant whose product contains mostly amosite. By the same token, if the plaintiff worked primarily with chrysotile and tremolite fibers are identified, the plaintiff may be able to implicate as the culprit a defendant who utilized chrysotile in its products.

On the other hand, a defendant may use a fiber analysis to exculpate itself from the case by demonstrating that the fiber type in its products is not present in the plaintiff's lung tissue, or that other fiber types, such as crocidolite, are present in excessive quantities. Ninety-five percent of all asbestos used in the United States in insulation products historically was of the chrysotile variety, and the remaining 5% was mostly amosite. Crocidolite was rarely, if ever, used in insulating materials in the United States,[59] and this fiber type was primarily imported into the United States for use in asbestos-cement pipes and certain specialty gaskets.[60] Nevertheless, lung burden analyses often reveal relatively little chrysotile, greater amounts of amosite, and, not infrequently, the presence of crocidolite. Tremolite, a contaminant of chrysotile, is often detected in lung tissue, and it is a marker of previous chrysotile exposure.[61] Chrysotile tends to dissolve in lung tissue and may be removed from the lung, whereas amphiboles, specifically crocidolite, are more durable and are retained. A brief crocidolite exposure may still be evident in lung tissue after decades have passed, whereas heavier chrysotile exposure may be undetected.

Differences in the methods of analysis by various laboratories may also result in different findings. Some investigators count all fibers, whereas some do not count those below five microns in length. In one case, lung tissue was evaluated by three investigators. One found an elevated amount of only chrysotile using transmission electron microscopy.[62] Another, also using transmission electron microscopy, identified crocidolite, amosite, tremolite, and chrysotile.[63] Finally, another, using scanning electron microscopy, identified tremolite.[64] The overall lung burden of asbestos also varied from laboratory to laboratory.[65] The variability between laboratories for fiber burden assessments often results in the parties having different investigators perform studies on the same lung tissue.

In no case is the pathologist's role greater than in the mesothelioma case. A pathologist is necessary in rendering the diagnosis, identifying asbestos in the lung tissue, and determining whether the type of asbestos found was responsible for the development of mesothelioma.

Although the diagnosis of mesothelioma is difficult, recent immuno-histochemical staining techniques are allowing more certainty in the diagnosis. The defense in most mesothelioma cases is centered on the difficulty in making a conclusive diagnosis. Even if the full battery of histochemical and immunohistochemical stains is performed, the defendants are usually able to find an "expert" to contest the diagnosis.[66] If the asbestos manufacturers are unable to present testimony that the tumor is not a mesothelioma, they may argue that a mesothelioma diagnosis cannot be made to a reasonable degree of medical certainty. From a plaintiff's perspective, it is certainly necessary in the mesothelioma case to have all possible diagnostic tests performed on the tumor tissue in order to ensure diagnostic certainty. Additionally, an autopsy of the patient is certainly advisable in order to defeat a potential defense claim that the mesothelioma was a metastasis from some other site.[67]

Once the diagnosis of mesothelioma is established, it is necessary to prove that asbestos was the cause. From a practical standpoint, asbestos is the only known cause of mesothelioma that exists in the American workplace.[68] The defendants, however, will engage in tactics of confusion by arguing that there are cases of mesothelioma caused by erionite, therapeutic radiation, certain drugs, and agents that are unknown.[69] These claims will be made even in cases where there is a significant occupational exposure to asbestos and where asbestos can be identified in the lung.

Finally, one of the most hotly contested issues in asbestos litigation is whether chrysotile asbestos can cause mesothelioma.[70] Because insulators are developing mesothelioma at an alarming rate and 95% of all asbestos used in insulating material was chrysotile, it would seem that chrysotile is certainly capable of causing mesothelioma. Nevertheless, certain studies of workers exposed only to chrysotile indicate that chrysotile may be a weaker cause of mesothelioma,[71] and the defendants maintain that these studies demonstrate that chrysotile in and of itself does not cause mesothelioma at all. Most authorities now accept that the amphibole, tremolite, is a cause of mesothelioma, and tremolite contaminates most of the chrysotile that has been used in this country.[72] If tremolite can be identified in the lung tissue, it is reasonable to assume that the source of the contamination was the chrysotile asbestos used by the plaintiff.

A few defense experts even contend that amosite is not a cause of mesothelioma and that all mesotheliomas are caused by crocidolite.[73] This position is untenable, and good evidence exists that the likelihood for exposure to crocidolite by most construction or insulation workers is nonexistent. In England, crocidolite was used for insulation purposes, and there is evidence that some British ships have been overhauled in U.S. shipyards. Consequently, in a mesothelioma case arising from an American shipyard exposure, the defendants argue that the potential for crocidolite exposure existed and this exposure is responsible. The defendants will strongly and consistently argue the potency of crocidolite in mesothelioma causation. And if the defendants can convince the jury that crocidolite was the likely cause, the manufacturers can usually succeed because few, if any, manufacturers utilized crocidolite in their asbestos-containing insulation materials.[74]

Pathology at Trial

To ensure success in a case where pathologic material is available, plaintiff's counsel should consult with a pulmonary pathologist who has knowledge of asbestos-related diseases, to establish the diagnosis, to identify asbestos in lung tissue, and to testify that asbestos was responsible for the disease process. When lung tissue is available, it is not enough to rely on clinical evidence alone. Plaintiff's counsel can be sure that, if pathologic evidence is available, the defendants will have it reviewed by a pathologist and will, in all probability, have a pathologist testify at trial. In many cases, the only tissue available is from a transbronchial biopsy, and the manufacturers will present evidence that the pathologic examination did not reveal the presence of either any disease process or asbestos bodies. It should be emphasized on cross-examination that, as explained by one prominent pulmonary pathologist, "transbronchial biopsy is totally unsuited for diagnosing asbestosis; diagnoses of asbestosis made on the basis of transbronchial biopsy are statistically equivalent to guessing, no matter how perfect the histologic pattern may be . . . [T]issue submitted for mineral analysis should be at least the size of a large open biopsy; analysis of transbronchial biopsies is to be avoided."[75]

When sufficient tissue is available, plaintiff's counsel should utilize the information to be gained from a pathologic examination to the greatest extent possible. The materials should be submitted for microscopic examination, and pictures should be taken that can then be presented in evidence. Visual evidence of asbestos in lung tissue is extremely persuasive to a jury, and pictures of asbestos bodies coupled with the pathologist's opinion that asbestos was responsible for the disease process may sway an otherwise indecisive jury. Additionally, a fiber burden analysis is extremely helpful in convincing a jury that asbestos caused or contributed to the disease process.

Conclusion

With the likelihood that future compensation for asbestos plaintiffs will be based on the extent of disease, without regard to the extent of wrongdoing by the defendants, plaintiff's counsel may not have the benefit of evidence of corporate misconduct when compensatory damages are decided. The plaintiff's lawyer must, therefore, emphasize to the decision maker, whether it is a jury, judge, or bankruptcy proceeding, the hazards of asbestos exposure and the numbers of preventable diseases that have been caused by asbestos exposure. The following points should be emphasized to the fact finder that will decide the extent of damage caused by asbestos exposure.

1. The extensive industrial use of asbestos throughout this century has caused an epidemic of asbestos-related diseases.

2. Asbestos-related diseases are man-made; that is, these are diseases that could have been prevented by the elimination of asbestos or through the use of proper respiratory protection.

3. Asbestos—and only asbestos—can cause an incurable, untreatable, irreversible, progressive, and often fatal disease known as asbestosis. It has been demonstrated beyond reasonable doubt that asbestos is a cause of human lung cancer, and asbestos alone is carcinogenic.[76] The combination of cigarette smoking and asbestos exposure is an explosive interaction, and an asbestos worker who smokes has a 50 to 90 times greater chance of developing lung cancer than the person who neither smokes nor is exposed to asbestos.[77]

4. Asbestos causes malignant mesothelioma, an incurable and invariably fatal tumor of the lining of the lung or abdomen. Mesothelioma is rare in the general population, but it is rampant among asbestos workers.[78]

5. After extensive hearings on the hazards of asbestos, the Occupational Safety and Health Administration of the U.S. government concluded that it was "aware of no instance in which exposure to a toxic substance has more clearly demonstrated detrimental health effects on humans than has asbestos exposure. The diseases caused by asbestos exposure are life-threatening or disabling. Among these diseases are lung cancer, cancer of the mesothelial lining of the pleura and peritoneum, asbestosis, and gastrointestinal cancer."[79]

6. After considering "45,000 pages of analyses, comments, testimony, correspondence and other materials," the U.S. Environmental Protection Agency banned the use of most asbestos-containing products.[80]

7. There is no known safe level for exposure to asbestos.[81]

8. Brief exposure to asbestos has caused mesothelioma in persons decades later, and persons have developed mesothelioma whose only exposure was living near an asbestos mine or plant or residing in the home of an asbestos worker.[82]

The fact finder must be informed that asbestos is by no means a benign substance, as the defendants would have it believe, and that

dangerous concentrations of asbestos can be invisible and unde-
tectable. Furthermore, asbestos fibers are inhaled into the lung, act like
tiny spears or splinters, and cause scarring of the lung tissue microscopically. This information must be presented visually, graphically,
and, most importantly, simply.

Asbestos litigation has created a major challenge for the American
judicial system. During the past thirty years, the growth of asbestos litigation has resulted in landmark court decisions and judicial innova-
tions. To ensure, however, that the hundreds of thousands of asbestos
victims or their families receive compensation within the next half-
century will require even more creative efforts by both lawyers and the
courts. The solution to the asbestos litigation crisis will not be easy. But
through national coordination and consolidation, the cases can be
resolved. Hopefully, the system that is created to solve the asbestos litigation crisis will remain as a blueprint for managing future complex
litigation.

References

1. First-century historians and authors Strabo and Pliny the Elder both
   observed adverse biological effects of asbestos in the lungs of slaves who
   wove asbestos into cloth. See Lee, DHK, Selikoff IJ, Historical background
   to the asbestos problem, *Environ Res* 18:300–314, 1979.
2. Murray HM: Departmental Committee on Compensation for Industrial
   Diseases—Minutes of Evidence. *Appendices and Index*. London: Wyman and
   Sons, 1907, pp. 127–28.
3. Cooke WE: Fibrosis of the lungs due to the inhalation of asbestos dust.
   Br Med J 2:147, 1924.
4. Merewether ERA, Price CW: Reports on effects of asbestos dust on lungs
   and dust suppression in the asbestos industry. H.M. Stationery Office, 1930.
5. W.C. Hueper, *quoted in*, Castleman B: *Asbestos: Medical and Legal Aspects*, 4th
   ed. New York: Harcourt, Brace, Jovanovich, 1996, p. xvii.
6. 36 Fed. Reg. 3031 (March 1971).
7. 38 Fed. Reg. 8820 (April 1973).
8. 40 Fed. Reg. 48299 (1975).
9. In October 1979, the EPA issued its Advanced Notice of Proposed Rule
   Making outlining EPA's intent to use section 6 of the TSCA to reduce the
   human health risk posed by asbestos. 44 Fed. Reg. 60061. In July 1982, EPA
   issued its reporting rule promulgated to collect information on industrial
   and commercial uses of asbestos. 47 Fed. Reg. 33207. In January 1986, EPA
   issued its Proposed Final Rule stating EPA's finding that asbestos exposure
   poses an unreasonable risk to human health. 51 Fed. Reg. 3738. In July 1989,
   EPA issued a Final Rule entitled Asbestos, Manufacture, Importation, Processing and Distribution in Commerce Prohibitions. 54 Fed. Reg. 29460. The
   EPA July 1989 TSCA regulations contain specific effective dates for various
   bans including the manufacture, import and processing ban, distribution
   in commerce ban, and the ban of different asbestos products banned in
   various stages.
10. 36 Fed. Reg. 10466 (May 1971).
11. In December 1971, OSHA issued an emergency temporary standard of
    5f/cc as an 8-hour time-weighted-average (TWA) and a peak exposure
    level of 10f/cc, 36 Fed. Reg. 23207. In June 1972, OSHA issued its final TWA

standard of 5f/cc and a ceiling limit of 10f/cc. The TWA automatically reduced to 2f/cc effective July 1976, 44 Fed. Reg. 11504. In June 1986, OSHA issued its reduced final standard of 0.2f/cc as a TWA. A short-term-exposure-limit (STEL) of 1.0f/cc was promulgated in September 1988, 51 Fed. Reg. 22612. In July 1990, OSHA proposed a reduction of the TWA to 0.1 f/cc, 55 Fed. Reg. 29712.

12. 51 Fed. Reg. 22615 (June 20, 1986).
13. Ibid., pp. 22628.
14. *Ortiz* v. *Fibreboard Corp.*, 527 U.S. 815, 821, 119 S.Ct. 2295 (1999) (stating that asbestos litigation "defies customary judicial administration" and "calls for national legislation." It is important to note, however, that all proposed national legislative solutions to date have been sponsored by manufacturing defendants and have been woefully inadequate in their terms in compensation to diseased individuals.)
15. *Borel* v. *Fibreboard Paper Products Corp.*, 493 F.2d 1075 (5th Cir. 1973), *cert. denied*, 419 U.S. 869 (1974).
16. *Jackson* v. *Johns-Manville Sales Corp.*, 750 F.2d 1314, 1335–36 (5th Cir. 1985) (*en banc*).
17. In 1995, a study concluded that the disposition of all then pending asbestos cases for both personal injury and property damages, if treated in the traditional course of litigation, would require approximately 150 judge years. See Jack B. Weinstein, Individual Justice in Mass Tort Litigation 140 (1995), *citing* Thomas Willging, History of Asbestos Case Management (Federal Judicial Center staff paper for June 25, 1990, National Asbestos Conference.)
18. Henderson, James A. Jr. and Aaron D. Twerski, Stargazing: The Future of American Products Liability Law, 66 N.Y.U.L. Rev. 1332, 1336 (1991).
19. 198 W. Va. 1, 4–5, 479 S.E.2d 300, 303–04 (1996).
20. *State of West Virginia* v. *MacQueen*, _ W. Va. _, _ S.E.2d _, W.L. 770899 (July 6, 2001) *citing* H.R. Comm. on Judiciary, The Fairness in Asbestos Compensation Act: Hearings on H.R. 1283, 106th Cong. (July 1, 1999).
21. *Georgine* v. *Amchem Products, Inc.*, 157 F.R.D. 246 (E.D.Pa. 1994).
22. *Amchem Products* v. *Windsor*, 521 U.S. 591 (1997).
23. Plevin and Kalish, What's Behind the Recent Wave of Asbestos Bankruptcies?, Mealey's Litigation Report: Asbestos, April 20, 2001.
24. Ibid. (noting that the stay is subject to a number of exceptions specified in the statute itself, such as regulatory actions by the government. See 11 U.S.C. § 362(b). The bankruptcy court can also terminate the stay, or modify its coverage, upon motion of a party in interest in the bankruptcy case. See 11 U.S.C. § 362(d).)
25. *Insurance Day* (September 13, 2001).
26. Testimony has been repeatedly taken from such industry consultants as Dr. Gerrit W.H. Schepers, former director of the Saranac Laboratory, and Dr. Thomas F. Mancuso, the consultant to the Philip Carey Corp., the predecessor of Celotex.
27. Paul Brodeur, The Asbestos Industry on Trial, *New Yorker*, June 17, 1985, at 45, 75.
28. Letter from F. H. Zimmerman, Director of Safety, National Gypsum Co., to C. L. Sheckler, Manager, Occupational Environmental Control, Johns-Manville Corp. April 17, 1968.
29. Motley, Ronald and Anne Kearse, Decades of Deception: Secrets of Lead, Asbestos, and Tobacco, *Trial Magazine* (October, 1999), citing Asbestos Textile Institute, Minutes of the Air Hygiene and Manufacturing Committee March 7, 1957.

30. Ibid. (which references further example that, in 1950, the Quebec Asbestos Mining Association, whose members included Canadian asbestos mining companies, contracted with Saranac to determine whether asbestos caused cancer. A 1952 report, which was never published, showed increased cancer in mice and suggested further study. In 1957, the Canadian association contracted with the Industrial Hygiene Foundation of American to study asbestos and cancer. The resulting report concluded that those with asbestosis had an increased occurrence of lung cancer. Nevertheless, attorneys and doctors hired by the Canadian association recommended those conclusions be omitted from the final report. The 1958 published report concluded that asbestos exposure did not lead to an increased statistical occurrence of lung cancer).

31. Letter from F. H. Zimmerman, Director of Safety, National Gypsum Co., to C. L. Sheckler, Manager, Occupational Environmental Control, Johns-Manville Corp., April 17, 1968.

32. Mathew M. Swentonic, Presentation by the Asbestos Information Association/North America to the Asbestos Textile Institute (June 7, 1973).

33. D. Ozonoff, Report concerning *Medical Literature Review* (1981).

34. W.C.L. Hemeon, Report of Preliminary Dust Investigation for Asbestos Textile Institute (*Industrial Hygiene Foundation*, 1947 unpublished).

35. Deposition of K. Smith in *Louisville Trust Co. v. Johns-Manville Corp.*, No. 174–922 (Jefferson Cir. Ct., 7th Div. Ky., April 21, 1976).

36. Castleman B: *Asbestos: Medical and Legal Aspects*, 2nd ed. New York: Harcourt, Brace, Jovanovich, 1986, pp. 164–79.

37. Memorandum from W.B. Hofferth to J.E. Zeller, January 17, 1962.

38. Compare *Roehling v. National Gypsum Co.*, 786 F.2d 1225 (4th Cir. 1986) with *Blackston v. Shook & Fletcher Insulation Co.*, 764 F.2d 480 (11th Cir. 1985).

39. Ad Hoc Committee of the Scientific Assembly on Environmental and Occupational Health: The diagnosis of nonmalignant diseases related to asbestos, *Am Rev Respir Dis* 134:363, 367, 1986.

40. Guidelines for the use of the ILO international classification of radiographs of pneumoconiosis In: *Occupational Safety & Health Series No. 22 (rev.)* Geneva: International Labour Office, 1980.

41. Compare Jones Pleural Plaques, In: *The Biological Effects of Asbestos* (Bogovski, ed.), Lyon: IARC Scientific Publication No. 8, 1972, pp. 243–48, with Schwartz: Determinants of restrictive lung function in asbestos-induced pleural fibrosis, *J App Physiol* 1932–37, 1990; Bourbeau: The relationship between respiratory impairment and asbestos-related pleural abnormality in an active work force, 142: *Amer Rev Respir Dis*, 837–42, 1990. Recent studies on the significance of pleural disease indicate that pleural thickening and plaques are not as benign as previously thought. They are associated with an impairment of lung function and they may predict future cancers. See Selikoff, IJ: Predictive significance of parenchymal and/or pleural fibrosis for subsequent death of asbestos-associated diseases. Exhibit 124A. Entered into OSHA docket at hearings. OSHA's Proposed Standard for Occupational Exposure to Asbestos, Tremolite, Anthophyllite, and Actinolite, January 1991. Washington, D.C.

42. Churg A: *Pathology of Occupational Lung Disease*, New York: Igaku-Shoin, 1988, pp. 251–253,

43. Andrion A: Pleural plaques at autopsy, smoking habits, and asbestos exposure, *Eur J Respir Dis* 65:125–30, 1984.

44. Surgeon General, *The Health Consequences of Smoking: Cancer and Chronic Lung Disease in the Workplace*, U.S. Department of Health and Human Services, 1985, pp. 241–254.

45. Ibid, pp. 241.

46. See cross-examination of Dr. Edwin Holstein in *Kulzer v. Owens-Corning Fiberglas*, No. 87-386T, p. 351 (W.D.N.Y., Rochester Div., April 24, 1990).

47. 51 Fed. Reg. 22621 (June 20, 1986).

48. Ibid. pp. 22616–17.

49. Although plaintiff may not be able to admit corporate documents in the medical phase of a consolidated trial to demonstrate suppression of scientific data, corporate memoranda are certainly admissible to prove that the manufacturers recognize that asbestos is a highly dangerous material. For instance, although the asbestos companies deny in a personal injury trial that asbestosis occurs prior to the development of clinical criteria, they take a quite contrary position in litigation against their insurance carriers. In order to prove an "occurrence" for purposes of product liability insurance policies, the manufacturers have argued in insurance litigation that asbestosis occurs on the inhalation of the fiber, and that one-third of the alveolar sacs must be affected before asbestosis is clinically diagnosable. Policyholders' Proposed Medical Findings of Fact, *In Re* Asbestos Insurance Coverage Cases, No. 1072, pp. 8–12 (Cal. Super. Ct., S.F. County, Jan. 26, 1987). Although the defendants minimize the hazards of asbestos exposure, internal corporate documents reveal their true concerns when litigation is not a factor. As stated by Dr. Jon Konzen on September 20, 1972: "Irreversible and progressive lung scarring will . . . occur in the overexposed [asbestos] workers before it is apparent to the man or on medical examination. Likewise, occupational exposure to asbestos is known to be causally related to carcinoma of the lung and malignant mesothelioma of the covering or pleura of the lung." J. Konzen to S. Mayer, Sept. 20, 1972. Finally, even though the defendants dispute that asbestos-containing construction materials are hazardous to building occupants, many of them are removing asbestos from their corporate offices.

50. Pneumoconiosis Committee of the College of American Pathologists and the National Institute for Occupational Safety and Health: The pathology of asbestos-associated diseases of the lungs and pleural cavities: diagnostic criteria and proposed grading schema, *Arch Pathol Lab Med* 106: 554, 559, 1982.

51. Churg: supra note 42, p. 260.

52. Ibid.

53. Ibid., pp. 262–263.

54. Ibid., pp. 262.

55. Ibid., pp. 262.

56. Ibid., pp. 285.

57. Doll R, Peto J: *Asbestos: Effects on Health of Exposure to Asbestos.* London: Her Majesty's Stationery Office, 1985, p. 32. The idea that . . . asbestos-induced cancers occur only secondary to the fibrosis of asbestosis has sometimes been expressed. The idea originated in the days before the discovery of DNA, when cancers were not thought to result from genetic variation in somatic cells, but from the repair of tissue damage that was macroscopically visible. In light of modern knowledge of carcinogenesis, such an idea does not seem plausible. No threshold for the carcinogenic effect of asbestos has been demonstrated in humans or in laboratory animals and, in the absence of positive evidence for a threshold, we have followed standard scientific practice and assume that none exists. One possible reason for thinking that asbestos-induced cancers might be secondary to asbestosis is the high incidence of cancer in the similar condition of cryptogenic fibrosing alveolitis. As, however, the aetiology of this disease is unknown,

the argument by analogy does not carry much weight and we have ignored it.

58. Warnock ML, Isenberg W: Asbestos and the pathology of lung cancer, *Chest* 89:20–26, 1986.

59. Selikoff I, Hammond E, Seidman H: *Cancer Risk of Insulation Workers in the United States,* IARC Scientific Publication No. 8, Lyon, 1972.

60. Hendry NW: The geology, occurrences, and major uses of asbestos, In: Biological Effects of Asbestos, *Ann NY Acad Sci* 132:12–19, 1965.

61. Doll and Peto: supra note 57, p. 17.

62. Report by Dr. Ronald Dodson, Dept. of Cell Biology and Environmental Sciences, University of Texas Health Center at Tyler, May 27, 1988.

63. Report by Dr. Fred Pooley, Dept. of Mining and Minerals Engineering, University College, Cardiff, Wales, June 23, 1988.

64. Report by Dr. Victor Roggli, Dept. of Pathology, Duke University Medical Center, December 4, 1987.

65. Dr. Dodson identified 3,025,082 chrysotile fibers per gram of dry lung tissue; Dr. Pooley identified 7,900,000 chrysotile fibers, 660,000 tremolite fibers, 64,000 crocidolite fibers, and 9,000 amosite fibers per gram of dry lung tissue; and Dr. Roggli found 6,120 fiber per gram of wet lung tissue. Dr. Roggli counted only those fibers whose length exceeded five microns, whereas Dr. Dodson and Dr. Pooley included all fibers in their counts.

66. Unfortunately, the defendants consistently rely on one or two pathologists, who, in the face of overwhelming evidence favoring the diagnosis, will testify that the tumor is not a mesothelioma.

67. In one case tried in Virginia federal court, the diagnosis of mesothelioma was confirmed by all pathologists except one who was retained by the defendants. This defense expert contended that the tumor was a metastasis from the thyroid, and the body was exhumed for further analysis. On exhumation, the thyroid gland was found to be free of tumor.

68. In approximately 20% of cases, the history of asbestos exposure was not taken in the occupational history. However, on further investigation, asbestos exposure can almost always be elicited when preparing the mesothelioma case for trial.

69. Pelnar, PV: Further evidence of nonasbestos-related mesothelioma *Scand J Work Environ Health* 14:141–44, 1988. The author is affiliated with the Asbestos Institute.

70. Churg: supra note 42, p. 289.

71. Berry G, Newhouse M: Mortality of workers manufacturing friction materials using asbestos, *Brit J Indus Med,* 40:1–7, 1983; McDonald JC, Fry, JS: Mesothelioma and fiber type in three American asbestos factories, *Scand J Work Environ Health* 8:53–58, 1982.

72. As stated by Doll and Peto: "It is not practicable to remove tremolite from chrysotile for commercial purposes and any distinction between the effects of chrysotile and tremolite may, therefore, be considered academic, unless supplies of chrysotile can be obtained in which little or no tremolite is present." Supra note 57, p. 17.

73. Wagner JC: Complexities in the evaluation of epidemiologic data of fiber-exposed populations, In: *Dusts and Disease,* (Lemen R, Dement J, eds., Park Forest South, IL: Pathotox, 1979, pp. 37–39.

74. In answers to interrogatories, all defendants maintain that they did not use crocidolite in their asbestos-containing pipe insulation.

75. Churg: supra note 42, p. 267.

76. McDonald, JC: Asbestos and lung cancer: Has the case been proven? *Chest* 78:374–376, 1980.

77. Surgeon General, *The Health Consequences of Smoking: Cancer and Chronic Disease in the Workplace*. U.S. Dept. of Health and Human Services, 1985, pp. 217–18.
78. Selikoff IJ: Asbestos-associated disease. In: *Public Health and Preventive Medicine*, 12th ed. (Maxcy-Rosenau, ed.), East Norwalk, CT: Appleton-Century-Crofts, 1986, pp. 523–534.
79. 51 Fed. Reg. 22615 (June 20, 1986).
80. 54 Fed. Reg. 19461 (July 17, 1989).
81. Selikoff: supra 78.
82. Ibid.

13

Medicolegal Aspects of Asbestos-Related Diseases: A Defendant's Attorney's Perspective

Albert H. Parnell

American Asbestos Litigation (1972–2004): A Perspective

The Development of Modern Asbestos Litigation in America

The basis for American asbestos litigation was formed during the pivotal 10-year period from 1960 to 1970. The physician, J.C. Wagner confirmed that malignant pleural mesothelioma was caused by crocidolite asbestos in 1960.[1] The New York Academy of Sciences led by Irving Selikoff, a physician, held a historic, course changing conference on the Biological Effects of Asbestos in 1964 that was attended by physicians, scientists, and industrial hygienists from around the world.[2] The Restatement, Torts, 2nd was published containing a new section on strict tort liability, 402A[3] that significantly changed product liability law and reduced the hurdles that people suing had to overcome to obtain a monetary recovery. These events of the 1960s came together when a Texas jury awarded damages in favor of a worker against manufacturers of asbestos containing insulation products that was affirmed as *Borel v. Fiberboard*[4] in 1972. These four seemingly disparate and separate events combined in a unique and almost invisible way to create the biggest and most expensive litigation that the United States has ever witnessed. The events started a process that has produced an avalanche of hundreds of thousands of lawsuits in virtually every state of the United States. The sheer number of cases has threatened to clog the American judicial system.

The legal activity in the 32 years since the *Borel* decision has spawned an incredible cottage industry. The asbestos litigation has created jobs for lawyers, and for physicians of almost every specialty. It thrives on the expert reports from scientific and medical consultants. It has created the need for jury consultants who specialize in asbestos jury selection. Many people from varied professions have acted as expert witnesses in asbestos cases. The asbestos litigation has supported a cadre of supporting industries that include court reporters, industrial hygienists, medical providers of multiple kinds, and software suppliers. There have been thousands of lawsuits tried, hundreds of thousands of personal injury and property damage claims settled, and billions of dollars distributed among plaintiffs, lawyers, and the cottage industry participants. It has also produced 27 bankruptcies among some of America's once proudest corporate names including Raybestos–Manhattan, Johns-Manville, Owens-Corning, W.R. Grace, Babcock and Wilcox, and the United States Gypsum Company (USG).

The Role and Use of Medical and Scientific Witnesses in Modern Asbestos Litigation

The tremendous number of case filings and the influx of cases into state and federal courts have produced a demand for scientific experts of all kinds. It is usual to see a combination of pathologists, oncologists, radiologists, pulmonologists, industrial hygienists, statisticians, mineralogists, and epidemiologists in any typical asbestos disease case. Witnesses in all medical specialties may give testimony about general medicine issues, the health effects of asbestos, anatomy, or the development of the medical knowledge about asbestos. The medical specialists also may give specific medical testimony. Pulmonologists generally act as medical examiners and offer opinions about the health of individual plaintiffs. Radiologists, particularly B-readers, are used for a variety of tasks, but often are the first, through screenings, to suggest that a person has asbestosis, cancer, or pleural changes. Pathologists are the arbiters of the presence or absence of asbestosis and cancer when sufficient tissue is present. These experts, some more expert than others, offer opinions on questions relating to diagnosis, causation, risk assessment, prognosis, and life expectancy. The expert witnesses testify about specific aspects of the total case, either affirming or refuting asbestos as a causative agent in the production of disease in a specific person.

The medical and scientific opinions that each witness is allowed to offer are governed by the trial judge's interpretation of the law that applies. The courts in each state and the courts of the federal court system have each developed specific rules of evidence that govern the evidence in every trial. The respective rules of evidence determine what is and is not relevant. Each judge determines how the rules of evidence are going to be applied in each case. The judge determines what documents may be introduced, the subject matter that each witness may testify about, and the scope of any expert's testimony. Each judge determines the substance of each witness' testimony. The rules of evidence and procedure are, in fact, different in each state court and the federal courts. The courts in each jurisdiction, state and federal, make little effort to be consistent.

It is important for the physician or medical expert to understand that there are many variables that can determine if, when, and what the expert may say. The judges and the attorneys have a role in determining what experts and others may say long before the actual trial begins. The judge has an important role because testimony is governed by the rules of evidence that apply to the specific case as applied and interpreted by that judge. The judges, even in the same states, do not always apply the rules equally, evenly, or consistently from county to county or even courtroom to courtroom. The lawyers also have rules to follow. Every jurisdiction requires some level of disclosure about the case before the case is tried so everyone knows the case. It is each lawyer's responsibility, depending on state laws, to comply with the disclosure requirements of the state or the court. These discovery requirements usually require the lawyers to disclose in advance of trial the names of all potential witnesses, the area or areas of expertise of each witness, and the limits of each witness' testimony. These disclosures usually have to be made within a specific time frame before trial. Lawyers in cases may not adequately anticipate testimony or witnesses and fail to timely notify the opposing counsel. The trial judge may exclude a witness or portions of a witness' testimony when the lawyers fail to comply with discovery orders. Therefore, the expert opinions of one expert may be allowed in a courtroom in Delaware and the same testimony disallowed in Iowa. The testimony in an asbestos case on both exposure and diagnosis may be far different in Delaware than in Iowa.

The Modern Asbestos Trial Procedure

The courtroom is the operating room of the tort litigation hospital. The judge presides over the trial (operation). The trial in the tort litigation hospital is led by at least two or more competing lawyers, each of whom differ significantly in their respective philosophy about the desired course of the trial and the desired end result. The judge, unlike the two lawyers, is usually a passive observer. The judge intervenes only when one of the trial lawyers presents a plan for the trial that is opposed and objected to by one of the other lawyers. One or more of the competing trial lawyers may propose a course of conduct or trial procedure that is experimental or that at least has not been adopted by multiple members of the profession. The judge may have to exercise discretion based upon the best available information. At least one set of the lawyers can be paid only if the trial is a success from the standpoint of that lawyer. That lawyer can receive no fee, a small fee, or a large fee depending on the value of the result. The other set of lawyers is paid irrespective of result. The jurors in the case determine whether the trial is or is not a success, depending on the perspective of the viewer.

The Makeup and Role of the Jury in the Modern Asbestos Trial

The American jury system is a highly competitive and leveraged advocacy system that depends, in part, on the skill and diligence of the lawyers presenting the case. Each case is different. There is no universal right. There is no universal result. Two different or twelve different juries in the same or different jurisdictions can reach disparate and vastly different conclusions based on what many observers consider to be essentially the same facts. The facts vary, to some degree, in every case. The lawyers and witnesses are different in each case. The juries are vastly different in each city and from court to court, jurisdiction to jurisdiction, and state to state. The jury is a product of geographic location and every location is different. There are gender, race, ethnic, political, religious, and educational differences in every locality and every jury. Thus, a jury in El Paso may be markedly different from a jury in Boston. The differences abound in every conceivable way.

The lawyers and the jurors are central to the American jury system, and it is important to understand the roles of the lawyers and the jurors in order to understand the role of the scientist in the American tort system. The lawyers are advocates. Each lawyer presents an opinion, a view. Theoretically, the lawyer presents the best possible facts for that opinion or view. The other lawyer advocates an opposite or different view. The trial, though a search for truth, is a search for truth within the context of the facts presented in each trial by the advocate lawyers through their witnesses. There is no universal truth because every case is different. There is only the truth of the case under consideration. Each lawyer, the plaintiff and the defendant, is proposing the truth that he or she advocates. Each lawyer may see some or all portions of the truth differently from the other. Therefore, each lawyer seeks to find jurors who are more likely than others to see the truth from that lawyer's perspective.

Prospective jurors are almost universally randomly selected from voting lists for the chance to be selected to serve on a specific case. At the moment of their initial selection they are the home of many gender, racial, religious, educational, and ethical opinions, bias, prejudices, known or unknown. The lawyers question a subset of these opinionated educated or uneducated prospective jurors. Each of the lawyer advocates has a profile of what he or she perceives is the "best" and "worst" juror for the specific facts of the case. The opposing lawyers can remove or eliminate a specific number of the potential jurors from the panel when the process is complete. It is typical to start with a panel of 24 prospective jurors when 12 jurors will ultimately be selected. Each lawyer then gets to remove the 6 jurors each believes is the 6 "worst" jurors from each lawyer's perspective. The remaining 12 are the jurors. The selected juries in most jurisdictions are racially, sexually, and ethnically diverse, have approximately a high school education, and have incomes in the lower third to half of incomes on a national average.

The Medical Witness and the Jury

The medical and scientific witness has to understand that the evidence has to persuade the jury to a given point or conclusion. The lawyers present medical and scientific evidence to this jury in accordance with the rules of evidence of the jurisdiction as interpreted by the sitting judge. The jury's ultimate verdict is based on the evidence that is presented in that courtroom, by those witnesses, and by those advocates. The jury cannot seek additional information on its own from the Internet or the local library. The jury cannot seek outside information to determine methodically whether the science it hears is representative of the science presented at medical seminars.

The "truth" of the medical science presented to any specific jury depends on many factors. The most expert doctor in a field may not offer an opinion. The most expert of doctors in a specific field may not want to be a part of the judicial process for any number of reasons. The medical and scientific witnesses may have their own separate agenda in testifying. The witnesses may be professional witnesses who make all or most of their incomes from the courtroom. The evidence that the jury hears may be less than optimum. The scientist who committed to attend the trial may not come because of schedule changes and may not be available at the date or time of the scheduled trial. All expert witnesses are not universally persuasive. Many witnesses who have inferior credentials, make better witnesses, communicate with jurors better, and are more persuasive than a witness with a superior background. In short, there are many witness factors that govern the result in a trial.

The Legal Requirements of Medical and Scientific Testimony

The introduction of medical evidence at a trial in the United States District courts is governed in general by the Federal Rules of Evidence, 701–705.[5] Most state courts have similar rules but there is variance from federal court to federal court and from state court to state court. Scientific testimony is generally allowed where the witness is an expert in the field of the prospective testimony, the evidence the witness is about to offer is reliable, the evidence is obtained in a usual and customary way, and the testimony will aid the jury in reaching a decision. These general rules govern all cases involving asbestos and disease.

The science and medical witness must testify within the parameters of the proposed specialty in order for the jury to consider the evidence. The proposed evidence must pass a number of evidentiary considerations before the jury hears it. In all U.S. District Courts, and in some state courts, the judge acts as a gatekeeper to screen out evidence that is ruled to be "junk science" or unsupported by the evidence. Appellate courts in *Daubert*,[6] *Havner*,[7] and similar cases have set rules governing the threshold standards that proposed scientific testimony must pass before the testimony can be presented to the jury. The threshold standards are not "litmus" test requirements but are considerations that judges must use in considering whether to admit or rule out specific questions or scientific positions or data.

The Role of the Medical or Scientific Witness at Trial

There are a number of different kinds of cases involving asbestos. The most numerous and most typical is the personal injury tort suit. The plaintiff in the tort suit claims that he or she suffers from an injury that was caused by exposure to asbestos. Each case is different. The chief medical questions are whether the person has an asbestos-related injury or whether the person's alleged asbestos disease was caused by a specific or several specific exposures. These causation questions involve an analysis of the type of exposure and the length of exposure. The causation answer may depend on the asbestos fiber type involved in the exposure. The answer may also involve an analysis of principles of epidemiology, pulmonology, oncology, and pathology. The jury may resolve the causation question by reliance on the credibility of one witness and one witness only. In most states the jury can rely on one witness and reject the testimony of every other witness who testifies. However, most lawyers are reluctant to present only one witness in an asbestos case. Consequently, the trial usually involves the testimony of multiple scientific witnesses from multiple specialties.

As an example, the exposure in a specific case may be weak, peripheral, or in an occupation that is not traditionally associated with asbestos disease. An industrial hygienist may testify about length and severity of exposures to this particular person with a conclusion that there is or is not sufficient exposure to cause the disease or insufficient exposure to a specific product or premises to have participated in the cause of the disease. Witnesses from other specialties may be used to make the exposure evidence of the industrial hygienist more or less credible. A radiologist may support high or low exposure through the presence or absence of radiographic evidence of plaques or asbestosis. The pulmonologist may support or refute the same propositions through an interpretation of pulmonary function tests (PFTs), x-ray readings, and the physical examination. The pathologist may support or reject exposure assessments through the presence or absence of plaques, asbestosis, the presence or absence of quantities of asbestos bodies, or the presence or absence of quantities of uncoated fibers. All disciplines come together in most cases to complement or confound the facts offered to the jury for belief.

The Role of the Pathologist at Trial

The pathologist is a very important witness in the trial of the appropriate asbestos case. The importance of the pathologist is enhanced because the pathologist examines actual tissue as opposed to a radiologist who examines shadows or the pulmonologist who interprets PFTs. Most lawyers believe that jurors attribute greater weight to the testimony of the pathologist. The belief centers on the thought that the pathologist is seen as having touched the inside or soul of the patient. Lawyers believe that jurors see the pathologist as the doctor who resolves diagnostic disputes. Most jurors understand that it is the pathologist who will likely determine their fate if they are in the hospital facing cancer surgery. It is because of this thought process that lawyers seek to expand the potential testimony of the pathologist at trial.

The lawyer in the asbestos trial is trying to convince the jury of a point of view or concept. The pathologist is a natural trial partner with the lawyer because the pathologist is, by nature, a visual person. The pathologist in everyday practice utilizes a number of diagnostic procedures that are visual in nature to affirm or reject a diagnosis. The pathologist physically examines the tissue under the microscope, and can, if necessary, demonstrate that process in the courtroom. The pathologist can take pictures or photomicrographs of the tissue and display them in court. The pathologist often stains the tissue as an aid to diagnosis and the pictures of the stains can be used to aid the lawyer in persuading the jury. The pathologist can order and supervise digestion studies and explain them in a way no other doctor can. The pathologist's photomicrographs can illustrate emphysema, idiopathic fibrosis, the presence or absence of asbestos bodies, and multiple other findings that cannot be demonstrated to juries to the same degree by other specialties.

The fundamental principle that a pathologist is credible in the eyes of the jury because he or she touches the tissue is very important in the trial process. The assumption of this concept allows the lawyer to elevate and extend the trial value of the pathologist. The lawyer seeks to capitalize on this credibility by attempting to get the pathologist to testify in areas that extend beyond the actual diagnosis or lack of diagnosis. The credibility acts as a springboard for other testimony. The concept is that if the pathologist can define disease, then *a priori*, the pathologist must be an expert on the dose required to produce the disease, how the dose was acquired, how the dose acted on the tissue and the cell structure, the relationship for determining causation, and the epidemiology of the disease.

The Asbestosis Case: The Defense Position

Did a Significant Number of Asbestosis Cases Exist in 2004?

The defense of an asbestosis case in 2004 rested on questioning whether the diagnosis of asbestosis is a correct diagnosis. The chief trigger for the question rested on the principle that asbestosis is a dose response disease. No one questions the fact that workers in particular occupations had the chance for very high doses of asbestos in the 1940s, 1950s, and even the 1960s. However, most people believe that OSHA lowered the regulations regarding doses of asbestos in 1972, and those regulations reduced exposures to asbestos in the workplace. If the dose of asbestos has steadily decreased since 1972, can workers exposed to post-1972 levels of asbestos develop asbestosis? Virtually all of the asbestosis reported by numerous authors in the 1960s and 1970s, but principally, the cohorts reported by Irving Selikoff and colleagues, resulted from high and significant exposures to asbestos in the 1930s, 1940s, and 1950s. Many scientists and reporters demonstrated high peak dust count exposures to shipyard workers,[8] some as high as 500 f/cc.[9] These exposures were significantly higher than the levels mandated by OSHA in 1972. The exposure picture began to change with the creation of OSHA and the promulgation of OSHA and EPA asbestos exposure standards, beginning in 1971.[10] The OSHA standard has steadily diminished from 5 f/cc to 0.1 f/cc. The steady decrease in exposure that has been forced on industrial and occupational setting since 1971 suggests that workers exposed after 1971 are either less likely to develop asbestosis or, if asbestosis is found, it takes longer to develop and is generally less severe. Consequently, the diagnosis requires more scrutiny as the legal and scientific community faces patients and plaintiffs whose majority exposure is post-OSHA.

The Modern Litigation Process as a Reason to Defend the Diagnosis of Asbestosis

There are valid social reasons to question the individual diagnosis of asbestosis in cases that appeared in 2001. The history of asbestos disease demonstrates that cases of asbestos-related disease were discovered and diagnosed differently in the years prior to the asbestos litigation explosion. In the 1950s, 1960s, and the 1970s, most of the plaintiffs with serious pulmonary conditions were exposed to asbestos during the heavy exposure years of the 1930s, 1940s, 1950s, and 1960s. They had worked in occupational trades that we now know were rife with heavy asbestos exposures. They saw their doctors because they were symptomatic and sought medical care. Those patients became plaintiffs as they gravitated to the litigation after they had received a diagnosis.

The usual plaintiff of today reaches the asbestos litigation in a far different way. They have not been exposed to the same levels of asbestos as plaintiffs in prior years. They are not symptomatic. They have never missed any time from work. They have never sought medical treatment of any kind, much less for asbestosis. Many unions in the 1980s and 1990s, and many law firms in the 1990s and 2000 began a process of x-ray screening of large numbers of people. Law firms today advertise screening in local newspapers for any individual who has an x-ray taken. The x-rays are obviously taken without a history, not in response to a complaint of a symptom, and offer a very temporal view of the subject. Any person who has an abnormal x-ray is a potential plaintiff based on that x-ray interpretation and nothing more. Most of the plaintiffs who enter modern asbestos litigation with a nonmalignant disease are discovered through screening of some nature. It is unlikely that any have pulmonary function studies or pathology. Consequently, most modern plaintiffs discover that they might have a diagnosis of asbestosis when they receive a letter from a union official, lawyer, or physician stating that there has been a suspicious finding on their x-rays.

The screening produces a plaintiff, a lawsuit, and a response. Once the screening has produced an x-ray, the plaintiff's lawyer typically sends the plaintiff to a physician selected by that lawyer or law firm. The doctor physically reviews the plaintiff. The doctor may or may not generate x-rays and/or pulmonary function studies. The usual post-1972 asbestos-exposed plaintiffs have a supporting screening x-ray reading of 1/0 on the ILO Scale (The most minimal positive finding). The PFTs are either normal, show a restrictive or obstructive component, or some other process. Since the PFTs are usually normal or nondiagnostic, the overwhelming majority of nonmalignant plaintiffs carry a diagnosis of asbestosis based on the original screening x-ray.

The plaintiff is then seen by physicians chosen by the defendants. The defense physicians almost always disagree with the findings of the physicians selected by the plaintiffs. The radiologist chosen by the defense invariably reads the screening film as normal or attributes any change to something other than asbestos. The pulmonologist selected by the defense does not report physical examination findings consistent with asbestosis. The defense PFTs are either normal or show obstructive disease. Thus, the usual clinical argument is between the pulmonologist and the radiologist without the benefit of the pathologist.

The Pathology of Asbestosis and Critical Standards

One of the severe difficulties in defending the disputed asbestosis case is the absence of a single standard to judge asbestosis. All of the medical experts who testify at trial recognize the seminal work of the College of American Pathologists[11] and the American Thoracic Society.[12] These standards, 20 years later, still serve as the base point for the clinical and pathological diagnosis of asbestos-related diseases in the courtroom. The pathological standard of the College of American Pathologists is more rigidly and universally applied than the suggestions of the American Thoracic Society standard, but they are only applicable in the rare case where pathology exists. The ATS standard is subject to significantly more interpretation in the clinical and courtroom setting than the suggestions of the College of American Pathologists. Many of the scientists at trial impose personal standards for the clinical diagnosis of asbestosis. They recognize the ATS standard as a starting point but they quickly either substitute or offer their own personal judgment about why the ATS applies or does not apply to their diagnosis or opinion.

The defense advocates a strict application of objective standards to make the diagnosis of asbestosis and would prefer a requirement of a lung tissue sample in every case. The litigation over asbestosis would likely stop or diminish significantly if lung tissue was required or if there was one objective standard to judge the presence or absence of asbestosis. However, the nature of the development of the case dictates that there will not have been a pathologist in the clinical history. Therefore, there are rarely tissue samples in the modern asbestosis case and no pathologic opinion. There is no concrete standard to apply. The diagnosis is subjective. Even the ATS standard does not require any rigid application. The result is that a jury determines which of the competing subjective views is most persuasive.

The defense always seeks pathology, and the opinion of the pathologist. The defense finds that having an opinion of a pathologist is very helpful in resolving the subjective disputes between the clinicians about whether a patient does or does not have asbestosis. The pathologic diagnosis, when available, can be used in a number of ways to either support or refute the clinical diagnosis of one or more of the physicians.

The Defense Position on Asbestosis and Coexisting Ailments

The clinical argument for and against asbestosis is clouded by the presence of confounding factors in the diagnosis, the presence of coexistent disease with symptoms similar to those exhibited by asbestosis, and the presence of major scientific differences between the published studies on asbestosis. The American Thoracic Society has noted a major problem in the differential diagnosis for asbestosis when the patient suffers from multiple disease processes.

Asbestosis rarely exists in a vacuum. Fibrosis rarely exists in a vacuum. Asbestosis and fibrosis coexist in most cases with emphysema, chronic obstructive pulmonary disease, asthma, heart problems, and multiple other ailments. The presence of coexisting ailments makes it difficult for all parties to evaluate the cause of the fibrosis because of the effect of the coexisting disease. Pulmonary function studies are always in conflict and are inconclusive in most cases. The existence of other diseases and drugs often provides a logical explanation for the presence of fibrosis of any kind. Therefore, a social history of cigarette smoking or a clinical history of heart disease and the use of some drugs sheds light on the question whether asbestos is the cause of the fibrosis in question.

The doctors agree in some cases that fibrosis is present. The question in those cases is whether the fibrosis is asbestosis. The conclusion is complicated for a number of reasons. First, the diagnosis is confounded if there is a history of significant cigarette smoking. There have been a number of articles suggesting that cigarette smoking produces the same types of small irregular opacities produced by asbestos and other dusts.[13] Second, there are often questions about the true occupational history of any significant asbestos exposure. There are many questions raised about whether a person can develop asbestosis at current occupational levels. Third, the diagnosis is confounded by the high incidence of idiopathic interstitial fibrosis. The existence of significant numbers of idiopathic fibrosis in the absence of documented exposure to occupational levels of asbestos forces the consideration that idiopathic fibrosis should be a part of the differential diagnosis.

The origin of the fibrosis and whether it is asbestosis, something else, or idiopathic fibrosis is important in the litigated case. Putting aside the issue of whether there is actual exposure to asbestos, many of the plaintiffs have a unique exposure to many substances and minerals in their occupational life. The defense urges the physician to consider the other causes of fibrosis to critically review whether the fibrosis is diffuse. The fibrosis could be focal, a response to some other stimuli in the particular plaintiff: idiopathic fibrosis, usual interstitial pneumonia, fibrosing alveolitis, a tumor, or some other factor.

The Defense of Lung Cancer Cases

The defense attorney in the defense of an alleged asbestos-related lung cancer case examines evidence from seven areas of our knowledge about asbestos and lung cancer to formulate whether a defense to the case is plausible: (1) Is there evidence that the carcinoma is of lung origin or is it a metastasis from another organ? (2) The general knowledge and agreement that cigarette smoking is bad for human health and causes cancer. (3) What was the extent and duration of the cigarette smoking history of the plaintiff? (4) Does the plaintiff have underlying asbestosis? (5) The strength or lack of strength of the association between this plaintiff's asbestos exposure and the development of lung cancer. (6) Does the plaintiff have exposures to other carcinogens that would explain the presence of the lung cancer? (7) Does fiber type exposure offer any defense to the causation issue?

Is the Carcinoma of Lung Origin?

The threshold question for the defense lawyer in an alleged lung cancer case is the origin of the cancer. Is it a lung primary or a metastatic tumor from another organ? The pathologist can play a significant role in making the determination and is generally better at assisting the lawyer than any other specialty. The first problem facing the defense attorney is that the clinicians are not necessarily interested in the question of what toxic agent caused the cancer. The physician's job for them is treatment. The issue of whether the tumor is metastatic is important in determining whether there is a course of treatment that will cure the cancer. However, because there is often insufficient information to determine if it is a metastatic tumor, it is not always of primary importance to the clinician.

The clinician or clinicians have taken a history. They have made a physical examination. X-rays have been reviewed. There may or may not have been an operation in which tissue was removed for analysis. Clinical, not legal, considerations are paramount. Consequently, there may be little or no tumor tissue available for review. Autopsy is not performed in most cases so that there is some conjecture as to whether the tumor was a lung primary.

The treating pathologist's opinion of the origin of the tumor is extremely important in cases where there is lung tissue. The jury usually sees the treating pathologist as an impartial participant who is above the fray. The treating pathologist was on the scene before the lawyers, was not visited by lawyers, and in theory, made an independent analysis. Therefore, the opinions of the treating physicians, and particularly, the treating pathologist, are analyzed by both sides. The lawyers who feel they have the most to gain usually attempt to solicit treating physicians for the case.

The plaintiff and the defense often hire an independent records review physician to look at all of the medical records, operative reports, x-rays, autopsy materials, and other reports to reach an independent conclusion as to the likelihood that the tumor originated elsewhere and was caused by some other agent. The defense radiologist will review the x-rays, magnetic resonance images (MRIs), and computed tomography (CT) scans to determine if there is any chance that the tumor originated in another source. The defense pathologist will review the records and the tumor to determine whether the cell type is capable of being a metastatic tumor. When the evidence points to another site of origin, the attorney will pursue that line of defense.

The General Knowledge About Cigarette Smoking and Human Health

The defense in the disputed lung cancer case assumes that the jury has become aware that cigarette smoking is dangerous to human health. It seeks to capitalize on the recent publicity about cigarette smoking, the ever-present warnings on tobacco products and some advertising, and the constant news references to the various tobacco lawsuits as a basis from which to develop information that the jury can process about cigarette smoking. Using that as a basis, the defense develops evidence that Oscar Auerbach and Alton Ochsner, two physicians, led science into study of the effect of cigarette smoking on human health in the mid-1950s.[14,15] It shows that Sir Richard Doll and Julian Peto followed with their epic study of British Physicians in 1955.[16] The defense presents evidence that the Surgeon General of the United States originally published its landmark piece on cigarette smoking in 1965,[17] followed with a number of updated studies,[18,19] and has just completed its most recent tome on cigarette smoking and women.[20]

These studies are a formidable weapon for the defense lawyer in a lung cancer case because they provide ample scientific data and information about the health effects of cigarette smoking. It builds upon the jury's existing knowledge. It supplies them with specific information that cigarette smoking and tobacco use are responsible for more than 30% of all cancer deaths, including cancers of the lung, larynx, oral cavity, pharynx, pancreas, kidney, bladder, and cervix. The Surgeon General reports that smoking is responsible for approximately 85% of the lung cancer cases in the United States.[21] The most recent Surgeon General's report documents the alarming increasing rates of cancer in females who smoke.

The defense relies on the presentation of data from Selikoff. It is hard to overestimate the effect that cigarette smoking has played in the health of the American worker who was employed between 1916 and 1965. Eighty-three percent of the insulation workers in Selikoff's 17,800 insulator study were present or former cigarette smokers.[22] Other studies of the American and North American worker show similar figures for the same or similar workers. Consequently, there is a strong suggestion, if not presumption, that cigarette smoking is at least a factor in almost every lung cancer case. The defense can use Selikoff's data to show that virtually every lung cancer in his asbestos-exposed cohort had a history of present or past cigarette, pipe, or cigar smoking.[23]

The defense will present evidence that there is extensive information supporting the significantly increased risk to lung cancer for all cell types in present and former cigarette smokers. The latest information from the American Cancer Society indicates that smoking males have a lung cancer relative risk of 22.36 which is increased from a relative risk of 11.35 reported in the September 1982, study.[24] The findings of this new study of 1.2 million men and women indicate that mortality risks among smokers have increased substantially for most of the eight major cancer sites and are causally associated with cigarette smoking.[25]

It continues to be clear that cigarette smoking is a significant factor in all cases of lung cancer and that lung cancer is rare in the absence of smoking despite the presence of other risk factors.

The Plaintiff's Smoking History, Knowledge of Danger, and History of Following the Advice of Physicians

The analysis and defense of the lung cancer case is complicated. There are many factors about the case that have to be discovered, assessed, and evaluated. The factors come from many sources including the plaintiff, the plaintiff's family, the medical records, and the tissue, if any exists. When taken together they form the basis for the personal defense of the lung cancer case.

There are two cornerstones of the defense of lung cancer cases in asbestos-exposed individuals: (1) the strong causative link between cigarette smoking and lung cancer, and (2) the extent and duration of the smoking history of the plaintiff. I have previously cited materials that suggest that virtually all asbestos-exposed lung cancer plaintiffs have a smoking history. It is important for several reasons to prove as extensive a smoking history as possible. The extent and duration of the smoking history is important socially as well as scientifically in an evaluation of the factors that jurors take into consideration when they make decisions about liability. The more the plaintiff smoked the more likely it is that the jury will consider cigarette smoking the total cause or the principal cause of the disease. The older the plaintiff the more likely that the smoking started early in life. The older the plaintiff the more likely that unfiltered cigarettes were smoked. The older the plaintiff the longer the smoking habit lasted. The more smoking the more likely that smoking was the cause.

There appears to be an underlying factor in jury decisions in lung cancer cases that is secondary to the amount of smoking. Juries judge knowledge and culpability. The juries seem to penalize people who do not take care of themselves irrespective of other factors. The establishment of the true number of pack years of smoking enhances the probability that smoking caused the cancer. The establishment of the true number of pack years smoked is also an indication to the jury of the number of years that the plaintiff avoided warnings and failed to exercise responsible conduct.

It is difficult to obtain an accurate measure of any individual's true smoking history. Every internist or pulmonologist will attest to the difficulty in getting an accurate account of a person's smoking history. No one keeps a smoking diary. The patient never kept accurate accounts of the smoking amounts that may have varied substantially over the lifetime. Every quantification is based on memory of ancient history. The plaintiff may have ceased smoking or cut down on consumption at various parts of the smoking years. The plaintiff may have smoked a combination of filtered and unfiltered cigarettes. The plaintiff may have smoked cigars and pipes during a period of the complete history. There are additional confounding factors. Litigants and non-litigants have social reasons for reducing their smoking history. Plaintiffs in litigation are schooled by their lawyers and are quite likely to increase their remuneration as their smoking history decreases.

Lawyers understand that the plaintiff may have reason to inaccurately quantify a smoking history. Lawyers understand that the physician currently treating the patient at the time of the litigation either may not have treated the patient before the litigation or may not have time to go back through records to see if there is conflicting information about smoking. Therefore, the search for information about smoking history does not stop with the plaintiff and the current physician. The extent and duration of the cigarette smoking history of the plaintiff has to be established by combining information from several different sources. The plaintiff, if alive, has to testify under oath and answer sworn questions about the cigarette smoking history. The relatives and friends of both living and deceased plaintiffs must testify as to their memories of the smoking habit. Lawyers and their staff review references in past medical records that predate the start of litigation to determine if a different smoking history was given before the lawsuit started. Lawyers search for conflicting information to and between the patient and their physicians. It is the composite picture that is important.

The inaccuracies in smoking also affect the science. All risk assessments are correlated to the amount of smoking that is or has been experienced by the cohort. The researcher develops information about a deceased cohort member from the next of kin who either does or does not have reliable information on the deceased's smoking history. Therefore, the inaccurate classification of smoking may also inaccurately report the risk of developing any specific disease. There is also no way to measure the amount or the effect of side stream smoke on the outcome.

The defense tries to demonstrate the influence that cigarette smoking has had on the body of the plaintiff in order to try to establish cigarette smoking as the dominant problem. The defense makes every attempt to engage the expertise of every medical specialty. The radiologist is utilized to visually demonstrate to the jury the presence of findings associated directly with cigarette smoking (emphysema, flattened diaphragms, and added translucency) or indirectly related to cigarette smoking (congestive heart failure, vessel disease, etc.). The pulmonologist is employed to explain physical examinations consistent with cigarette smoking (wheezes) and the presence of obstructive lung disease evidence by PFTs. The pulmonologist may also reinforce the x-ray finding testimony of the radiologist. The pathologist will be called to testify about the tissue. The testimony will cover the presence or absence of emphysema, the cell type, the appearance, location, the cancer origin, and the cancer development.

Cessation of smoking is also a factor for several reasons. First, if the record reveals that a plaintiff failed to cease smoking after warnings by the attending physician, juries have a tendency to blame the plaintiff. If the plaintiff stopped smoking, the jury will evaluate the length of time between the smoking cessation and the development of the cancer. The defense will present evidence of the cell doubling times of the specific cell types in an effort to offset the psychological effect that smoking cessation has on causation issues. In general, juries are less likely to penalize the plaintiff as more years have passed since the plaintiff stopped smoking.

Does the Plaintiff Have Underlying Asbestosis?

The most critical asbestos issue for the defense is the presence or absence of asbestosis in the plaintiff. Virtually all physicians and scientists who testify in asbestos cases agree that where there is confirmed underlying asbestosis, asbestos is considered to at least be a contributing cause of the tumor. Therefore, where asbestosis is present, the only defenses available to a specific defendant are exposure issues.

The defense actively and aggressively pursues the presence or absence of an asbestosis diagnosis in lung cancer cases to determine whether there is a plausible defense. The defense relies heavily on the opinions of the pathologist about the presence or absence of asbestosis or pleural plaques in the available tissue. The presence of pleural plaques is not scientifically associated with the presence of asbestosis or the cause of lung cancer but its presence makes it emotionally more difficult for the jury to discount a contribution by asbestos exposure. If the pathological diagnosis is against the existence of asbestosis, that defense is pursued. Both plaintiffs' lawyers and defense lawyers have considerable more difficulty in the absence of sufficient tissue for pathological diagnosis or a disagreement between qualified pathologists. The same difficulties in the diagnosis discussed in the section on asbestosis apply to this controversy.

The defense asserts that the presence of underlying asbestosis is required before medical causation can be attributed to asbestos. The defense engages that position from the considerable debate in the scientific community about whether there is any attributable risk to lung cancer from exposure to asbestos in the absence of underlying asbestosis. The question is whether the lung cancer develops from exposure alone or from the asbestosis. Medical science and epidemiology have been unable to completely differentiate between the rates at which, if any, lung cancers occur in asbestos-exposed individuals who do not have underlying asbestosis. The seminal studies of Selikoff, Hammond, and Seidman,[26,27,28] did not report the numbers of their cohorts with lung cancer who also had underlying asbestosis. These authors confounded the problem by defining their nonsmoking population as "never smoked regularly." Their study included people who did smoke cigarettes but who did not meet their definition of regular smoking. It is clear that at least one study by Selikoff's colleagues at Mt. Sinai found underlying pathological asbestosis in every case of lung cancer in their series.[29]

The Strength or Lack of Strength in the Association Between Asbestos Exposure and the Development of Lung Cancer

The lawyers must assess the medical and scientific data regarding studies that demonstrate a link between asbestos exposure and the existence of lung cancer. It is clear that there are a number of articles that do associate the presence of asbestos with the occurrence of lung cancer. However, there is clearly a debate among medical people about the strength of the association and the incidences where that association takes place. The defense witnesses testify about the differences between the various articles and the existence of what they consider to be flaws in the methodology.

1. Does the plaintiff have exposures to other lung cancer carcinogens that would explain the presence of the lung cancer?
In some cases, the plaintiff clearly had sufficient exposures to ambient asbestos to amply connect the asbestos exposure with the lung cancer. In other cases, the exposure to asbestos is less precise or less substantial. The defense lawyer examines every aspect of the plaintiff's life and the lives of parents and siblings to attempt to discover other exposures to toxic agents that are associated with lung cancer to determine if the exposures are causative. That evidence is presented by expert witnesses if the exposure to other carcinogens is sufficient to produce doubt.

The defense can be used that the plaintiff had exposures to lung cancer causing agents sufficient to be the sole cause of the cancer or if the other exposures acted in combination with cigarette smoking to produce the lung cancer. The analysis of the success of the defense under these circumstances is very similar to the analysis of the success of the defense in the presence of cigarette smoking. The jurors have to be convinced that the lung cancer was caused, in whole or in part, by an agent other than asbestos. The asbestos defendant, depending on the occupational and environmental setting of the plaintiff's workplace, implicates all of the other workplace and occupational contaminants that have caused lung cancer in animals or humans. These other agents include ionizing radiation, arsenic, and a host of chemicals and other agents.

2. Does fiber type exposure offer any defense to the causation issue?
The chrysotile issue is very prominent in the lung cancer case as well as the mesothelioma case. The defendant who manufactured a product from chrysotile or who had chrysotile products on the premises uses the defense to attempt to convince the jurors that chrysotile did not produce the lung cancer or was less likely to produce the lung cancer. The defense attempts to demonstrate the concept that chrysotile is less likely to reach the lungs and that once in the lungs is removed much more rapidly than amphiboles. The ultimate position is that the chrysotile is much less likely to produce the underlying asbestosis because of chemical and physical factors.

The Defense of Pleural and Peritoneal Mesothelioma Cases

The Changing Course of Mesothelioma Cases from 1977 to 2004

The quality and number of defenses of pleural mesothelioma cases have changed significantly in every respect from the early litigation of

1977 to the 2004 cases. The changes have occurred because everything about the litigation has changed. The nature and work processes of both the current plaintiffs and the current defendants have changed. The length and intensity of exposures of the current plaintiffs to the products and premises of current defendants has changed. The number of the mesothelioma cases has multiplied. The ratio by sex of the patients has changed. The occupations have changed. Many of the changes are directly related to the advances in medicine and diagnosis but not all of the changes can be explained in this fashion. The changes encompass many aspects of societal change and reflect the changing landscape of the litigation in 2004. It is a view of contrasts.

The Numbers of Pleural Mesotheliomas Have Changed
The number of diagnosed mesotheliomas has increased significantly since 1977. The asbestos defense lawyer practicing in 1977 rarely saw a mesothelioma case in a year. The defense lawyer today is called upon to defend the filing of between 1000 and 1500 cases a year. The defense of mesothelioma cases has become the biggest challenge for the asbestos defense lawyer and defendants in the 21st century.

There are more cases because more asbestos-exposed people are living long enough to develop the disease. The 1977 asbestos lawyer handled cases resulting from extremely high exposures that occurred in the 1930s, 1940s, 1950s, and 1960s. These heavily exposed people developed severe asbestosis and other respiratory complications early and died BEFORE they could develop mesothelioma. These heavily exposed persons suffered premature deaths, but as their numbers diminished and others lived longer, the incidence rate for pleural mesothelioma began to rise.

Mesothelioma was a rare disease (about 1 per 300,000 deaths) in 1977. The disease was not widely known within the broad medical community. There was significant controversy and disagreement between pathologists about whether the disease existed and how to correctly define the diagnosis. The U.S.–Canadian Mesothelioma Panel was organized to assist physicians in resolving disputes about the pathological diagnosis and to help make correct diagnoses. Many of the stains and tests for mesothelioma that existed in 2004 did not exist in 1977. Many of the early cases were not properly diagnosed. Many of the diagnosed cases did not get to lawyers because the connection between mesothelioma and asbestos was not as well recognized.

Today, lawyers handle almost every case of pleural mesothelioma. Most pathologists in 2004 are aware of pleural mesothelioma and its association with asbestos exposure. There are improved diagnostic techniques that increase the chances of a correct diagnosis. Further, every physician, not just pathologists, knows, at a minimum, that asbestos has some potential connection with many, if not most, mesotheliomas. Most of the diagnosed cases of mesothelioma are referred to attorneys. When the physician does not directly refer a case of mesothelioma, the patient who turns to the Internet to find out more about the disease and treatment cannot escape the proliferation of lawyer Internet Web sites promising monetary resolution and monetary recovery. It is estimated that the new pleural mesotheliomas will cost in the area of $3 billion annually through 2015.

The Defendants Are Different

Today's defendants are different from yesterday's defendants. The traditional pipe covering manufacturers of amosite and crocidolite products are virtually gone from present litigation. The absence of these manufacturers from the lawsuits does not mean that their products did not cause or contribute to the current development of disease. It means that as the traditional pipe covering defendants have filed for bankruptcy, lawyers have sought to replace them with new, nontraditional defendants. The plaintiff of today has to prove that the disease was caused in whole or in part by a defendant that still has assets to get any money. This requirement has caused more than one tenuous allegation of exposure.

The new defendants did not make pipe covering products that produced massive exposures similar to the pipe covering and cement exposures of the past. These new defendants made different products. Many of the products contained less asbestos on a percentage basis than pipe covering and cement products. Many used exclusively chrysotile asbestos. These defendants made joint compound, floor tile, and roofing materials. They made gaskets. They made brake linings. They made encapsulated products. They are premises owners who did not make any products but had asbestos on their premises. The defenses for these defendants are substantially different from the defenses that could have been urged by the pipe covering defendants because the exposure levels have been significantly lowered from earlier exposures.

The Exposure Levels Are Different

The traditional exposures of insulators, pipefitters, sheet metal workers, and other direct users of asbestos-containing products in the shipyards and power houses before 1972 were extremely high. The exposures were often uncontrolled and consisted of exposure to amosite, crocidolite, and mixed asbestos exposures. It was very difficult for the traditional pipe covering manufacturers to advance any defenses based upon low exposure or asbestos fiber type.

The new, nontraditional defendants all seem to have plausible arguments that their products did not release any (much) asbestos to the ambient air or that exposures were controlled on their premises. Many of the products of the current defendants release little or insignificant amounts of asbestos to the ambient air. Often, if they release asbestos, they release ambient asbestos at levels orders of magnitude lower than that associated with pipe covering materials. In many instances the releases of asbestos are at levels well within OSHA requirements and at levels that even the most liberal investigator believes would not cause asbestosis or pleural plaques. Most of these products were made almost exclusively of chrysotile asbestos raising fiber type and fiber burden questions that were never thought in 1977.

The Occupations of the Plaintiffs Are Different

The occupations of the current plaintiffs are different from the occupations of earlier plaintiffs. The current plaintiffs are not and never have been involved in the traditional asbestos-exposed populations. The current plaintiffs often never directly used asbestos themselves. When they directly used asbestos they did so on a fleeting basis. Many do not have an independent idea of if, where, or how they were exposed. Even the current plaintiffs who have jobs that carry such traditional occupational titles as insulator, pipefitter, and sheet metal worker have never knowingly worked with or removed asbestos. The current plaintiffs are also building occupants, homemakers, and children. In most cases, it is hard to suggest that their doses are anywhere near the doses upon which past epidemiology is based.

The Sex of the Plaintiff Is Different

The early cases of mesothelioma were almost all men. Men were employed as insulators and in other direct asbestos trades. This is no longer the case. A significant number of the current plaintiffs are female. They are family members of former employees in the asbestos insulation industry and allied trades. They are workers who became involved in industry after 1972. They are homemakers who have little or no known extensive exposure to asbestos.

The Diagnosis of Pleural Mesothelioma in the Defense Case

The first threshold in the defense of the pleural mesothelioma case is to confirm or dispute the diagnosis of mesothelioma. Almost every current plaintiff has had a complete thoracic and pathologic workup. The plaintiff has undergone a radical pleuropneumonectomy in some cases. The clinicians have already made all the judgments between adenocarcinoma, metastatic tumor, benign pleural fibrosis, and other tumors and processes. There are some differences of opinion between pathologists but disagreements have become rare. It is only occasionally that there fails to be complete agreement. Consequently, disagreement in diagnosis ceases to be a major defense issue.

Asbestos Causation as a Defense to Pleural Mesothelioma Cases

Many modern cases do not have clear and distinct exposures to high levels of asbestos. Plaintiffs no longer worked exclusively with insulation products nor did they always work in jobs that are traditionally known for heavy asbestos exposure. These plaintiffs often did not work in industrial settings. Exact exposures to asbestos are not easy to find. There is often little documentation of the level or duration of asbestos exposures. The absence of clean and precise knowledge of asbestos exposure enhances the defense of asbestos as the culprit in the development of the tumor. Therefore, there is less compelling evidence that asbestos is or was the cause of the plaintiff's tumor.

The fact that all mesotheliomas are not caused by asbestos coupled with the lower and less certain exposure creates doubt as to whether this product or this exposure is the real cause in each specific case. It is clear that many substances and agents have been identified in producing mesotheliomas in animals and humans.[30] Spirtas has written that approximately 80% of the pleural mesotheliomas in men and 20% of the pleural mesotheliomas in women are conclusively related to asbestos exposure.[31] Other authors have given similar numbers,[32,33] although there are some authors who believe that all pleural mesotheliomas are caused by asbestos.[34] There are studies that demonstrate that there are nonasbestos agents and other occupational associations that are implicated in the cause of mesothelioma.[35,36,37] Scarring of the pleura, chronic inflammation, chemical carcinogens, viruses, hereditary predisposition,[38] chronic empyema, and therapeutic pneumothorax[39] have been implicated in mesothelioma. Chemical carcinogens,[40] genetic factors,[41] and therapeutic irradiation[42,43,44] have also been implicated. These other potential and proven causes of mesothelioma offer jurors alternative causes in asbestos cases.

Fiber Type Defenses in Mesothelioma Cases

The vast majority of defendants in cases in 2004 made, sold, or used products that were composed of Canadian chrysotile. These defendants can defend causation based on lack of exposure evidence as well as based on the fiber type of exposure. The reduced, limited, or ambient exposures to asbestos in current cases usually dictate that the plaintiff will not have underlying clinical pleural plaques or any medical consensus as to the presence of asbestosis. The judgment on causation will have to come from the mere presence of the tumor without tissue confirmation. The connection must come from the presence of the tumor and anecdotal evidence of sufficient exposure to cause disease.

The substantial controversy among the most esteemed asbestos authors on whether, and the extent to which, chrysotile asbestos causes malignant pleural mesothelioma provides a healthy fact issue in any mesothelioma case. The controversy is twofold: Does chrysotile cause mesothelioma? If so, what is the threshold level of exposure required?

It is a given that amphibole asbestos is the principal or main cause of pleural mesothelioma,[45,46] and, as late as 1978, Chris Wagner reported his opinion that all of the cases of asbestos-related mesothelioma were caused by exposure to crocidolite.[47] There seems to be no dispute that the amphiboles, crocidolite and amosite, have a more significant association with pleural mesothelioma than does chrysotile.[48,49,50] There have been several theories advanced to explain the lower relative risk for mesothelioma for chrysotile than for amosite and crocidolite. Some suggest that the shorter lung biopersistence of chrysotile is a factor.[51] The evidence is clear that the half-life of the amphiboles in the lung is consistently[52] significantly longer than that of chrysotile. The chrysotile fiber changes more in the lung than do the amphiboles.[53] The increased presence in the lung may provide a longer and more important time for the amphiboles to be in contact with target cells to create DNA changes. It seems that chrysotile is, at the most, a weak carcinogen for mesothelioma.[54] Some authors have questioned whether chrysotile causes mesothelioma or any increased health risk at today's occupational exposure levels.[55,56,57]

The developments in the knowledge about chrysotile and its relation to mesothelioma present a new dynamic for the trial of mesothelioma cases where the sole or principal exposure is to chrysotile asbestos.

Fiber Burden in the Defense of the Pleural Mesothelioma Case

Scientific studies by Roggli, Warnock, Churg, and others since 1977 have shed considerable light on the amount of exposure to various fiber types of asbestos that is required to produce pleural mesothelioma. These same studies have provided information on fiber burden and fiber type comparisons between asbestos-related diseases. Fiber burden studies and their techniques have been identified.[58] The important points from a litigation standpoint center on those that suggest a presence or absence of a causal relationship between exposure to asbestos and pleural mesothelioma from a fiber standpoint. It is clear that individuals who live in urban populations carry a substantial lung burden of asbestos without developing any asbestos-related disease.[59] Churg has suggested that the general population of Vancouver (Canada) has as many as 40 million fibers of chrysotile, 40 million of tremolite, and 400,000 fibers of amosite or crocidolite in each pair of dried lungs weighing approximately 40 grams.[60] Roggli and his colleagues have studied the lungs of occupationally and nonoccupationally exposed people. They have determined that there is a background incidence among their cohort that would be classified as having fewer than 20 asbestos bodies (ABs) per gram of wet lung.[61] Further, Churg and Mossman report on some of Churg's earlier published data that demonstrate lung burden differential for amphiboles versus chrysotile for both mesothelioma and asbestosis.[62] Churg compared lungs from shipyard workers exposed to amosite and mixed dusts with those of chrysotile miners and millers. His results showed that mesothelioma occurred in the amosite-exposed shipyard workers at fiber burdens, on average, almost 220 times less than the average fiber burden of the lungs of the chrysotile miners and millers. He also found that asbestosis occurred in the amosite-exposed shipyard workers at fiber burdens, on average, almost 17 times less than the average fiber burden of the lungs of the chrysotile miners and millers.

The defense lawyer has several options in using the fiber burden studies as a defense to the claim that the mesothelioma was caused by asbestos. First, a fiber burden study that showed the absence of asbestos or asbestos below the established background levels for the laboratory lends weight to the argument that the mesothelioma was not caused by asbestos. This result follows whether the product was an amphibole or chrysotile. In fact, it may argue more strongly for amphibole products because the amphiboles stay in the lung significantly longer than chrysotile. The results also may aid the manufacturer of the chrysotile products if either no chrysotile is found in the lung fiber burden and/or amphiboles are found.

A.H. Parnell

Retrospective Exposure Assessments in the Defense of Mesothelioma, Lung Cancer, and Asbestosis Cases

The advances in knowledge about levels of exposure and the onset of disease allow the lawyer to use other scientific methods to support or attack the proposition that any asbestos disease is related to a specific exposure, series of exposures, or specific product use. Retrospective exposure assessments (REAS) use scientific methods and facts to recreate the exposure to a lifetime of agents, a specific agent or product, or a comparison between products and exposures. REAS are particularly helpful in asbestos litigation in mesothelioma causation cases and in nonmalignancy cases where there is a clinical dispute about whether there is asbestosis and there is a question about the sufficiency of the exposure.

The purpose of REAS is to define the limits of a past exposure. It begins with identifying who is or was exposed. The method looks at the agent under investigation. It attempts to quantify the types of exposure to the products by using a number of approaches including actual records or exposure levels doing similar jobs in similar ways. It looks at the era in which the exposure took place and the impact that the evolution of occupational health standards may have had on exposure. It incorporates preexisting scientific and medical reports that examine past exposures, exposure levels, and the development of disease. REAS develop a model for assessing the data in a scientific way. Finally, the method reports a quantitative description of the exposure and real time assessments of the amount of exposure. REAS are traditionally and often used in the industrial hygiene profession.

There are several examples that illustrate the use of REAS in litigated matters. Assume an alleged chrysotile exposure to a 46-year-old woman with pleural mesothelioma who alleges that her only exposure to asbestos was when she was with her father when he was changing brakes on his car 6 times in her early childhood. There is substantial data on the amount of dust generated during a brake change and the length of time of the average brake change. The industrial hygienist calculates this exposure as a time weighed average (TWA) and determines, as an example, that the combined exposure was between a range of .003 fiber/cc-years and .001 fiber/cc-years. Both of these exposure levels are in the range of ambient exposure and the lawyer would use this comparison to urge the lack of asbestos causation. In another example, assume that an REA of a pipefitter with mesothelioma had a combined occupational exposure of 150 f/cc-years. The pipefitter had 147 f/cc-years of amosite exposure and 3 f/cc-years of chrysotile exposure. The defense will ask the jury to compare the exposures and determine that the chrysotile exposure was not a *"substantial factor"* in the production of the disease. The defense lawyer might also argue that exposure levels of 3 f/cc-years of chrysotile would not exceed the threshold for mesothelioma causation.[63]

References

1. Wagner JC, Sleggs CA, Marchand P: Diffuse pleural mesothelioma and asbestos exposure in North Western Cape Province. *Br J Ind Med* 17:260–271, 1960.
2. Selikoff IJ, Churg J: Biological effects of asbestos. *Ann NY Acad Sci* 132:1–766, 1965.
3. Restatement (second) Torts Section 402A.
4. *Borel v. Fibreboard Paper Products Corp.*, 493 F. 2d 1076 (5th Cir. 1973), *cert. denied*, 419 U.S. 869 (1974).
5. Fed. R. Evid. 701–705.
6. *Daubert v. Merrell Dow Pharmaceuticals, Inc.*, 509 U.S. 579, 113 S. Ct. 2786, 125 L. Ed. 2d 469 (1993) (Daubert I), on remand, *Daubert v. Merrell Dow Pharmaceuticals, Inc.*, 43 F. 3d 1311 (9th Cir.), *cert. denied*, 133 L. Ed. 2d 126, 116 S. Ct. 189 (1995)(Daubert II).
7. *Merrell Dow Pharmaceuticals, Inc. v. Havner*, 953f S. W. 2d 706 (Tex. 1997.)
8. Fletcher DE: A mortality study of shipyard workers with pleural plaques. *Br J Ind Med* 29:142–145, 1972.
9. Cross AA: What to do about the asbestos currently in ships and industry. *Ann NY Acad Sci* 330:379–381, 1979.
10. 29 USCS Section 651, et seq.
11. Craighead JE, et al.: The pathology of asbestos-associated diseases of the lungs and pleural cavities: Diagnostic criteria and proposed grading schema. *Arch Path Lab Med* 106:541–596, 1982.
12. American Thoracic Society: The diagnosis of non-malignant diseases related to asbestos. *Am Rev Respir Dis* 1336:1205–1209, 1986.
13. U.S. Department of Health, Education and Welfare. *Smoking and health: A report of the surgeon general*. U.S. Department of Health, Education and Welfare, Public Health Service, Office of the Assistant Secretary for Health, Office on Smoking and Health, 1979 DHEW Pub. No. (PHS) 79–50066.
14. Auerbach O: Changes in the bronchial epithelium in relation to cigarette smoking and cancer of the lung. *N Engl J Med* 256:97–104, 1956.
15. Ochsner A: *Smoking and Your Life*. Julian Messner Pub., 1954, rev. 1964.
16. Doll R, Peto R: Mortality in relation to smoking: 20 years' observations on male British doctors. *Br Med J* 2:1525–1536, 1976.
17. *Ibid*.
18. U.S. Department of Health, Education and Welfare: supra 13.
19. U.S. Department of Health and Human Services. *The health consequences of smoking: The changing cigarette. A report of the surgeon general*. U.S. Department of Health and Human Services, Public Health Service, Office of the Assistant Secretary for Health, Office on Smoking and Health, 1981 DHEW Pub. No. (PHS) 81–50156.
20. U.S. Department of Health and Human Services. *Women and Smoking: A Report of the Surgeon General*. U.S. Department of Health and Human Services, Public Health Service, Office of the Assistant Secretary for Health, Office on Smoking and Health 2000.
21. U.S. Department of Health and Human Services: *The health consequences of smoking: Cancer: A report of the Surgeon General*. U.S. Department of Health and Human Services, Office of the Assistant Secretary for Health 1982 (PHS) 82–50179.
22. Hammond EC, Selikoff IJ, Seidman H: Asbestos exposure, cigarette smoking and death rates. *Ann NY Acad Sci* 330:481, 1979.
23. *Ibid*.

24. U.S. Department of Health and Human Services: supra 21.
25. *Ibid.*
26. Selikoff IJ, Hammond EC, Churg J: Asbestos exposure, smoking and neoplasia. *JAMA* 204:106–112, 1968.
27. Hammond EC: Relation of cigarette smoking to risk of death of asbestos-associated disease among insulation workers in the United States. In: Biological effects of asbestos. (Bogovski P, Gilson JC, Timbrell V, Wagner JC eds.), IARC Scientific Publications, Lyon, 1973, pp. 312–317, 1973.
28. Seidman H: Short-term asbestos exposure and delayed cancer risk. In: *Prevention and detection of cancer.* (Neisburgs HE, ed.) New York: Marcel Dekker, Inc., 1976, pp. 943–960.
29. Selikoff IJ, Churg J, Hammond EC: The occurrence of asbestosis among insulation workers in the United States. *Ann NY Acad Sci.* 330:132–155, 1979.
30. Petersen JT Jr, Greenberg SD, Buffler PA: Nonasbestos-related malignant mesothelioma. *Cancer* 54:951–960, 1984.
31. Spirtas R, Beebe GW, Connelly RR, Wright WE, Peters JM: Recent trends in mesothelioma incidence in the United States. *Am J Ind Med* 9:397–407, 1986.
32. Browne K: The epidemiology of mesothelioma. *J Soc Occup Med* 33:190–194, 1984.
33. Kane MJ, Chahinian AP, Holland JF: Malignant mesothelioma in young adults. *Cancer* 65:1449–1455, 1990.
34. McDonald JC: Health implications of environmental exposure to asbestos. *Environ Health Perspect* 62:319–328, 1985.
35. Kelsey KT, Yano E, Liber HL, Little JB: The in vitro effects of fibrous erionite and crocidolite asbestos. *Dr J Cancer* 54:107–114, 1986.
36. Baris YI, Artvinli M, Sahin AA: Environmental mesothelioma in Turkey. *Ann NY Acad Sci* 330:423–432, 1979.
37. McDonald JC: Cancer risks due to asbestos and man-made fibers. *Cancer Res* 120:122–130, 1990.
38. Riddell RH: Peritoneal malignant mesothelioma in a patient with recurrent peritonitis. *Cancer* 48:134–139, 1981.
39. Petersen JT Jr, et al.: supra 30.
40. Hueper WC: Cancer induction by polyurethane and polysilicone plastics. *J Natl Cancer Inst* 33:1005–1027, 1964.
41. Martensson G, Larsson S, Zettergren L: Malignant mesothelioma in two pairs of siblings: Is there a hereditary predisposing factor? *Eur J Respir Dis* 65:179–184, 1984.
42. Stock RJ, Fu YS, Carter JR: Malignant peritoneal mesothelioma following radiotherapy for seminoma of the testis. *Cancer* 48:134–139, 1979.
43. Maurer R, Egloff B: Malignant peritoneal mesothelioma after cholangiography with thorotrast. *Cancer* 36:1381–1385, 1975.
44. Antman KH, Corson JM, Li FP, Greenberger S, Sytkowski A, Henson DE, Weinstein L: Malignant mesothelioma following radiation exposure. *J Clin Oncol* 1:695–700, 1983.
45. McDonald AD, Fry JS, Woolley AJ, McDonald JC: Dust exposure and mortality in an American chrysotile friction products plant. *Br J Ind Med* 41:151, 1984.
46. Churg A, Wiggs B, Dipaoli L, Kampe B, Stevens B: Lung asbestos content in chrysotile workers with mesothelioma. *Am Rev Respir Dis* 130:1042–1045, 1984.
47. McDonald AD, et al.: supra 45.
48. Becklake M, Case B: Editorial *Am J Resp Crit Care Med*, 1994.

49. Gibbs A: Review, *Thorax*, 1990.
50. Doll R, Peto J: Asbestos—effects on health of exposure to asbestos. London: Health & Safety Commission.
51. Attanoos and Gibbs: Pathology of Malignant Mesothelioma, Invited Review.
52. Churg A, Vedal S: Fiber burden and patterns of asbestos-related disease in workers with heavy mixed amosite and chrysotile exposure. *Am J Respir Crit Care Med* 150:663–669, 1994.
53. Boutin C, Dumortier P, Rey F, Viallat JR, DeVuyst P: Black spots concentrate oncogenic asbestos fibers in the parietal pleura. *Am J Respir Crit Care Med* 153:444–449, 1996.
54. Dr. Alan Gibbs: Review, *Thorax*, 1990.
55. Mesothelioma and chrysotile; William Weiss, 1983.
56. Churg A: Malignant mesothelioma. Ch. 10 In: *Pathology of Occupational Lung Disease*, New York: Igaku Shoin Medical Publishers, 1998.
57. Mossman B, Bignon J, Corn M, Seaton A, Gee JB: Asbestos: Scientific developments and implications for public policy. *Science* 247:294–301, 1990.
58. Roggli VL, Pratt PC, Brody AR: Asbestos content of lung tissue in asbestos associated diseases: A study of 110 cases. *Br J Ind Med* 43:18–28, 1986.
59. Churg A: supra 56.
60. *Ibid*.
61. Roggli VL, McGavran MH, Subach J, Sybers HD, Greenberg SD: Pulmonary asbestos body counts and electron probe analysis of asbestos body cores in patients with mesothelioma. A study of 25 Cases. *Cancer* 50:2329–2423, 1982.
62. Mossman A, Churg A: Mechanisms in the pathogenesis of asbestosis and silicosis: A state of the art review. *Am J Respir Crit Care Med* 158:1666–1680, 1998.
63. Browne K: A threshold for asbestos related lung cancer. *Br J Indus Med* 43:556–558, 1986.

Appendix

Tissue Digestion Techniques

Victor L. Roggli

Method A

The digestion procedure used by the author[1] is a modification of the sodium hypochlorite digestion technique described by Williams et al.[2] The details of the procedure are as follows:

Materials

0.4 μm pore-size, 25 mm diameter Nuclepore® filters
Nuclepore® filtering apparatus, including cylindrical funnel (10 cc), fritted glass filter support, and 250 cc side-arm flask
Vacuum source, vacuum tubing, trap
20 cc plastic screw-top scintillation counter glass vials
Aliquot mixer for blood tubes (Miles Laboratories)
Two-sided sticky tape
Scalpel handle, clean scalpel blades
Forceps (coarse and fine tip)
25 mm diameter rubber "O"-rings for filters
Pasteur pipettes with rubber bulbs
Rectangular plastic weighing dishes
Analytical balance

Reagents (all reagents prefiltered through 0.4 μm pore size filter)

5.25% sodium hypochlorite solution (commercial bleach)
8.0% oxalic acid solution
Absolute ethanol
Deionized water
Chloroform (caution: cannot filter through Nuclepore filter, as it will dissolve the filter!)

Methods

Step 1: Selected specimen (up to approximately 0.3 gm) is weighed wet in plastic dish on an analytical balance after gently blotting excess fluid with a paper towel.

Step 2:   Tissue is minced into 1 or 2 mm cubes within plastic dish using fresh scalpel blade and coarse-tip forceps.

Step 3:   Two Pasteur pipettes full of filtered sodium hypochlorite solution are added to plastic dish, and tissue in hypochlorite solution is carefully transferred into a 20-cc plastic screw-top scintillation counter vial.

Step 4:   An additional aliquot of hypochlorite solution from a Pasteur pipette is used to rinse the weighing dish, and this is added to the vial. Two more aliquots (total of 10 cc) of hypochlorite solution are added directly to the vial.

Step 5:   The vial is labeled for identification and placed on an aliquot mixer with double-sticky tape (Figure A-1). Digestion proceeds until tissue fragments are no longer visible to the naked eye (usually 20–25 minutes for a 0.3 gm sample; however, more time may be required for severely fibrotic or deparaffinized specimens).

Step 6:   The digested suspension is transferred into the glass cylinder of the assembled filtration apparatus (Figure A-1). It is best to add no more than approximately 25% of the suspension to the filter at any one time.

Step 7:   As the filtration slows, aliquots of 8.0% oxalic acid, absolute ethanol, and fresh hypochlorite solution may be added to the filter surface with a Pasteur pipette to reduce buildup of any

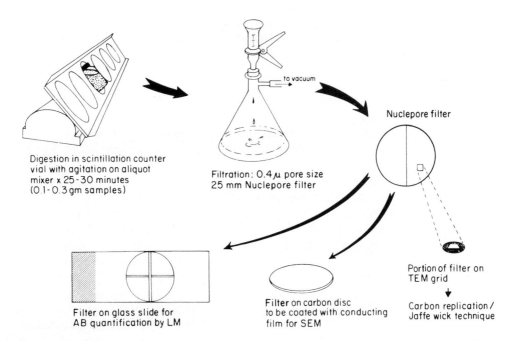

Figure A-1. METHOD A: Technique for extracting mineral fibers and other inorganic particulates from lung tissue. Tissue is first digested in sodium hypochlorite solution (commercial bleach) and the residue collected on a Nuclepore® filter. The filter may be mounted for light, scanning electron, or transmission electron microscopy. See text for details.

organic residues. An aliquot of deionized water should be added between additions of oxalic acid, ethanol, or hypochlorite solution to prevent crystal deposition on the filter surface.

Step 8: After the final portion of the suspension has passed through the filter and a final rinse with oxalic acid, ethanol, and hypochlorite solution has been effected, then a final aliquot of absolute ethanol is washed through the filter.

Step 9: The filter is transferred from the filtering apparatus onto the surface of a glass slide using fine-tip forceps. The periphery of the filter should be attached to the surface of the slide with small, torn portions of white, lightly adhesive tape (to prevent folding and buckling of the filter when chloroform is added).

Step 10: After the filter has completely dried, chloroform is added drop-wise to the filter surface with a Pasteur pipette until the filter is covered and cleared. The tape securing the edges of the filter can now be removed with fine-tip forceps before the chloroform dries.

Step 11: After the chloroform dries, a coverslip can be added to the slide in a suitable mounting medium (e.g., Permount), and the slide is now ready for viewing by light microscopy.

Step 9a: If one wishes to examine the filter by scanning electron microscopy (SEM) rather than light microscopy, the filter can be mounted on a 25mm carbon disc with colloidal graphite and sputter-coated with gold, platinum, or carbon (Figure A-1).[3] If the examiner wishes to employ transmission electron microscopy, then a small portion of the filter can be cut out and transferred onto a TEM grid and the filter material removed by chloroform using the Jaffe wick technique.[4,5]

Notes Regarding Digestion Procedure

In selecting tissue for digestion, one should avoid areas of tumor, congestion, or consolidation as much as possible. These would affect the denominator in calculations of asbestos fiber or body concentrations, and thus would tend to falsely lower the calculated value. The author prefers formalin-fixed tissue, although fresh lung tissue works just as well. An adequate sample is at minimum an open lung biopsy; lobectomy, or pneumonectomy. Autopsy tissue is even better. Transbronchial biopsies are inadequate to give meaningful results.[6] For lobectomy or pneumonectomy specimens, the author generally prepares two or three filters, and for autopsy cases, four filters (one from the upper and lower lobes of each lung). One filter is typically examined by SEM for asbestos bodies and uncoated fibers; the rest are examined by light microscopy for asbestos body content.

In some cases, only paraffin-embedded lung tissue is available. In such cases, a portion is selected from the block, deparaffinized in xylene, and rehydrated through absolute and 95% ethanol. The usual times for deparaffinizing tissue are doubled to maximize paraffin removal, because residual paraffin clogs the pores of the filter, obscuring fibers and bodies. The wet weight is obtained from the specimen in 95% ethanol. A correction factor has to be applied to deparaffinized specimens because of lipids removed at the time the tissue was originally processed[6] (See below).

There may be some variability in Steps 6 and 7 (filtration) depending upon the individual sample. Some samples pass readily through the filter and require little rinsing with oxalic acid, ethanol, or hypochlorite solution to remove residues. Other cases may sharply decrease their rate of filtration and require considerable effort to remove organic residues. Sometimes ethanol most readily restores the filtration rate, while in other cases oxalic acid is more effective. The use of warm water rinses helps to reduce crystal accumulation on the filter surface. If there is systematic slowing of filtration on multiple samples, this may be due to clogging of the fritted glass filter support. This can be rinsed with acetone or hot double deionized water to remove such residues.

Method B

In some cases, the asbestos body content is too low to obtain an accurate estimate from a 0.3 gram sample. If an accurate quantification is desirable in such cases, then the original method of Smith and Naylor[7] employing a larger sample size may be preferable. The details of the procedure are as follows:

Materials

0.4 µm pore-size, 25 mm diameter Nuclepore® filters
Nuclepore® filtering apparatus, including cylindrical funnel (10 cc), fritted glass filter support, and 250 cc side-arm flask
Vacuum source, vacuum tubing, and trap
300-cc glass jar with lid
Scalpel handle, clean scalpel blades
Forceps (coarse and fine tip)
25 mm diameter rubber "O" rings for filters
Pasteur pipettes with rubber bulbs
50 cc screw-cap conical centrifuge tubes
Rectangular plastic weighing dishes
Analytical balance
Desktop centrifuge

Reagents (filtration optional)

5.25% sodium hypochlorite solution (commercial bleach)
Chloroform
95% ethanol
50% ethanol

Methods

Step 1: Selected specimen (approximately 5 gm) is weighed wet in plastic dish on an analytical balance after gently blotting excess fluid with a paper towel.

Step 2:   Tissue is minced into 2- or 3-mm cubes within plastic dish using fresh scalpel blade and coarse-tip forceps.

Step 3:   Tissue is transferred from dish into glass jar with scalpel blade. The dish is rinsed with a 2-cc aliquot (one Pasteur-pipette-full) of sodium hypochlorite solution which is added to the jar. Approximately 250 cc of hypochlorite solution are then added to the jar (approximately 50-cc hypochlorite solution per gram of tissue).

Step 4:   The glass jar is allowed to sit for several days to allow time for the tissue to digest and for the asbestos bodies to settle to the bottom (Figure A-2).[8]

Step 5:   The supernatant is removed by gentle aspiration using a Pasteur pipette attached to the vacuum system, being careful not to disturb the sediment at the bottom of the jar.

Step 6:   A 20-cc aliquot of chloroform is added to the jar to suspend the asbestos bodies embedded in the sticky layer on the bottom of the jar. After swirling the chloroform to dissolve these residues, a 20 cc aliquot of 50% ethanol is added to the chloroform suspension. The ethanol chloroform mixture is then transferred to a 50-cc screw-cap conical centrifuge tube.

Step 7:   The centrifuge tube is labeled for identification and placed in a table-top centrifuge. A tube from another sample or a tube filled with water is used as a counterbalance. The specimen is centrifuged at 200 g for 10 to 15 minutes.

Step 8:   The supernatant is removed by gentle aspiration using a Pasteur pipette attached to the vacuum system, being careful to remove pigment and lipid residues at the chloroform–ethanol interface and leaving approximately 5 cc

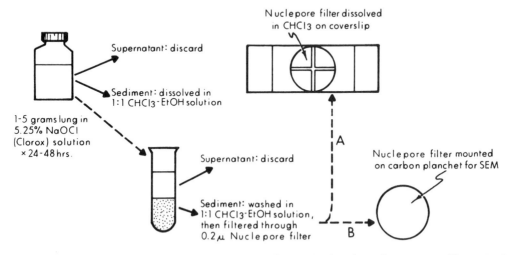

Figure A-2. METHOD B: Technique for extracting asbestos bodies from lung tissue. Tissue is first digested in sodium hypochlorite solution (commercial bleach), followed by a centrifugation step to separate the inorganic particulates from inorganic carbon and undigested lipid residues, the latter remaining at the chloroform–ethanol interface. The residue is recovered on a Nuclepore® filter, which may then be mounted on a glass slide for examination by light microscopy. See text for details. (Reprinted from Ref. 8, with permission.)

of chloroform and sediment at the bottom of the tube (chloroform is heavier than ethanol and settles to bottom).

Step 9:   If the sediment remaining after Step 8 is black, then an additional 20 cc aliquot of chloroform and 20 cc of 50% ethanol may be added to the centrifuge tube and Steps 7 and 8 repeated. Otherwise, approximately 15 cc of 95% ethanol are added to the sediment and residual chloroform.

Step 10: The sediment is suspended in the 95% ethanol, using vigorous shaking or a vortex mixer, if necessary. This suspension is then transferred into the glass cylinder of the assembled filtration apparatus (Figure A-2), and the sediment collected on the filter surface.

Step 11: The filter is transferred from the filtering apparatus onto the surface of a glass slide using fine-tip forceps. The slide is then prepared for examination by light microscopy as described in Steps 9 to 11 under Method A (see above).

Notes Regarding Digestion Procedures

Tissue selection guidelines are similar to those outlined for Method A above. Generally, a lower lobe sample abutting the pleura is used. The values obtained for asbestos bodies per gram of wet lung using Method B are generally quite comparable to those obtained with Method A. In a study of 10 cases in which both methods were used to quantify the asbestos body content, the average ratio of the results obtained by Method B to those obtained by Method A was 1.1 (range, 0.3–3.5).[9] Although filters prepared by Method B can also be examined by analytical electron microscopy, the author does not recommend this because there is evidence of a significant uncoated fiber loss at the chloroform–ethanol interface during the centrifugation step (unpublished observations). Others have also reported fiber losses with each sequential centrifugation step.[10]

It is important to emphasize the necessity for maintaining scrupulously clean glassware. Studies have shown that asbestos bodies and fibers adhere to glassware surfaces and may be removed with difficulty.[11,12] Such loss of fibers or bodies may give a falsely low count. Of greater concern, however, is the contamination of glassware with carryover of bodies or fibers from a case with a heavy burden to a case with very low tissue asbestos content.[13] A new scalpel blade, centrifuge tube, or glass vial should be used for each case. The cylindrical glass funnel and the glass jars are carefully cleaned with warm soapy water and a scrub brush between cases, rinsing with copious amounts of deionized water. Cleaning with acetone in an ultrasonicator is recommended after cases with a particularly heavy asbestos burden.

Filtration of reagents is optional for Method B because asbestos bodies derive only from biological systems and do not contaminate these reagents. (Uncoated fibers, on the other hand, may contaminate many different reagents and give falsely elevated fiber counts by electron microscopy. This is especially problematic for small chrysotile fibers, which are ubiquitous. Reagent blanks should be prepared and examined to control for this possibility whenever electron microscopic techniques are employed for asbestos fiber quantification.)

Bronchoalveolar Lavage Fluid

In some circumstances, it may be of interest to analyze the asbestos content of bronchoalveolar lavage fluid (BALF). This procedure is typically performed by digesting the BALF pellet in sodium hypochlorite solution and collecting the residue on a Nuclepore® filter. For this purpose, we typically use a 13 mm filter, which further concentrates the specimen since this filter has only 25% of the area of the 25 mm filter used for lung digests. The filter may be mounted on a glass slide for asbestos body quantification by light microscopy or on a carbon planchet for examination in the scanning electron microscope. Counting rules are the same as for lung digest samples (see below). The results may be reported per ml of BALF or per million (10^6) cells.[13]

Counting Rules and Calculations

The morphologic features of asbestos bodies are described and illustrated in detail in Chapter 3. Asbestos bodies, which have thin translucent cores, are to be distinguished from pseudoasbestos bodies, which have broad yellow sheet silicate or black cores. The author enumerates the true asbestos bodies and pseudoasbestos (nonasbestos ferruginous) bodies separately. Except in rare cases, true asbestos bodies are more numerous than pseudoasbestos bodies. Indeed, asbestos bodies are identified in more than 90% of cases, whereas pseudoasbestos bodies are observed, in the author's experience, in approximately 25% of cases. Identification of asbestos bodies by scanning electron microscopy is dependent upon morphologic features in combination with elemental composition as determined by EDXA, since one cannot appreciate the additional information regarding the color of the core fiber that is available from light microscopic observations.

Fibers are defined as particles with a length to diameter (aspect) ratio of at least 3:1 and roughly parallel sides. The author does not count particles with aspect ratio less than 3:1 or with sides that are nonparallel or excessively irregular. Clumps of fibers are seldom encountered with the digestion procedures described above. Both asbestos and nonasbestos fibers are counted together (total uncoated fiber count). Although there is considerable morphologic overlap, most of the fibers that are 10 μm or greater in length with aspect ratio greater than 10:1 are asbestos, whereas nonasbestos mineral fibers tend to be shorter than 10 μm in length and have aspect ratios less than 10:1. Asbestos fibers are distinguished from nonasbestos mineral fibers on the basis of their morphology and elemental composition as determined by energy dispersive spectrometry (see Chapter 11). Asbestos fibers must also be distinguished from crystals that may form on the filter surface, which often have pointed ends. Such crystals are not included in the total fiber count.

Quantification of the asbestos body content of a lung tissue sample requires a determination of the numbers of bodies per unit area of filter surface. This can usually be accomplished by counting the number of bodies in a portion of the filter of known area, and multiplying this value by the total effective surface area. The author usually counts the number of bodies in two perpendicular strips at a magnification of 400× (Figures A-1 and A-2). In cases with a low asbestos body burden, the entire filter surface may need to be counted to obtain accurate results. In quantifying the asbestos body and uncoated fiber burdens by scanning electron microscopy, the author counts 200 fibers or 100 consecutive 1000× fields, whichever comes first. The latter amounts to approximately 1% of the surface area of the filter. The total numbers of bodies or fibers on the filter can then be determined by multiplying the number of bodies or fibers per mm^2 of surface area by the total effective surface area of the filter. Determination of asbestos body or fiber concentration can then be accomplished by dividing the numbers per filter by the amount of wet tissue digested in preparing that particular filter. For paraffin blocks, the value must be multiplied by 0.7 for the results to be comparable to wet fixed lung tissue[9] (see above). Some investigators prefer to report their results in terms of bodies or fibers per gram of dried lung. In this circumstance, a portion of lung adjacent to the one actually digested should be weighed wet and then dried to constant weight in a 60 to 70°C oven. Then the asbestos body or fiber concentration per gram of wet lung can be multiplied by the wet-to-dry weight ratio, yielding an asbestos body or fiber concentration per gram of dried lung (see also Chapters 3 and 11).

Sample Calculations

Example 1: Light Microscopy

Sample weight: 0.308 gm
Total effective filter area $= \pi r^2 = \pi\,(10.5\,mm)^2 = 346\,mm^2$
Asbestos bodies counted in two perpendicular strips of filter (see Figures A-1 and A-2) = 423
Area of two perpendicular strips $= 2 \times 21\,mm \times 0.42\,mm$ (empirically determined diameter of one 400× field) $= 17.6\,mm^2$
Asbestos bodies (AB) per $mm^2 = 24$
Therefore,

$$AB/gm = \frac{(24/mm^2)(346\,mm^2)}{0.308\,gm}$$
$$= 27,000\ AB/gm$$

Example 2: Scanning Electron Microscopy

Sample weight = 0.299 gm
Uncoated fibers counted in 100 fields = 35
Total area of 100 fields $= 2.3714\,mm^2$
Effective area of filter $= 346\,mm^2$ (See above)

Fibers/mm^2 = 14.76
Fibers/filter = (14.76 fibers/mm^2) (346 mm^2) = 5110
Fibers/gm = (5110 fibers/filter)/0.299 gm = 17,100 fibers/gm

References

1. Roggli VL, Brody AR: Changes in numbers and dimensions of chrysotile asbestos fibers in lungs of rats following short-term exposure. *Expl Lung Res* 7:133–147, 1984.
2. Williams MG, Dodson RF, Corn C, Hurst GA: A procedure for the isolation of amosite asbestos and ferruginous bodies from lung tissue and sputum. *J Toxicol Environ Health* 10:627–638, 1982.
3. Roggli VL: Scanning electron microscopic analysis of mineral fibers in human lungs, Ch. 5 In: *Microprobe Analysis in Medicine* (Ingram P, Shelburne JD, Roggli VL, eds.), New York: Hemisphere Pub. Corp. 1989, pp. 97–110.
4. Churg, A: Quantitative methods for analysis of disease induced by asbestos and other mineral particles using the transmission electron microscope, Ch. 4 In: *Microprobe Analysis in Medicine* (Ingram P, Shelburne JD, Roggli VL, eds.), New York: Hemisphere Pub. Corp. 1989, pp. 79–95.
5. Churg A, Sakoda N, Warnock ML: A simple method for preparing ferruginous bodies for electron microscopic examination. *Am J Clin Pathol* 68:513–517, 1977.
6. Roggli VL: Preparatory techniques for the quantitative analysis of asbestos in tissues. Proceedings of the 46th Annual Meeting of the Electron Microscopy Society of America (Bailey GW, ed.), San Francisco: San Francisco Press, Inc., 1988, pp. 84–85.
7. Smith MJ, Naylor B: A method for extracting ferruginous bodies from sputum and pulmonary tissues. *Am J Clin Pathol* 58:250–254, 1972.
8. Roggli VL, Shelburne JD: New concepts in the diagnosis of mineral pneumoconioses. *Sem Respir Med* 4:138–148, 1982.
9. Roggli VL, Pratt PC, Brody AR: Asbestos content of lung tissue in asbestos associated diseases: A study of 110 cases. *Br J Ind Med* 43:18–28, 1986.
10. Ashcroft T, Heppleston AG: The optical and electron microscopic determination of pulmonary asbestos fibre concentration and its relation to the human pathological reaction. *J Clin Pathol* 26:224–234, 1973.
11. Corn CJ, Williams MG, Jr., Dodson RF: Electron microscopic analysis of residual asbestos remaining in preparative vials following bleach digestion. *J Electron Microsc Tech* 6:1–6, 1987.
12. Gylseth B, Batman RH, Overaae L: Analysis of fibres in human lung tissue. *Br J Ind Med* 39:191–195, 1982.
13. Roggli VL, Piantadosi CA, Bell DY: Asbestos bodies in bronchoalveolar lavage fluid: A study of 20 asbestos-exposed individuals and comparison to patients with other chronic interstitial lung disease. *Acta Cytolog* 30:460–467, 1986.

Index

ISBN 0-387-20090-8

EAN

9 780387 200903 >